FAMILY HEALTH CARE

Volume One
General Perspectives

Second Edition

FAMILY HEALTH CARE

Volume One
General Perspectives

Editors

Debra P. Hymovich
Professor, School of Nursing
University of Colorado

Martha Underwood Barnard
Faculty and Nurse Clinician
School of Nursing and School of Medicine
University of Kansas College of Health Services and Hospital

McGraw-Hill Book Company

New York   St. Louis   San Francisco   Auckland   Bogotá
Düsseldorf   Johannesburg   London   Madrid   Mexico
Montreal   New Delhi   Panama   Paris   São Paulo
Singapore   Sydney   Tokyo   Toronto

twin

NOTICE

Medicine is an ever-changing science. As new research and clinical experience broaden our knowledge, changes in treatment and drug therapy are required. The editors and the publisher of this work have made every effort to ensure that the drug dosage schedules herein are accurate and in accord with the standards accepted at the time of publication. Readers are advised, however, to check the product information sheet included in the package of each drug they plan to administer to be certain that changes have not been made in the recommended dose or in the contraindications for administration. This recommendation is of particular importance in regard to new or infrequently used drugs.

FAMILY HEALTH CARE
Volume One   General Perspectives

Copyright © 1979, 1973 by McGraw-Hill, Inc. All rights reserved. Printed in the United States of America. No part of this publication may be reproduced, stored in a retrieval system, or transmitted, in any form or by any means, electronic, mechanical, photocopying, recording, or otherwise, without the prior written permission of the publisher.

1234567890 DODO 7832109

Library of Congress Cataloging in Publication Data

Hymovich, Debra P
    Family health care.

    Includes bibliographies and index.
    CONTENTS: v. 1. General perspectives.—v. 2.
Developmental and situational crises.
    1. Nursing. 2. Family medicine. 3. Family.
I. Barnard, Martha Underwood, joint author.
II. Title. [DNLM: 1. Community health nursing.
2. Family. WY106 F198]
RT41.H94 1979   362.8′2   78-18495
ISBN 0-07-031675-9 (v. 1)
ISBN 0-07-031676-7 (v. 2)

This book was set in Times Roman by The Book Studio Inc. The editor was Mary Ann Richter and the production supervisor was Milton J. Heiberg.
R. R. Donnelley & Sons Company was printer and binder.

To
Our Families

CONTENTS

Part 2   Factors Affecting the Family

Part 3   Approaches to Assessment and
Intervention

LIST OF CONTRIBUTORS

BEVERLY HENRY BOWNS, R.N.,
   Dr. P.H.
Dean, College of Nursing, Rutgers
University, Newark, New Jersey

CAROLYN BROSE, R.N., M.S.
Dean of Nursing and Director of
Nursing Service, Baptist Memorial
Hospital, Kansas City, Missouri

MAXINE CADENA R.N., M.S.
Nurse Educator, San Antonio, Texas

KATHRYN ELLEN CHRISTIANSEN,
   R.N., M.A.
Assistant Professor, Department of
Community Health Nursing, School
of Nursing, University of Kansas,
Kansas City, Kansas

EDWARD R. CHRISTOPHERSEN,
   Ph.D.
Associate Professor of Pediatrics and
Director, Pediatric Research Institute,
University of Kansas Medical Center,
Kansas City, Kansas

JOY PRINCETON CLAUSEN,
   R.N., Ph.D.
Associate Professor, School of
Nursing, Duke University,
Durham, North Carolina

NANCY L. DIEKELMAN, R.N.,
   M.S.
Lecturer, School of Nursing,
University of Wisconsin, Madison,
Wisconsin

GEORGIA S. DUDDING, R.N., C.
Pediatric Nurse Practitioner,
Ambulatory Pediatrics, and Teaching
Associate, School of Nursing, College
of Health Sciences and Hospital,
University of Kansas Medical Center,
Kansas City, Kansas

CHARLES L. DUNLAP, D.D.S
Professor, Department of Oral
Pathology, School of Dentistry,
University of Missouri, Kansas City,
Missouri

LEE J. DUNN, JR., J.D., LL.M.
General Counsel, Northwestern
Memorial Hospital, Chicago, Illinois

CAROLYN E. EDISON, R.N., B.S.N.
M.W.
Independent clinical nurse specialist
and Instructor, William Jewell
College, Liberty, Missouri

MICHAEL P. FARRELL, Ph.D.
Associate Professor of Sociology and
Director, Family Study Center,
Department of Sociology, State
University of New York at Buffalo,
Amherst, New York

LORETTA C. FORD, R.N. Ed.D.
Dean and Director of Nursing,
University of Rochester Medical
Center, Rochester, New York

JEAN HUFF GALA, R.N., M.S.N.
Assistant Professor, Public Health
Nursing, College of Nursing–
Peoria Branch, University of Illinois,
Chicago, Illinois

GERALD HANDEL, Ph.D.
Professor of Sociology, The City
College and The Graduate School,
City University of New York, New
York, New York

DEBRA P. HYMOVICH, R.N.,
Ph.D.
Professor, School of Nursing,
University of Colorado Medical
Center, Denver, Colorado

ELLEN H. JANOSIK, R.N., M.S.
Assistant Professor, College of
Nursing and Health Care, Alfred
University, Alfred, New York

NORGE W. JEROME, Ph.D.
Professor, Department of Community
Health, School of Medicine,
University of Kansas College of
Health Sciences and Hospital,
Kansas City, Kansas

MIRA L. LESSICK, R.N., M.S.
Assistant Professor of Pediatric
Nursing and Clinician, School of
Nursing, University of Rochester,
Rochester, New York

ROSEMARY J. McKEIGHEN,
R.N., M.S.
Associate Professor, Clinical
Specialist, Psychiatric Mental Health
Nursing; Marriage, Family, and Child
Counselor, College of Nursing,
University of Iowa, Iowa City, Iowa

JED B. MAEBIUS, JR., LL.B.,
LL.M.
Attorney, San Antonio, Texas

JEAN R. MILLER, R.N., Ph.D.
Assistant Professor, School of
Nursing and Department of
Sociology, University of Rochester,
Rochester, New York

HELEN REISCH MOORE, R.N.,
M.A.
Coordinator, Undergraduate Public
Health Nursing, University of Illinois
Medical Center, Chicago, Illinois

ORA RIOS PRATTES, R.N., M.S.
Director, Barrio Comprehensive
Child Health Care Center, San
Antonio, Texas

PETER T. ROWLEY, M.D.
Professor of Medicine, Pediatrics,
and Genetics, School of Medicine,
University of Rochester, Rochester,
New York

MADELINE H. SCHMITT, R.N.,
  Ph.D., F.A.A.N.
Associate Professor of Nursing and
Sociology, School of Nursing,
University of Rochester, Rochester,
New York

JEAN L. SPARBER, M.S.,
  A.C.S.W. (deceased)
Medical Social Worker, Children's
Hospital, Morristown, New Jersey

MELINDA M. SWENSON, R.N.,
  M.S.N.
Clinical Coordinator, Planned
Parenthood of South Central Indiana,
Bloomington, Indiana

CAROL TAYLOR
Anthropologist-in-Residence, College
of Nursing, University of Florida,
Gainesville, Florida

MICHAEL A. VIREN, Ph.D.
Director of Utilities, Missouri Public
Service Commission, Jefferson City,
Missouri

PREFACE

Professional personnel concerned with today's health delivery systems are seeking improved methods of providing health care to the masses while attempting to keep this care personal and individualized. Nurses play a key role in delivering this individualized health care. Nurses have an advantage in developing and utilizing unique and innovative methods of delivering health care, because in all health care settings, they are with individuals and their families a greater majority of time than are other professionals. One method being developed for improved health services is the emphasis on the entire family unit rather than on just one individual member.

We believe, as nurses, educators, and citizens, that this trend to emphasize the entire family unit is a realistic and reasonable one. It is one that emphasizes the dignity and personality of the family as well as the dignity and personality of the individual. It is a realistic approach to helping people help themselves, because they can avail themselves of the resources and strengths of their nuclear, extended, or other family type. Therefore, it seems only fitting that a book should be compiled to bring together selected original multidisciplinary references that are applicable to the nursing of members of family units.

It is imperative that nurses become informed, and inform others, of how health care can be practiced by considering the family unit. We have, therefore, compiled original contributions from nurses working with family units, and from other professionals from whom nurses obtain basic knowledge related to families.

We do not pretend to give you all the concepts and theories related to working with the family. We want you, whether students or practicing health team members, to use this material as a basis for application in your individual health care situations and as a stimulus for ideas related to new and effective roles for delivering health care to families. We encourage you to share your ideas and opinions with us and we welcome all feedback.

Since the first edition of *Family Health Care* was published in 1973, there has been an ever-expanding emphasis on the family as a unit of care. Consequently, we have found it useful to expand this edition into two volumes. Volume I contains introductory information regarding theories, frameworks, and approaches useful in providing high quality care to families. Volume II contains selected concepts and interventions related to developmental and situational crises at various points in the family life cycle.

Volume I, *Family Health Care: General Perspectives,* provides a general background that can be applied by health care providers caring for families in a variety of settings and situations.

Part 1, Introductory Considerations, presents a number of conceptual and theoretical approaches to viewing the family that can be applied in planning and delivering health care. In addition, an historical perspective of the American family is provided along with a discussion of current and emerging family systems. Part 2, Factors Affecting the Family, is concerned with selected variables that affect family development and interaction. Specific areas covered include legal, economic, cultural, environmental, dental, and nutritional factors impinging upon the family. Also included is the effect on the family of a career mother. Part 3, Approaches to Assessment and Intervention, covers a variety of considerations useful in the delivery of health care to families. Included in this section are suggestions for family assessments, counseling, and education. In addition, the development of family nursing, the concept of community health family nursing, and the means of humanizing health care are discussed along with the legal aspects of nursing and medicine.

Volume II, *Family Health Care: Developmental and Situational Crises,* provides a variety of perspectives for working with families facing developmental and situational crises. Part 1 of this volume, Expanding and Contracting Families, covers the family life cycle from expectant parenthood through senescence, along with selected aspects of parenthood. Part 2, Situational Family Crises, covers crisis situations that have been selected to provide a variety of physical and psychosocial problems spanning the life cycle.

ACKNOWLEDGMENTS

The development of a book such as this can occur only with the cooperation and encouragement of family, friends, and colleagues. We would like to acknowledge the support and assistance of those who made this book possible.

The authors are especially grateful to both of their faculties, who made many important suggestions. Thanks also go to those nurses, physicians, and members of other disciplines who contributed so much of their time and effort to the writing of these chapters. We would also like to express our appreciation to the many students and readers of the first edition who offered their suggestions for these books. This type of cooperation narrows the communication gap and serves to make the content more relevant.

Special thanks go to Lucretia McClure, Librarian, University of Rochester, for her magnificent support and assistance. Thanks also to Gloria Hagopian, R.N., M.S., for doing some of the tedious proofreading and the indexing and to Barry Pless, M.D., for his support and belief in this book.

We would like to thank the many authors and publishers who have given permission to use their data and publications. It is this type of cooperation that will make it possible to unite the efforts of a variety of individuals to share their knowledge in order to strive for quality care for many families.

We are especially grateful to Nancy Kita, not only for her fine secretarial assistance, but for keeping the project organized. We are also grateful to Kathie Barnes, Zelma Bicknell, and Betty Phelps for their secretarial assistance. They helped us meet our deadlines.

We would also like to thank the McGraw-Hill Book Company for making this book possible and especially Sally Barhydt and Mary Ann Richter for their cooperation.

Our warmest and sincerest appreciation goes to Lillian Hymovich and Howard, Amanda, and Rebecca Barnard for their kindness and patience during the development of these books.

Debra P. Hymovich
Martha Underwood Barnard

FAMILY HEALTH CARE

Volume One
General Perspectives

PART ONE

INTRODUCTORY CONSIDERATIONS

This section presents a variety of conceptual and theoretical perspectives that can be applied in the delivery of health care to families. It is important for all members of the health team to be aware of a variety of approaches when working with families, as awareness can make it possible to use knowledge from specific disciplines in order to deliver optimum health care.

The first chapter, *Theories of Family Development,* provides an overview of frameworks based on psychoanalytic, general systems, developmental, interactional, and role theories. Chapter 2, *Family Epidemiology: An Approach to Assessment and Intervention,* shows how the epidemiological triad of host-agent-environment can be applied in providing families with primary, secondary, and/or tertiary levels of prevention. Chapter 3, *Sociological Aspects of Parenthood,* provides us with an understanding of reproduction and child-rearing behaviors from a sociological perspective. Parenthood is discussed from the standpoint of social class and ethnic differences and the impact of social change. Chapter 4, *The American Family: An Historical Perspective,* traces the development of American family life and suggests implications for family health care. Among the topics covered are husband-wife, parent-child, and extended family relations; marital formation; and divorce rates. An overview of crisis theory and crisis intervention is presented in Chapter 5, *Theories of Family Crisis.* The final chapter of this section examines *The Development of Family Nursing.*

1

THEORIES OF FAMILY DEVELOPMENT

ELLEN H. JANOSIK AND JEAN R. MILLER

NEED FOR A THEORETICAL FRAMEWORK

Theoretical frameworks are inductive structures within which specified knowledge can move from speculation toward sound, definable concepts. Although not a complete theory, a theoretical framework is a set of concepts, connected in hypothetical terms, that must be tested and proved through empirical investigation if a theory is to emerge. An hypothesis may be intuitive, but objective evidence is required for the theoretical framework to be reliable and durable. Furthermore, widespread application of tested hypotheses within a theoretical framework permits an investigator to adopt a unifying terminology in which to present and contrast observations. Utilization of a theoretical framework to the study of families represents an attempt to produce order from the disorder of family life. What is required then for real understanding of families is a theoretical framework that acknowledges the commonalities of all families while recognizing the uniqueness of each.

Theory has been described poetically as "the net man weaves to catch the world of observation—to explain, predict, and influence it." The same source justified theories as "intellectual tools for organizing data in such a way that one can make inferences or logical transitions from one set of data to another; they serve as guidelines to the investigation, organization, and discovery of matters of observable fact" (Deutsch and Krauss, 1965, p. 6).

A theoretical framework applicable to families provides a comprehensive structure that identifies and defines the relationships within the family. Having selected a theoretical framework, the health professional can begin to select circumstances in which observations are made, to outline enabling procedures, and to connect the observed phenomena to the concepts that comprise the theoretical framework. Professionals seeking effective ways to assess family resources, plans, and implementation of therapeutic stratagems may choose one theoretical framework or devise an approach drawn from several schema. The manner in which assessment, planning, and intervention progress, the inclusion or exclusion of salient factors, the choice of family goals, and the establishment of the therapeutic contract all constitute procedures determined by the therapeutic framework used to analyze family interaction and development. Whether the theoretical framework is applied in a pure or modified form, its use permits the selection and organization of discrete observations into meaningful constructs that facilitate assessment, planning, and therapeutic intervention.

PSYCHOANALYTIC THEORY

A broad approach to family study might begin with Freud's postulates, which were based on clinical observation but were not subject to rigorous testing of hypotheses. Freud outlined three premises that, if developed further, might have contributed to the development of family theory. These premises stated that there exists a collective psychological life within the family shared and created by each member. In addition, there is a transmitting of attitudes and feelings from one generation to the next, plus an unconscious process of assimilation. Freud considered the family to be a natural group that embodied a collective psyche comparable to the individual psychological processes of persons comprising the family. According to this formulation, it is the intrapsychic life of the family that enables older members to transmit values to younger generations so that there is always a continuity of emotional life within the family that renders the unconscious experiences of one generation comprehensible to the succeeding one. Although Freud was writing specifically of the transmission of neurotic behaviors and of the dissemination of family pathology, his postulates do not exclude a collective psychological life inherent in every family system, functional or otherwise (Anthony, 1971).

According to Freud, ambivalence and conflict are inherent in family life, perhaps as an outcome of the continuous, fluctuating level of tension that results from family bonding, caring, and involvement. The preponderance of dependent members within any family predisposes to fragility and a state of precarious equilibrium. Yet this same dependency of younger family members on powerful parent figures fosters identification with the parent of the same gender and eventual internalization of prevailing family standards.

GENERAL SYSTEMS FRAMEWORK

A theory that health professionals are applying with increasing frequency to the study of families is general systems theory. According to this theory, families are viewed as systems comprised of subsystems that interact around collective concerns and purposes. In addition, the family system also interacts with other social systems such as schools, churches, and political institutions. The family is an open system to the extent that external cultural factors greatly affect the sequence and development of family life. However, the permeability of family boundaries varies from family to family. There are many families that do not replicate community normative systems but rather adapt norms to conform to family preferences. Often such families reject more of community values than they accept, so that there are dimensions of family life that are not readily revealed except by the application of a theoretical framework. Moreover, parental influence is not absolute. Even the most effective parents are instruments of the community in the sense that their behaviors are supplemented by input from siblings, grandparents, teachers, clergy, and various sociolegal figures. These external agents occasionally impose contradictory expectations on the family, or demand conformity to standards that are unacceptable to families that resist change.

Each system has characteristic properties, structure, functions, boundaries, and feedback mechanisms. As systems, families are characterized by wholeness, nonsummativity, and equifinality. A family has wholeness or unity because it is made up of interdependent rather than independent parts. Family members depend upon one another in varying degrees for a number of purposes. Children are dependent on the family for food, shelter, and for socialization and emotional support, whereas parents may be dependent upon the children for emotional gratification and possible assistance in old age. Incipient resentments that might arise from the prolonged dependence of weak family members on the strong is somewhat moderated by the interdependence of family members on each other and on the family as a functioning system.

The concept of *interdependence* of family members is interpersonal, since it includes not only intrapsychic needs that foster interdependence, but interactional processes as well. Interdependence allows nurturing parents to experience vicarious pleasure in witnessing the accomplishments of their children, and to savor the approval of the community as reward for their efforts. Interdependence also necessitates careful monitoring of aggression within the family so that moderate amounts can be tolerated but excessive amounts may be controlled. Families impose certain constraints on all members and must endeavor to maintain acceptable levels of spontaneity without jeopardizing the well-being of any member. The problem of reconciling the needs of all members is never easy, for satisfying one person may occur at the expense of another. This is often the pattern when the needs of one family member may appear more acute at a particular time, or when the attributes of one member are more highly valued than the attributes of another.

A second characteristic of family systems, *nonsummativity,* defines the degree of interrelatedness among the system parts. Family assessments must include the connecting or interactional patterns between and among the parts. For instance, an accurate picture of interrelatedness of family members cannot be obtained by taking a measurement of individual members on a certain dimension. Rather, the assessment would have to include a measurement of each potential interaction between members. In a family of two members, this might constitute only one measurement; but in a family of four, six measurements would be included. A system in which a change in one member does not greatly cause change in other members is a system with a low degree of interrelatedness or nonsummativity. Families do not function very well without considerable interdependence among the members, and total absence of interdependence may cause the family to cease existing in any meaningful sense.

A third characteristic of family systems is *equifinality,* a term that describes the progressive complexity of interactional patterns in the family. Equifinality means that assessment of a family's interactional patterns can be approached from various vantage points. Health practitioners need not be overly concerned with simple causal relationships, since the assessment of interactional patterns is likely to be the same regardless of the content or the cause of the interaction. This means that the practitioner need not trace dissension within the family to a specific cause or a specific consequence. What is more useful is to ascertain the reciprocal nature of the interaction that contributes to the maintenance of dysfunctional patterns within the system. Consideration of equifinality means that process or *the how* of interactions is more relevant than content, which deals with *what* is occurring.

Structure exists within each family system. This refers to the organization of relationships between and among members. Within families, patterns are established over time regarding how, when, and to whom family members should relate. According to systems theory, this organization of relationships is sufficiently flexible for the system to function effectively when changes occur within and outside the family unit. Structural organization makes it possible for members to interact with a minimum of frustration, since they know what interactions are possible and to what extent. Structural flexibility is important when family members are added or subtracted, since new patterns of relating must emerge to carry on the functions of the system.

The structure of families is manifested through subsystems that are formed to carry out the functions of the system. These subsystems develop not only through function, but also through age, sex, generation, and interests. An example is the parental subsystem that evolves from the marital dyad and is joined eventually by the sibling subsystem. There are a large number of other complementary relationships such as mother-daughter, aunt-niece, older sister-younger sister, and sister-brother subsystems. Any one family member is a part of several subsystems in which the members have different functions and levels of power and influence.

Boundaries exist around the family and around each subsystem to protect the subsystem. These boundaries are inclusionary or exclusionary, and state who may participate in the family system and in subsystems. Clarity of boundaries is important for effective family functioning, since this allows family members to perform their functions with a minimum of ambiguity. Boundaries vary in several respects. Some families have inappropriately rigid boundaries; others have diffuse boundaries. Rigid boundaries imply separation and disengagement. This means that there is little communication between subsystems and that members do not get involved sufficiently in times of equilibrium or disequilibrium. A highly enmeshed family with diffuse boundaries is characterized by excessive involvement on the part of family members. In times of stress, the enmeshed family responds quickly, with great reactivity, but no particular efficiency. The optimum middle range where boundaries are clear to all members allows healthy conditions for differentiation of family functions and growth of individual members.

The functions of each subsystem and of the family as a whole are influenced by family values and purposes, which vary according to sociocultural backgrounds. A common purpose of the family is the socialization of children, who incorporate such values as expressiveness, education, religion, and materialism. On an optimum level, subsystems within the family perform various activities congruent with these values. Recognition and understanding of family values are important to the health professional, since interventions designed to change aspects of family functioning are unlikely to be followed unless the suggestions are concordant with family values and norms.

Functioning of family systems and subsystems is affected by a process called *feedback*. This is a process whereby the system of subsystems takes in information (input) through permeable boundaries and puts out information or behavior (output) according to a set level of functioning. If family output deviates above or below this level, a process called *negative feedback* serves to alert the system to return to the usual level. This process is similar to the regulation of temperature by a thermostat. Changes can be made in the level of family functioning through the process of *positive feedback,* which, once initiated, may proceed to the point of making the family system dysfunctional. Positive feedback encourages activity in one direction, which, if continued, may proceed to an inappropriate extreme. An untoward effect of positive feedback may be that historically inappropriate behavior is continued past the point of functionality. Usually, however, health professionals use regulated amounts of positive feedback to bring the family to a more effective level of functioning.

The health professional can use concepts from general systems theory to assess family functioning. Aspects that must be considered in this framework are the degree of interrelatedness among the family members, the organizational structure of relationships, the nature of boundaries between subsystems and other social systems, and the extent to which the functions of the family meet individual and community needs. There is an optimal level of family functioning, so that marked deviation is dysfunctional and must be adjusted by the family either through its own resources or with the help of health professionals.

DEVELOPMENTAL THEORY

The developmental framework is a relative newcomer to the list of theoretical formulations applied to family life. Its introduction to family study began about 1930, but it has become widely used only within the last two decades (Duvall, 1977). A primary advantage of the developmental approach is that it sees families as changing, not only from day to day but also from year to year. Basic to this framework is the definition of a developmental task as one that must be accomplished at a crucial point in time if the individual is to experience success with later tasks. Conversely, failure to accomplish a developmental task at the time of its ascendence leads to difficulty or failure with subsequent tasks. Thus, the developmental framework assumes that there are successive tasks that families confront over the years, in the same manner as individuals who advance, through mastery of the preceding task, from one developmental stage to the next.

Applying the developmental framework permits family life to be divided into various chronological stages. The simplest division merely categorizes families into expanding or contracting systems, with the expanding stage lasting from the establishment of the marital dyad until the children are grown. The stage of the contracting family begins when the first child leaves the parental home and ends with the death of the surviving spouse (Duvall, 1977). A more complicated developmental scheme

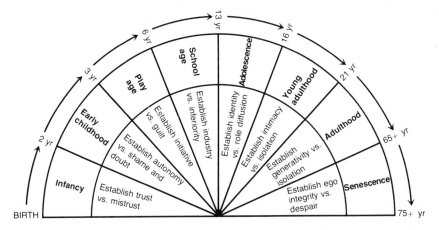

Figure 1-1   Stages in the life cycle of man. After Erikson, 1950.

divides the family into twenty-four stages (Rogers, 1973) and includes not only the progression of older children in the family, but also the concurrent influences of the younger children. Although the two-stage division of family life is inadequate for most purposes, the twenty-four stage categorization suffers from excessive detail. A useful compromise can be found in the eight-stage categorization of family life (Duvall, 1977), which can be contrasted effectively with the eight-stage categorization of individual development of Erikson (1963), and is comprehensive enough to permit sufficient differentiation of cyclic family stages of development (see Figure 1-1).

The basic assumption of the Eriksonian scheme is that each developmental task is related to the others; the tasks are accomplished sequentially with allowance being made for variations in rate and efficiency. The eight stages in the life cycle of the family formulated by Duvall (Figure 1-2) offer an interesting corollary and provide insight into the complexity of the family's developmental tasks that are interrelated with the developmental tasks of the family members comprising the family system.

It is sometimes difficult for the family to reconcile the egocentric demands of every member in a way that minimizes conflict but still allows the developmental tasks of individual members to be accomplished. Ascendence of a developmental task is often accomplished by a sense of urgency that arises from the (1) physical maturation of the individual, (2) cultural pressure and expectations for the individual, (3) internal aspirations and values of the individual (Duvall, 1977). For example, the developmental task of an adolescent is to resolve an identity crisis and avoid role diffusion. This struggle to free oneself from parental bonds may take place at a time when parents are still unready to relinquish their roles as parents of a busy Teen-Age Family in order to accept less dominant roles

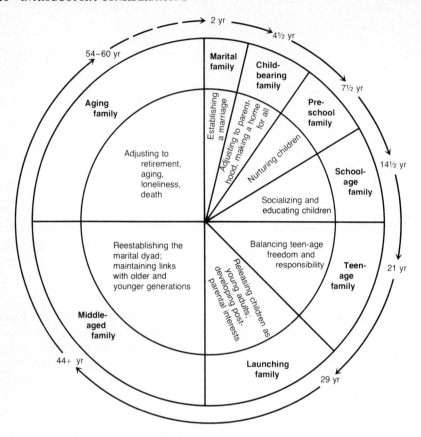

2 yr

4½ yr

54–60 yr

Marital
family

Child-
bearing
family

7½ yr

Aging
family

Pre-
school
family

Establishing
a marriage

Adjusting to parent-
hood, making a home
for all

Nurturing children

Adjusting to
retirement,
aging,
loneliness,
death

School-
age
family

14½ yr

Socializing and
educating children

Reestablishing the
marital dyad;
maintaining links
with older and
younger generations

Balancing teen-age
freedom and
responsibility

Teen-
age
family

21 yr

Releasing children as
young adults;
developing post-
parental interests

Middle-
aged
family

44+ yr

Launching
family

29 yr

Figure 1-2   Stages in the family life cycle. After Duvall, 1977.

as parents of a Launching Family. On the other hand, adult children who
have moved through the Eriksonian stages of Adolescence and Young
Adulthood and have established the generativity of Adulthood may find
themselves ultimately confronted by parents in Senescence, whose infir-
mities encroach on the lives of mature children. This problem can be expressed as easily in Duvall's family life cycle, since senescent parents
represent an Aging Family that is no longer self-sufficient but requires
help from children who now constitute a Launching or Middle-Aged Family with developmental tasks of its own.

One of the responsibilities of the family is to create an environment in
which each member can undertake the task crucial to their life stage. At
the same time the family is engaged in meeting the individualistic demands
of each member in a way which allows the family to survive and function.
The developmental framework uses the notion of cyclic stages because of
the intergenerational nature of family development. As the family founded

by the marital dyad moves from an expanding to a contracting phase, its grown children embark on their own cycles of family expansion followed by contraction. During periods of expansion, the number of family members increases but the number of relationships within the family is greater than the number of members since individual members simultaneously occupy multiple roles. It must be noted that periods of family expansion occupy far less time than do periods of contraction, although attention given to early stages in the family life cycle has in the past received disproportionate attention from investigators and from representatives of the media and the helping professions.

At times the developmental tasks of the family and of individual members move harmoniously toward completion. The small child learning trust through the nurturing of a child-bearing family is accomplishing its own developmental task, assisted by parents who have accepted the enactment of that time-appropriate role. A short time later the same child, moving toward autonomy over its own person, is assured of support and understanding from parents who have now undertaken performance of a later family developmental stage. Over the course of time task accomplishment may be endangered by lags that create conflict as the crucial task of one member meets with reluctance of other members to move to the next stage in the family life cycle. Therefore, the unwillingness of parents to accommodate to changes in their growing children, or their wish to continue child-bearing functions in order to forestall their own progression to later stages of family life, is sometimes apparent, to the detriment of family efficiency. The developmental framework considers changes in family systems over time. As individual members move from one life stage to the next, family life is marked by changing relationships, with family functions of one stage superseded by responsibilities of the next.

INTERACTIONAL THEORY

Family interaction occurs in the present, is oriented toward the future, but is also modified by memories of events in the past. What this implies is that for most families the current situation is seen in light of future consequences and that the perception of the present and future is altered by the early life experiences of family members, especially the parental dyad. This means that the quality of family interaction is affected by a vast number of variables that are subtle and complex.

George Herbert Mead is considered the originator of the theory of symbolic interaction (Mead, 1934). The contributions of Mead that are relevant to the study of the family include his definition of "meaning" and his analysis of the "act." *Meaning* refers to the relationship between an individual and the events in the environment. The individual must respond to environmental events in the form of acts that have meaning to the responding individual. Within the family an environmental event may occur, such as the birth of an infant. To a 2-year-old in the home, the meaning of such an event may be a fear of a reduction in motherly cherishing. A 2-year-old's response to the event may assume the form of a hostile "act" if insecurity is habitually expressed by tormenting the baby or making excessive demands on mother. With continued reassurance regarding mother's love, the anxiety of the 2-year-old is allayed. As an understanding grows of mother's ability to nurture both her children, and as hostility is gradually replaced by acceptance the child again feels secure. The basic assumptions derived from Mead's two concepts (meaning and act) are (1) that human beings live in a world of meanings, and (2) that humans are capable of being socialized into acting in different ways according to the environmental context in which they find themselves.

It is through interaction with the family and with the larger community that individuals attain a sense of selfhood or identity. The reactions that individuals receive from others and that they process in idiosyncratic ways give substance to feelings and attitudes about the self that ultimately become the self system. The capacity of individuals to assume the perspective of others in respect to themselves causes them to experience themselves both as subjects and objects. What this means is that the developing self system creates an awareness that allows one to be actor and audience simultaneously and to see oneself as one is seen by other participants in interpersonal transactions. This concept of self develops cognitively from social interactions, which in time are organized into consensually validated relationships that have external origins but eventually become internally integrated. Although all interactions are influential to some extent, the self system is derived from the attitudes and reactions of "significant others" in the family (Sullivan, 1953) and "generalized others" (Mead, 1967) representing the community. In explaining the evolving self system, Mead wrote that individuals experience themselves both from the specific standpoint of individual members of the small groups to which they belong and from the standpoint of their larger reference groups.

ROLE THEORY

Life in the parental family has been depicted as a time of emergence of the self system when family interaction molds the personality through its effect on the children. By means of the self-concept the individual chooses from the roles available those that can be enacted adequately and with some assurance of reward. The world of the child is organized into pairs of roles, one of which he or she enacts, with the complementary role being enacted by another. Such complementarity has been termed *prototype role differentiations,* inasmuch as the self-concept develops through learning in sequence different ways of role enactment. For example, the child of a domineering parent may incorporate into its self system the submissiveness that experience has taught it to portray. Through the same experience the child has been introduced to the parent's dominant role, which may be found to be enviable, in spite of having never practiced it. The child, when allowed to interact in the absence of the father, may choose the role of bully toward others, having already learned domineering behaviors through interactions with the father. On the other hand, discomfort with the unfamiliar role of dominator may persuade the child to continue a usual posture of submissiveness even in the absence of the father. A simpler way of expressing this is that the child of a domineering parent may identify with the aggressor, or, by assuming a submissive role, choose to identify with the victim.

The first role differentiation is the experience of fusion with the mother, which is later disrupted as the infant learns of the separateness of the mother. At this point the infant does not differentiate clearly between mother and father, since both are all-powerful in relation to the child. In time the child learns to enact one distinctive role with mother and another with father. The loss of fusion with the mother is based on the infant's perception of itself as powerless and mother as omnipotent. As the child moves out into the community, it learns that the relationships it had with its parents are less useful with outsiders, and that the same role may be enacted with many different persons outside the family. With teachers the child need only play the role of schoolchild and with shopkeepers the role of customer. Having learned this, the child is able to distinguish unique relationships that can be enacted with only one person from those that can be enacted with many categories of persons. Eventually the child is able to distinguish ascribed status from achieved status, with all that this implies. Ascribed status is that position that chances to fall to individuals, and is based merely on belonging to a certain family, school, or neighborhood. Achieved or acquired status refers to earned rank or position such as that held by the President or the class cheerleaders. An individual who can make all such distinctions has mastered role choice and role repertoire to the point where a role appropriate to most situations that will be encountered in everyday life can be assumed. This complicated process has its origins in the interactions taking place from moment to moment in the family.

Consistent parental roles in the family are essential if children are to identify and internalize the roles they must someday assume. Parental roles are socially rewarding and usually earn the approval of the community and the previous generation, unless norms are transgressed. Therefore, the functions of nurture, protection, and guidance that are bestowed on children are not relinquished easily or willingly by parents who have grown accustomed to these interactions. At the time when children are demanding greater independence, the emotional and financial investment of parents is often at a peak. Realizing that the passage of time has altered the enactment of their parental roles and unsure of what is left for them, parents are often reluctant to accept any lesser involvement with their maturing children. Lives that were crowded and active suddenly seem empty, and parents are faced with the realization that they have only each other. Thus, the empty-nest syndrome is made more frightening by children who depart just when parents are facing mid-life crises of unfulfilled hopes and waning powers.

Role enactment requires a balancing of interpersonal transactions against intrapersonal needs. In role taking, family members negotiate compromises based upon the goals of some members, as these are affected by the working consensus reached by the family as a whole. Negotiation proceeds through repeated interactions that mediate between role expectations and role performances of family members.

NEED FOR AN ECLECTIC APPROACH

Each conceptual framework offers a particular focus for studying family development. Focusing on one aspect of family life reveals that aspect but may ignore others of equal or greater importance. To adopt a single framework is unnecessarily restrictive, because it discounts the multiple aspects of family life and confines itself to a reductionistic point of view. Every conceptual framework is advantageous in some respects, but consigning all observations into one theoretical framework results in emphasizing some details at the expense of the others.

The psychoanalytic framework has the advantage of stressing early childhood experiences as modifiers of instinctual traits. The family is considered a natural group that is dominated by parental figures with whom the child identifies and whose values are gradually internalized by the child.

The general systems approach has been widely used in family study. This framework has applicability to individual family members, to family subsystems, and also includes the family in relation to external influences and institutions. It deals with reciprocal relationships and with family structural organization and patterns.

Usefulness of an eclectic approach to family study has been enhanced by the developmental framework, whose perspective is chronological. This approach is inward looking to the extent that functions, roles, and tasks of family members are examined as these change over time. As the family life cycle progresses, activities change and relationships of family members with each other and with larger social institutions alter qualitatively and quantitatively. The developmental approach provides a structure in which these alterations can be defined and assessed. In addition, the developmental approach employs a sweeping or historical view that deals with stages in family development rather than immediate occurrences.

An interactional framework employs an internal perspective that examines behaviors and transactions of family members. This framework permits the observation of how family roles are enacted and how role performance is perceived within the family. The interactional framework and general systems theory give little attention to antecedent events, but deal largely with a here-and-now content.

Role theory provides a framework whereby specific norms of the family guide family members in interpreting explicit and implicit messages regarding expected behavior, in learning the skills of role-playing, and in performing overt role behavior. Families provide the opportunities and impetus for members to assume new roles as members make transitions from one developmental stage to the next.

In eclectic terms the family represents a system of interacting personalities that does not depend for its survival on the harmonious relations of its members, but endures even in the presence of long-standing conflict. As long as family members are involved and interacting, the family is viable and enduring.

A related series of concepts that are generally accepted, communicated, and understood form the basis of any theoretical framework. Although devised for a specific framework, such concepts tend to overlap. Some concepts formulated for one framework can be expanded to facilitate understanding of general family observation and research. Yet these statements do not refute the argument for an eclectic approach in studying families. Since there is no one theoretical framework at this time that is extensive enough to encompass all facets of family life, the family must be seen from many perspectives so that all dimensions are apparent. Each theoretical framework can best reveal only that aspect of family life that it purports to examine. Utilizing an eclectic framework permits an illumination of family life that is truly comprehensive.

REFERENCES

Anthony, J. E. History of group psychotherapy. In H. I. Kaplan & B. J. Sadock (Eds.) *Comprehensive group psychotherapy.* Baltimore: Williams and Wilkins, 1971.

Auger, J. R. *Behavioral systems and nursing.* Englewood Cliffs, N.J.: Prentice-Hall, 1976, 1–47.

Biddle, B. J., & Thomas, E. J. (Eds.) *Role theory: Concepts and research.* New York: John Wiley and Sons, 1966.

Bradin, C. J., & Herban, N. L. *Community health: A systems approach.* New York: Appleton-Century-Crofts, 1976.

Chin, R. The mobility of systems models and developmental models for practitioners. In W. G. Bennis, K. D. Benne, & R. Chin (Eds.), *The planning of change* (2d ed.). New York: Holt, Rinehart and Winston, 1969, 297–312.

Deutsch, M., & Krauss, R. M. *Theories in social psychology.* New York: Basic Books, 1965.

Duvall, E. M. *Marriage and family development* (5th ed.). Philadelphia: J. B. Lippincott, 1977.

Erikson, E. *Childhood and society.* New York: W. W. Norton, 1963.

Foley, V. D. *An introduction to family therapy.* New York: Grune and Stratton, 1974.

Ford, F. R., & Herrick, J. Family rules: Family life styles. *American Journal of Orthopsychiatry,* 1974, *44*(1), 61–69.

Glennin, C. Formulation of standards of nursing practice using a nursing model. In J. P. Riehl & C. Roy (Eds.), *Conceptual models for nursing practice.* New York: Appleton-Century-Crofts, 1974, 234–246.

Gray, W., Duhl, F. J., & Rizzo, N. D. (Eds.) *General systems theory and psychiatry.* Boston: Little, Brown, 1969.

Hall, J. E., & Weaver, B. R. *Distributive nursing practice: A systems approach to community health.* Philadelphia: J. B. Lippincott, 1977.

Mead, G. H. *Mind, self and society.* Chicago: University of Chicago Press, 1934.

Minuchin, S. *Families and family therapy.* Cambridge, Mass.: Harvard University Press, 1974.

Nisbet, R. A. *The social bond.* New York: Alfred A. Knopf, 1970.

Pratt, L. *Family structure and effective health behavior: The energized family.* Boston: Houghton Mifflin, 1976.

Robischon, P., & Scott, D. Role theory and its application in family nursing. *Nursing Outlook,* 1969, 52–57.

Rogers, R. H. *Family interaction and transaction: The developmental approach.* Englewood Cliffs, N.J.: Prentice-Hall, 1973.

Skynner, A. C. R. *Systems of family and marital psychotherapy.* New York: Brunner/Mazel, 1976.

Sullivan, H. S. *The interpersonal theory of psychiatry.* New York: W. W. Norton, 1953.

Von Bertolanffy, L. *General system theory.* New York: Braziller, 1968.

Wertheim, E. S. The science and typology of family systems II. Further theoretical and practical considerations. *Family Process,* September 1975, *14*(3), 285–309.

Yura, H. *The nursing process: Assessing, planning, implementing, evaluating* (2d ed.). New York: Appleton-Century-Crofts, 1973.

CHAPTER TWO

FAMILY EPIDEMIOLOGY: AN APPROACH TO ASSESSMENT AND INTERVENTION

KATHRYN ELLEN CHRISTIANSEN

Epidemiology, traditionally and historically, is considered to be the study of outbreaks of infectious disease or epidemics. Modern-day epidemiologists, however, are concerned with the distribution of human health problems. They attempt to define the cause of these problems as they try to identify effective preventive measures.

"The etymological derivation of the word 'epidemiology' suggests its purview: epi = upon, demos = people, logos = study—the study of what (comes upon) the people" (Omran, 1974, p. 675). With this derivation in mind, the following more encompassing definitions of epidemiology are offered. Cassel (1962) concludes that, "Epidemiology is one of the sciences concerned with the study of the processes which determine or influence the health of people (health includes social as well as physical and mental health). People live in groups and it is with their health in relation to their behavior in social groups that epidemiology is primarily concerned." Leavell and Clark (1965, p. 40) also define epidemiology in a broad sense as a "field of science which is concerned with the various factors and conditions that determine the occurrence and distribution of health, disease, defects, disability and death among groups of individuals."

The "factors and conditions" referred to in Leavell and Clark's definition are identified as host, agent, and environment in the epidemiologic triad (see Figure 2-1). Since the host, agent, and environment are constantly interacting with one another, they are often represented schemati-

H = Susceptible host

    The particular individual or
    group of immediate concern.

A = Causative agent

    Disorder is created
    by its presence of
    absence.

E = Environment

    All that is external to the
    agent and host.

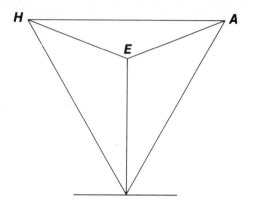

Figure 2-1 The epidemiologic triad.

cally as a three-sided figure. In this case, however, they are diagrammed as the base corners of a pyramid that is inverted and balanced on its apex.

The key to understanding the interaction and the interdependence of the host, agent, and environment is to visualize them in dynamic equilibrium. While balanced there is no disorder. Minor imbalances can be tolerated, and adjustments made, within the triad. It is easy to see from the diagram that failure to compensate for changes at any point will cause the pyramid to topple. It will stay out of balance until changes can be made to regain the equilibrium.

The *epidemiologic method* consists of a series of steps to be followed when dealing with disorder or triad imbalance.

1. Define the problem or disorder. Consider the nature, extent, and significance of the health problem. Ask the question: How does this group differ from others?
2. Appraise existing information. Identify and categorize data under the respective headings of host, agent, and environment. Acknowledge gaps in data.
3. Formulate plans for intervention. This will include objectives for primary, secondary, and tertiary prevention.
4. Institute the plan of health promotion, specific protection, early diagnosis and prompt treatment, disability limitation, or rehabilitation.
5. Determine the success of the approach. Evaluate the extent to which objectives were met.
6. Apply the findings to similar disorders. Share results with the family, groups, and colleagues.

This method can be applied to all human disorders—anything that is a problem to the people and the groups in which they live.

WHY FAMILY EPIDEMIOLOGY?

The family is the most basic societal group. Freeman (1970, p. 110) states that,

> The health problems of families are interlocking. The health of any one member of the family is highly likely to affect the health of others. Each individual affects the family environment by his own presence. That is, each person serves either to reinforce or to contest the values or attitudes held by others, to preserve or to modify the existing physical environment, and to strengthen or to weaken the cohesiveness of the family as an operating unit.

Very often it is the family that influences decisons of its members, particularly in relation to health-related decisions. If there is family disorder, it frequently becomes a family task to set it right or to conceal it from the outside world.

Utilizing the epidemiologic approach to family disorders, one must proceed from the known to the unknown. By looking at the family with a health disorder and comparing it to families without the problem, it is possible to analyze group similarities and differences. The question of why one family manifests certain problems, and other families do not, must always be asked. Consideration must also be given to (1) the effect of disorder on each family member, and the family's effect on the community; (2) the distribution of family health problems; (3) the causes of family health problems; (4) the interaction of causative factors; and (5) the prediction of further occurrence.

The next step is to identify and classify attributes of the host, agent, and environment. Listed below are examples of various characteristics of the host, agent, and environment that can be present in, or have an influence on, the family unit. The lists are not all-inclusive, merely representative of the variety of possibilities. It would be difficult to identify all the influencing variables of most disorders as many are concealed, obscured, or latent. It is suggested that the reader add to the lists as other attributes are uncovered or come to mind.

Attributes of the host, whose susceptibility or resistance to (a) causative agent(s) will affect the occurrence and distribution of a condition or disorder.

1. Habits, customs, characteristic manner of living, personal cleanliness, food preferences, sanitation practices, extent of personal contacts.
2. Demographic data: age, sex, ethnic group, marital status, height, weight.
3. Socioeconomic indicators: occupation, income, role, how viewed by the community.

4. Defenses: immunity, anatomic structures, use of defense mechanisms, level of nutrition.
5. Physiologic processes: coughing, temperature regulation, tolerance.
6. Personality: appearance, heredity, birth order.
7. Constitutional make-up: ability to learn from past experiences, handling of stress, motivation, attitude toward self, attitude toward others (family, friends, acquaintances), approximation to expectations of self or others, level of sophistication or naiveté.
8. Degree of power: internally or externally controlled.

Attributes of the agent, or factor whose presence or absence *causes* the occurrence of a condition.

1. Physical agents: mechanical forces or frictions that may cause injury, atmospheric abnormalities, extremes of temperature and other adverse weather conditions, excessive radiation, noise.
2. Chemical agents: dusts, gases, vapors, fumes, presence of a lethal substance (drugs, lead, plants).
3. Nutritive agents: lack or overabundance of one or more of the basic dietary elements (vitamins, minerals, cholesterol, protein, CHO, fat, water).
4. Biologic agents (living organisms): insects, worms, protozoa, fungi, bacteria, rickettsiae, viruses, humans, animals.
5. Intangible agents: love, hate, ambivalence, self-esteem, availability of support systems.

Attributes of the environment, which, depending upon their characteristics, help to suppress the occurrence of a condition or assist it to thrive.

1. Physical: geography (climate, season, time, weather), soil.
2. Biologic: food supply, water supply, number of living animals, insects, plants.
3. Social and economic: attitudes, beliefs, behavior, customs, culture, transportation, housing, degree of crowding, availability of health services and health providers, occupation, role-status, activities, political climate, family, neighbors, community, city, state, nation, world, mobility.

Some characteristics may easily fit under more than one of the triad components. The degree of crowding, for instance, is listed as an environmental factor. The host's personal reaction to crowding, however, will determine the extent of susceptibility to disorder. Crowding, therefore, could also be identified as the causative agent creating disorder in the host. Actually, how the attribute is originally classified, in and of itself, is not of utmost importance. How the host, agent, and environment are presently affecting one another is a question of greater significance.

At this point the assessor has defined the problem and the nature, extent, and magnitude of the health disorder. In addition existing information has been organized into the classifications of host, agent, environment. The next step in the epidemiological process is to plan an approach to regain triad equilibrium. This approach must include objectives for primary, secondary, and/or tertiary prevention. The following list contains a few representative general goals that one may strive to achieve:

1. Reduce *host* susceptibility.
2. Reduce exposure of the *host* to the causative agent.
3. Increase the positive attributes of the *host*.
4. Provide the *host* with additional knowledge, skills, and defenses.
5. Decrease the *agent* effectiveness.
6. Modify the *agent*.
7. Provide the *agent* with other means of interaction.
8. Remove the *agent* temporarily or permanently.
9. Increase the number of support systems within the *environment*.
10. Modify and/or reduce the factors in the *environment* that contribute to the disorder.
11. Change *environments*.

Leavell and Clark's (1965) classic model, "Levels of Application of Preventive Measures in the Natural History of Disease" (see Table 2-1), provides a format that can be used to identify and categorize prevention measures for any family disorder. What is being proposed in this chapter is that one consider the problems or disorders of individual families within the framework of the epidemiological triad and the following prevention levels of Leavell and Clark: health promotion, specific protection, early diagnosis and prompt treatment, disability limitation, and rehabilitation. Child abuse, as a family disorder, can serve as a prototype to help demonstrate this proposal.

Consider the following:

Mrs. X always wanted a career. She married but wanted no children. When she did become pregnant—an unplanned accident—she was angry and unhappy. She was moralistically opposed to abortion, but hoped that she would spontaneously miscarry. She did not. When the baby was born it was irritable, cried a great deal, kept her awake at night, spit up milk, and resisted her efforts at comfort. It physically reminded her of her mother from whom she had been estranged for years. Her mother had been harsh with her as a child and had disciplined her severely for minor infractions of arbitrary rules. She left home as soon as she was able to support herself, and never returned.

Table 2-1 Levels of application of preventive measures in the natural history of disease

THE NATURAL HISTORY OF ANY DISEASE OF MAN

Interrelations of agent, host, and environmental factors → Production of *stimulus* ——→ Reaction of the *host* to the *stimulus* → Early pathogenesis —→ Discernible early lesions —→ Advanced disease —→ Convalescence

Prepathogenesis period		Period of pathogenesis		
Health promotion	**Specific protection**	**Early Diagnosis and prompt treatment**	**Disability limitation**	**Rehabilitation**
Health education	Use of specific immunizations	Case-finding measures, individual and mass	Adequate treatment to arrest the disease process and to prevent further complications and sequelae	Provision of hospital and community facilities for retraining and education for maximum use of remaining capacities
Good standard of nutrition adjusted to developmental phases of life	Attention to personal hygiene	Screening surveys	Provision of facilities to limit disability and to prevent death	Education of the public and industry to utilize the rehabilitated
Attention to personality development	Use of environmental sanitation	Selective examinations		As full employment as possible
Provision of adequate housing, recreation and agreeable working conditions	Protection against occupational hazards	Objectives:		Selective placement
Marriage counseling and sex education	Protection from accidents	To cure and prevent disease processes		Work therapy in hospitals
Genetics	Use of specific nutrients	To prevent the spread of communicable diseases		Use of sheltered colony
Periodic selective examinations	Protection from carcinogens	To prevent complications and sequelae		
	Avoidance of allergens	To shorten period of disability		

Primary prevention		Secondary prevention		Tertiary prevention

LEVELS OF APPLICATION OF PREVENTIVE MEASURES

Source: R. H. Leavell & E. G. Clark, *Preventive medicine for the doctor in his community,* New York, McGraw-Hill, 1965, p. 21. Reprinted by permission of McGraw-Hill.

Mr. X was of little or no help. He was a passive man who was delighted with the baby, but wanted to have no responsibility for its care. Shortly after the birth he changed jobs and traveled extensively, necessitating that he be away from home many nights of the week. There were no relatives close by and none came to visit. Mrs. X had made no friends outside her office, and, since her colleagues were not social friends, they now made no contact with her.

Mrs. X wanted to return to work but was of the belief that a mother should stay with her child until it is able to be in school. Her husband reinforced this idea.

Using the epidemiological approach to family disorder, more specifically child abuse, let us consider the case of Mrs. X. Below are some of the data known about the characteristics of child abuse (Kempe and Helfer, 1972). The starred items apply to the X family (Table 2-2).

Table 2-2 Characteristics of child abuse

Susceptible *Host* (a special child)	Causative *Agent* (mother/father/boy friend with potential to abuse)	*Environment* (a combination of events that occur in the right order, and at the right time)
*Seen differently by parent or parents	*Abused as a child	*Offers no support systems
*Fails to respond in expected manner	*Unable to deal effectively with stress	*Stress-producing situations
*Seen as bad, willful, stubborn, spoiled, demanding, or slow	*Isolated—cannot trust others	*Ambiguity of the parent role
*Was not a wanted child	*Unrealistic expectations of child or children	*Crisis or series of crises (major and/or minor)
Really is different (retarded, too smart, hyperactive, has a birth defect)		

*Applies to X family. (Adapted from C. H. Kempe and R. E. Helfer, *Helping the battered child and his family,* Philadelphia: J. B. Lippincott, 1972.

With this approach, one first considers the host, agent, and environment in evaluating the potential for child abuse within a family. If the professional was working with the X family (agent) before they had the child (host), they would still have every potential for abuse, and the environment would also contain contributing factors. No child abuse would occur, however, because all three elements of the triad were not present and interacting. The action of the professional, in this situation, would be to strongly encourage birth control methods until the environment changed or until the agent could be counseled regarding this potentially dangerous situation. Advice against this person's becoming involved with day care, or care of the children of friends, would also be appropriate.

With the birth of the child (host), the triad is complete. If, somehow, the host-agent-environment triad were in equilibrium, that is, no abuse was occurring, it would still be necessary to be constantly aware of changes that could upset the balance. The husband being layed off at work, cold weather causing unexpected heating bills, a major illness, the family moving, or the child becoming a behavior problem, are a few of the changes that could occur at any time and cause the triad to become imbalanced.

In working with the X family, one begins to formulate a plan for prevention. Table 2-3 demonstrates the use of Leavell and Clark's model in the identification of various preventive approaches to the family problem of child abuse.

After the data has been gathered, identified, and categorized, and a plan for prevention has been formulated, one has a guide for intervention. This, as we all know, requires time, energy, and patience. In most cases, this task cannot be embarked upon in isolation. It is necessary to enlist the aid of the family, colleagues, and, in many instances, other professional and lay groups within the community. The guide for intervention will involve periodic review to determine the current status of the host-agent-environmental equilibrium. It will also necessitate reevaluation of the prevention objectives to determine if they are being met. Various levels of prevention may be simultaneously invoked. Depending upon the family's progress and motivation, they may attain levels of primary prevention for future problems when they might not previously have been cognizant of those actions as alternatives.

As interaction with the family unit continues, evaluation of the success of the intervention approach is taking place. Concurrently, this knowledge can be applied to similar situations or disorders identified as occurring within other families.

The predictive knowledge that accompanies this approach to family disorder cannot be stressed enough. Ideally, professionals should be identifying host, agent, and environmental factors leading to disorder within every family unit and comparing this knowledge to every other family with whom they have contact.

There are several important points to remember, however. Those factors responsible for the onset of disorder and those responsible for recovery or return to order may be very different. Once one becomes involved with a family, one is a part of the environment and a consultant to the host and/or agent. This presence may assist in the restoration of triad balance, or may cause continued disequilibrium. The professional strives to influ-

Table 2-3 Levels of prevention for child abuse and neglect

Epidemiologic triad of host-agent-environment in equilibrium		Epidemiologic triad of host-agent-environment out of equilibrium		
Period of prepathogenesis		Period of pathogenesis		
Health promotion	**Specific protection**	**Early diagnosis and prompt treatment**	**Disability limitation**	**Rehabilitation**
Use of media and existing groups to describe problem of child abuse while being sensitive to the abuser and the abused	Identifying support systems within a family	Case finding	Removal of children from home	Return to home and family as early as is safe
Advertising parents anonymous groups	Identifying potential in individual or self	Reporting by lay public and professionals	Assignment of a case worker to work closely with family	Involve individuals and/or family in a therapeutic program
Health education re: parenting, child development, discipline, and realistic expectations.	Work toward keeping host, agent, and environment in equilibrium	Recognizing predisposing factors and early patterns of abuse	Supportive and understanding approach by professionals	Continued follow-up
Mental health promotion for parents	Providing an outlet to the potential abuser	Early involvement of agencies		
Assistance to individuals and families to recognize and cope with stress	Counseling children and adults who were abused to the risk of being future abusers	Less punitive judicial system		
Community support of agencies and professionals to treat an abusing family	Attempts to reduce own stress	Assisting existing support systems to be more effective		
		State-to-state retrieval system		
		Assisting abuser to be less alienated		
		Assisting abused to understanding		
		Treatment of abused and/or neglected		
Primary prevention		Secondary prevention		Tertiary prevention

ence positive health choices on the part of the family, and this presence *must* be recognized as a factor.

The epidemiological method can be used quite effectively to analyze the family disorder of child abuse. Can it be used as well, however, to study and intervene in those problems that cause confusion and frustration because of their multifaceted and complicating circumstances? The following two examples, one of isolation problems of the elderly (see Tables 2-4 and 2-5) and the other of multiple crises in crisis-prone families (see Tables 2-6 and 2-7), have been outlined as to common host-agent-environment interaction and levels of prevention. The reader should apply the information to situations encountered to make the disorder more applicable to personal practice. The lists are not all-inclusive and should be supplemented by the reader.

Table 2-4 Social isolation problems of the elderly

Susceptible Host	Causative Agent	Environment
Elderly persons living alone or with one other	Social system	Large home
Isolated	Decreased interest in knowledge or values of the elderly	Older, established section of town
Proud		Decreased property values
Previously independent, now more dependent on others or on system	Nuclear families living away from home	Few acceptable alternatives; home, with children, retirement housing, or nursing home
Chronic conditions and health problems	Retirement	
	Lack of transportation	
Living in past	Lack of activity	Fast-paced living
Fixed income	Lack of proper nutrition	Madison Avenue emphasis on youth, beauty, activity
Target of a hoax or a con-man		
Not enough money set aside for adequate living		Move from downtown to distant shopping centers
		Old friends dead or ill

SUMMARY

Although there is no easy way to investigate family problems, the need for an organized approach to family assessment and health problem management is paramount for the health professional. There is not, nor should there be, one right or best way to approach individual or multifactor family disorders.

Table 2-5 Levels of prevention of social isolation of the elderly

Epidemiologic triad of host-agent-environment in equilibrium		Epidemiologic triad of host-agent-environment out of equilibrium		
Period of prepathogenesis		Period of pathogenesis		
Health promotion	Specific protection	Early diagnosis and prompt treatment	Disability Limitation	Rehabilitation
Teaching health for the life span	Careful selection of individuals for provision of health care	Case finding	Seeking therapy for mental or physical problems	Utilize therapy regimes at place of residence
Emphasis on lifetime sports and recreation	Utilization of flu immunization programs	Multiphasic screening clinics for hypertension, diabetes, glaucoma, cancer, etc.	Hospitalization when indicated	Determine what services are available and utilize them
Counseling before retirement	Exercise	Recognition of isolation behavior and/or depression	Move when indicated to retirement home	Return to home if realistic
Development of hobbies and leisure-time activities	Assistance with some routine but taxing jobs	Regular health care	Realistic plans for self as conditions change	Seek help when needed
Good standard of nutrition	Become aware of organizations for elderly	Awareness of risk factors and warning signals of disease	If nursing home is indicated, pick one with good staff and reputation	Utilize community help for rehabilitation
Effort to stay in touch with all ages	Development of support systems outside of family and friends of same age	Consultation with lay or professional groups regarding plans and decisions	Attempt to make friends with those around, but don't allow them to influence your activities or your mood	Assist others to manage
Consideration of housing location on bus route and close to people of all ages	Avoidance of isolation		Utilize community agencies such as VNA, Meals-on-wheels, Bus '62, Council on Aging	Join foster grandparents
Early planning and saving for retirement	Travel			Find an outlet for any special skills and hobbies
Active participation in community and group work	Develop new interests			
	Read/continue education			
	Obtain enough insurance			
	Institute safety protection around home			
	Be careful of salesmen and get-rich schemes			
	Consider a roommate (same or opposite sex) or boarders			
Primary prevention		Secondary prevention		Tertiary prevention

Table 2-6 Crisis-prone families

Susceptible Host	Causative Agent	Environment
Suspicious	Crisis or series of crises	Poorly administered welfare system
Often low-income or minority families	Poor education	
	Poverty	Distrust and/or dislike of low-income and minority groups
Lack of ability to set priorities	Not being able to plan ahead	
Wants override needs	No support systems	Host seen as lazy, undesirable and undeserving
Lacks of ability to manage money	Attitudes	
	Unexpected extremes of weather conditions	Allows for limited access to the health care system
No adequate role model		
Poor self-concept	Poor level of nutrition	High unemployment
Users of community resources	Community apathy	Decreased neighborliness
Not an active member of community		Inadequate public transportation
Unskilled worker		Risking standard of living— food, rent, utilities
Lack of education		Seen by police as potential law breaker
Work short time and then quit		Unresponsive landlords
Low level of motivation		
Increased health risk		
History of being unable to meet obligations		
Frequent moves		
No telephone		
Unwilling or unable to learn from past experience with crisis		

The use of the epidemiological method is one way to systematically gather data. It allows one to sort out and categorize the factors involved in causation, and, thereby, to visualize the interaction. Once the chain of interaction is established, one can hypothesize how the chain can be broken and how the weak links can be strengthened.

Unfortunately, there are some family groups who do not want change, and who will resist attempts to assist them toward order. There are also some professionals who do not have the time nor the energy to see the epidemiological process through to fruition. For professionals, and the

Table 2-7 Levels of prevention of multiple crises in crisis-prone families

Epidemiologic triad of host-agent-environment in equilibrium		Epidemiologic triad of host-agent-environment out of equilibrium		
Period of prepathogenesis		Period of pathogenesis		
Health promotion	Specific protection	Early diagnosis and prompt treatment	Disability limitation	Rehabilitation
Adequate housing, sanitation, nutrition, and recreation facilities	Assisting families to gain access to the health-care system	Case finding	Communication between public agencies to reduce the chance of "loosing families"	Job training on request
Education of community to needs of poor and minority groups	Day care facilities	Reduce the school drop-out rate	Follow-up referral	Work incentives
Value clarification to learning individual differences	Nutrition programs for those in need	Early prenatal care	Anticipate crisis and become a support system	
Promote self-esteem	Revised welfare system that allows families to stay together	Assistance from community agencies		
	Routine immunizations	Reduce the "do gooders"		
	Provide young with positive role models	Assist families to learn and grow from crisis		
	Educational system that teaches family living	Increasing family counseling services		
	Birth control education	Use crisis as a time of teaching and learning		
		Assist families to make and achieve realistic goals		
Primary prevention		Secondary prevention		Tertiary prevention

more motivated families, the epidemiological method not only offers a means of assessment, but also directs the approach needed to interrupt and rehabilitate the current disorder and to prevent further disorder within the family unit.

Not all family disorders can be easily identified. Many are multifactorial and deep-rooted. The professional must continually ask the questions: What is the host-agent-environment interaction that is causing disorder in this family? How does this family differ from others who have no evidence of the disorder? What can be done to restore equilibrium in the epidemiologic triad? What levels of prevention are appropriate for this family disorder?

REFERENCES

Benson, E. R., & McDevitt, J. Q. *Community health and nursing practice*. Englewood Cliffs, N.J.: Prentice-Hall, 1976.

Cassell, J. C. *The potentialities and limitations of epidemiology*. Presented at a Public Health Seminar, Princeton, N.J., March 6, 1962.

Freeman, R. B. *Community health nursing practice*. Philadelphia: W. B. Saunders, 1970.

Kaplin, B. H., & Cassell, J. C. *Family and health: An epidemiological approach*. Chapel Hill, N.C.: Institute for Research in Social Science, 1975.

Kempe, C. H., & Helfer, R. E. *Helping the battered child and his family*. Philadelphia: J. B. Lippincott, 1972.

Leavell, R. H., & Clark, E. G. *Preventive medicine for the doctor in his community*. New York: McGraw-Hill, 1965.

Omran, A. R. Population epidemiology: An emerging field of inquiry for population and health students. *American Journal of Public Health*, 1974 *64*(7), 674–679.

CHAPTER THREE

SOCIOLOGICAL ASPECTS OF PARENTHOOD[1]

GERALD HANDEL

Sociology,[2] like psychology and psychiatry, is concerned with understanding human behavior, thought, and feeling. Its distinctive task, however, is to understand how these phenomena are shaped by group life, a term whose scope encompasses a range from society in the large to two-person or dyadic relationships. Whereas psychology differentiates and elaborates upon the components of personality, studying behavior as the outcome of interrelationships among these components, sociology differentiates and elaborates upon the components of group life. To be sure, psychology attends to and investigates factors or environmental conditions that shape personality components, but it is not systematically concerned with the order that obtains among these extrapersonal conditions, treating them, rather, as discrete variables. In contrast, the guiding con-

---

[1]This chapter is a revision of "Sociological Aspects of Parenthood" by Gerald Handel originally appearing in Anthony & Benedek (Eds.), *Parenthood*, (Boston: Little, Brown & Company, 1970).
[2]Sociology shares an indistinct boundary with social psychology. I have tried to adhere to a strictly sociological presentation in order to highlight the effects of large-scale social forces on parenthood. For this reason and also because of space limitations, I do not discuss many topics that form part of the sociology of parenthood and that are of a more social psychological nature. For one approach on the other side of the boundary see G. Handel (Ed.), *The Psychosocial Interior of the Family,* second edition (Chicago: Aldine, 1972). Thanks are expressed to my wife, Ruth D. Handel, for editorial suggestions that have helped to sharpen the presentation.

ception of sociology is that humankind lives in a socially ordered world, and that behavior is to be understood as a product of that order.

Sociologically considered, parenthood is a position in a social structure. To say this is immediately to state that it is tied to other positions in a set of interconnected groups of institutions. To be a parent is to occupy a position that is connected in socially defined ways to such other social positions as parent of the opposite sex, child, neighbor, teacher, pediatrician. Each position is socially defined in terms of a set of expectations. The expectations that define a position in one group differ from those that define the same position in another group. Thus, for example, a teacher in a school serving a working-class neighborhood is expected by the parents to be more of a disciplinarian than is the case among parents in an upper-middle-class neighborhood. The latter, being generally more articulate and better educated, expect to have more influence in the curriculum content than would working-class parents. More generally, upper-middle-class parents expect to exert more direct influence on their children's schooling than do working-class parents.[3]

From this illustration it can be seen that parenthood is definable not only in reference to such institutionalized positions as teacher, but also in terms of more embracing, though noninstitutionalized, aspects of social order such as social class. The way in which the position of parent is enacted is shaped, then, not only by the expectations deriving from other institutionally based positions, but, more importantly, by more pervasive aspects of the social order. The structure of the society as a whole is one such pervasive shaping factor. Thus, in an industrial society, a father does not typically teach his son an occupation. In an agricultural society, a father who is a farmer will teach his son to earn his living by farming. In the two types of society, the position of father is defined by different expectations concerning preparation of the child for an occupation.

While the structure of society as a whole sets certain general expectations, no society of any size is homogeneous. It is, rather, differentiated into a variety of different kinds of segments, of which the most significant are social class and (in our society) ethnic group. Other segmentations that have some importance are religion, occupation, and type of community (e.g., suburban vs. urban). These social segmentations cut across each other in multifarious ways, and one task of sociology is to identify what kind of importance each type of segmentation has upon the way in which

[3]The author has studied one school system in which upper-middle-class parents succeeded in pressing the Board of Education to provide foreign language instruction in elementary schools in upper-middle-class neighborhoods, over the opposition of the Board's own professional staff of educational administrators. The administrators spoke more approvingly of parents in lower-middle-class and working-class neighborhoods who "support" the schools but don't "interfere."

parenthood is performed. This task has not yet been carried out so comprehensively and systematically that we can, say, differentiate the parental performance of the upper-middle-class, Irish Catholic, suburban mother married to a professional man from an upper-middle class, Irish Catholic, suburban mother married to a businessman, or from an upper-middle-class black or Jewish mother married to either a professional or businessman and living in either a suburb or in a city. In other words, each of these segmentations (social class, ethnicity, religion, community type) has been shown to have some effect on how parenthood is performed, but not enough work has yet been done to provide a comprehensive and composite picture of how they all interact. In addition, it must be noted that the significance of each type of segment changes through time so that the relative importance of different kinds of segmentation changes. Thus, for families of a given social class level, but diverse in ethnic origin, who have moved to the suburbs, the fact of being suburban probably has a greater effect on how parenthood is enacted than the fact of being Irish or Swedish in ethnic origin. A conclusion of this kind, is, however, somewhat inferential, based on the general knowledge that ethnic origin among whites is somewhat less important in the suburbs than it was in the areas of earlier settlement in the city.

So far as the study of parenthood and child-rearing is concerned, more concentrated attention has probably been given to the importance of social class than to other types of social segmentation. This is due, in part, to the fact that attention was emphatically drawn to the existence of social classes in America by a series of researches during the 1930s, particularly those conducted by W. Lloyd Warner and his associates. Although Warner's particular approach to social class became the subject of some dispute, sociologists thereafter generally had no difficulty recognizing the importance of this type of segmentation in America. Even so, the emphatic enunciation of the existence of social classes in the United States challenged the vague but prevalent ideas of universal equality of opportunity. If social classes exist, children start out in life with systematically different preparation. Indeed, the notion that children were starting out in life with equal opportunity to participate in a wide-open race in which they were all running had to be modified in two major respects. Investigation began to suggest not only that they did not start out with equal opportunity, but that they were not even being prepared for the same race. It became evident, rather, that parents in each social class were primarily preparing their children to become adult members of the same social class into which they were born, rather than to compete in a kind of free-for-all in which the members of each succeeding generation would sort themselves out independent of their origins.

Prior to Warner's work, students of child development had discovered that children's mental development was affected by their socioeconomic status. But these earlier studies did not examine parental behavior, attitudes, and values. Two of Warner's principal co-workers, Allison Davis and Robert J. Havighurst, applied his concepts of social class to the study of parental behavior (Davis and Havighurst, 1946). This study stimulated various efforts first to replicate it, then to improve upon it, and thus played an important part in setting the problem for a whole series of later studies.

Over time, the most sustained attention, then, has been given to social class as a factor influencing parental performance. This dimension has emerged as the most enduringly significant large-scale social influence on parenthood in the United States. The importance of rural-urban differences has shrunk, in view of the increasing urbanization of the American people. With the decrease in immigration, ethnic differences became less important, although some remain important. Religion as a segmenting factor retains some importance, as will be suggested, but its significance is attenuated. In any case, it has not attracted the same concentration of interest that social class has. For these reasons, the reader will find more frequent references to social class than to other large-scale social factors in the balance of this chapter. However, it should also be noted that as knowledge has grown, some efforts have been made to draw distinctions within social class and also to locate smaller-scale social groupings that mediate the effects of social class.

THE SOCIOLOGY OF REPRODUCTION

Every society seeks in various ways to maintain itself, to preserve its continuity. It does this by such means as fashioning legends of its past, which it then cherishes and transmits to its young. It seeks to preserve its territorial boundaries against encroachment from other societies. Not the least important, it recruits new members through reproduction. Parents are, then, society's agents for replenishing its population. Society reveals its interest in this process through various official means that encourage or discourage the rate of reproduction: programs to limit family size when overpopulation threatens, programs to stimulate reproduction when the net reproduction rate is insufficient to maintain the population at its existing size or to sustain a desired growth rate. Most fundamentally, society declares its interest in reproduction by establishing norms for the legitimacy of unions and their offspring. Certain unions and their offspring are defined as illegitimate; these are, at the very least, denied the honor that society accords to legitimate unions and births. Often, illegitimacy is subject to additional penalty beyond dishonor. Various legal and social disabilities still attach to illegitimacy; efforts to moderate or abolish these continue in the United States at the present time. The social significance of illegitimacy is highlighted in these observations by Vincent:

> Because of their greater visibility, and consequently their greater threat to the value judgments sustaining marriage, illicit births are given far greater attention than is given to the more generic problem of *unwanted pregnancy*—licit and illicit. Not all illicit births are unwanted and pose a social problem; and not all licit births are desired and problem-free. This becomes evident when we consider whose value judgments determine which births are unwanted by whom. *Illicit pregnancies* may be unwanted by the mothers and society, as in cases of rape and incest; they may be wanted by the mothers but not by society, as in some cases of very low-income unwed mothers receiving public assistance; and they may be unwanted by the mothers but highly desired by other couples, as in cases of unwed mothers who release their children for adoption and enable childless couples to establish families. Similarly, *licit pregnancies* may be unwanted by the mothers and society, as in cases involving severe genetic abnormalities or economic deprivation; they may be unwanted by the mothers but desired by childless couples, as in the case of the estimated 15% of adoptions that involve children relinquished by married couples; and *licit pregnancies* may be wanted by the mothers but not by society, as in some cases of extreme economic deprivation, or unwanted by the mothers but wanted by society as in some cases of affluent and brilliant parents. . . .
>
> The far greater public concern about illegitimacy than about the more generic problem of unwanted pregnancy is consistent with the value judgments and social mores involved in the following: (1) The amount of public (and research) interest in a social problem is closely related to the visibility and public expense of the problem; unwed parenthood not only is the most visible of the various alternatives in coping with unwanted pregnancy, but in cases of very young and poor females it imposes the greatest cost upon the public. (2) The "principle of legitimacy" is maintained by censuring the unwed mother. . . . Censuring her is believed to serve as an object lesson to prevent these mores from "dying out in the conscience" of society. (3) The greater concern with illegitimacy is also consistent with the mores which prescribe that the sexual relationship be a private, covert experience (Vincent, 1966, pp. 22–23).

The biological route to parenthood is the same for all parents, but the social route is not. Whether or not an act of sexual intercourse that has a high probability of resulting in a pregnancy will occur is influenced by various social factors that operate at various junctures in the time sequence between mental concept and biological conception. The most comprehensive study of this problem is that by Rainwater; in what follows we draw upon his study except where otherwise indicated (Rainwater, 1965). The study is of interst also because it reveals the complex interplay of social factors in parenthood.

The general problem to which Rainwater addresses himself is that of family size—how families come to have the particular number of children that they do. As Rainwater phrases it: "Each couple is confronted with the twin goals (and necessities) of having 'enough' children and not having 'too many.'" Most generally, the number of children that a couple has is a function of (1) the number of children that they desire, and (2) the effectiveness with which they practice contraception. The first, second, third, or nth child may be the result of a planned effort to conceive in order to realize some ideal concerning family size or it may be the result of failure in the use of contraception and thus a defeat in the effort to realize a goal. The inquiry follows these two proximate determinants of family size to *their* determinants; that is, the study investigates the factors influencing number of children desired and the factors influencing effectiveness of contraceptive practice. From a summary of some of the main findings of the study, it will be evident that conception has social as well as biological and psychological determinants.

The research is based on interviews with 409 persons—152 couples plus fifty men and fifty-five women not married to each other. The sample included members of four social classes—upper-middle class, lower-middle class, working class, and lower class; it also included Catholics and Protestants, and whites and blacks, since it was anticipated that family size would reflect these three aspects of social segmentation. Since the investigator was interested not simply in showing the existence of a relationship between these large social groupings and family size, but also in indicating how membership in such groupings was related to marriage, the data gathered included information on conjugal role relationships[4] and on sexual relations. These five major factors—social class, religion, race, type of conjugal role relationship, and social psychological aspects of sexual relations—significantly affect the number of children a family will have, because they affect both the number of children desired and the effectiveness with which contraception is practiced.

The Rainwater study yields a great number of specific findings that are not readily summarizable in brief compass. A short statement of cer-

---

[4]This concept was introduced by Elizabeth Bott in *Family and Social Network* (London: Tavistock Publications, 1957). As adopted by Rainwater, it refers to "those aspects of the relationship between husband and wife that consist of reciprocal role expectations and the activities of each spouse in relation to each other." Three types of role relationship are distinguished: (1) *Joint:* the pattern is one in which most husband-wife activities are either shared or interchangeable; (2) *Segregated:* husband's and wife's activites are separated and different, sometimes carried out with minimum, day-to-day articulation, sometimes fitted together to achieve coordination; (3) *Intermediate:* sharing and interchangeability of task performance are valued, but more formal division of household tasks is maintained than in the joint conjugal role organization.

tain highlights will, however, indicate the complex interplay of social de-terminants of parenthood: Protestants tend to want fewer children than do Catholics at all social class levels except the lower class, where there is no difference between the two religious groups. (In a study of the effects of religion on family life, Lenski (1963) found that Protestant mothers are somewhat more likely than Catholic mothers to feel that children are bur-densome. Family size preferences tend to shift during the course of mar-riage, with middle-class couples often wanting fewer children than when they were first married and lower-class couples wanting more (as a passive adaptation to the larger number actually born to them because of ineffec-tive contraception). But within the middle class, couples who have a joint conjugal role organization, with much husband-wife sharing and inter-changing of activities and responsibilities, are more likely to want a smaller family than couples with a lower level of husband-wife involvement. But irrespective of social class or religion, large families tend to be more often desired by those couples in which both members consider sexual relations very important than by those couples in which one or both partners say sexual relations are not very important.

Effective use of contraception (regular and consistent use of a method that has a high degree of effectiveness when used appropriately) varies according to the same general factors as does desired size of family. To begin, middle-class Protestants are more optimistic than other groups studied that the size of family they want can be achieved. Middle-class Catholics and working-class whites and blacks are hopeful but less confi-dent. Lower-class whites and blacks are passive and fatalistic; they do nothing because they do not think anything will help, or they go through the motions of using a method in which they have little confidence and thus do not use it consistently. As would be anticipated from such basic attitudes, among the middle-class Protestants alone, of the groups studied, there is much serious discussion of family planning between hus-band and wife early in the marriage. Not surprisingly, middle-class Prot-estants are most likely to use effective contraceptive practices before the birth of the last child they want. After the birth of the last wanted child, this contraceptive superiority is maintained by middle-class Protestants, although an increased number of couples in all groups learn to use the methods more effectively (98 percent of middle- and working-class Prot-estants, 73 percent of middle- and working-class Catholics; 50 percent of working-class blacks; 33 percent of lower-class Protestants, and 13 per-cent of lower-class blacks and Catholics use contraception effectively after the birth of the last wanted child). Within the lower class, after the birth of the last wanted child, effective contraception practice is more likely in couples maintaining joint or intermediate conjugal role relation-ships than segregated, and in couples in which the wife finds sexual rela-tions gratifying and important to the marriage.

It can be seen from the summary of Rainwater's study that the likelihood of a couple's becoming the parents of yet another child is not a chance event but is influenced by the particular position of the parents in the social structure. Conception of a child has societal determinants as well as biological and psychodynamic ones.

INFANT CARE AND CHILD REARING

From a sociological point of view, the principal task of parents is to prepare their children to become adult members of society. This involves various kinds of care, the inculcation of values and norms, training in certain specific kinds of behavior, provision of models of adult roles upon which the child can draw in forming a concept of self and one's place in society, and the fostering of appropriate self-regard—all of which are summed up in the concept of socialization.

Although socialization begins with the birth of the child, the earliest days of life have been little, if at all, studied by sociologists; the field has essentially been left to psychologists and psychiatrists, so that we do not as yet have a sociology of the neonate. Sociological attention has been directed to that point in the infant's development at which the explicit imposition of "discipline" begins. The control of feeding has been regarded as the first major socializing experience, followed by toilet training. Recognition of the importance of these activities had been stimulated by psychoanalysis, and efforts were then made to place their significance in a larger social context.

The Davis-Havighurst study mentioned above aroused particular interest. The studies that followed in its wake resulted in various findings that seemed incompatible. Bronfenbrenner has endeavored to integrate results obtained from fifteen studies done over a 25-year span from 1932 to 1957 (Bronfenbrenner, 1958). Over time, he finds that whereas the middle-class mothers were previously more strict than working- and lower-class mothers, they have become more permissive. Middle-class mothers, in contrast to their earlier practice and in contrast to working- and lower-class mothers, now more often allow self-demand feeding and wean later from the bottle, although breast-feeding is apparently becoming less common in all social classes. As part of the same overall trend toward increased permissiveness, middle-class mothers at the end of the period reviewed were instituting bowel and bladder training later than were working- and lower-class mothers, reversing the situation that existed at the beginning of the period.

The basic trend that Bronfenbrenner identifies is an increase in middle-class permissiveness, although he finds also a less marked trend in the same direction for the working and lower classes. An interesting aspect of his analysis is his relating of his survey to Wolfenstein's survey of successive editions of the U.S. Children's Bureau bulletin on infant care (Wolfenstein, 1943). Her study showed that over substantially the same time period the advice issued by this publication changed from an emphasis on domineering and "taming" the child to an emphasis on meeting the child's needs. Research has indicated that middle-class mothers have been more likely to read not only this bulletin, but other child-care literature such as Spock's *Baby and Child Care*. Bronfenbrenner concludes: "Taken as a whole, the correspondence between Wolfenstein's data and our own suggests a general hypothesis extending beyond the confines of social class as such: *child rearing practices are likely to change most quickly in those segments of society which have closest access and are most receptive to the agencies or agents of change (e.g., public media, clinics, physicians, and counselors).* From this point of view, one additional trend suggested by the available data is worthy of note: rural families appear to lag behind the times somewhat in their practices of infant care" (Bronfenbrenner, 1958).

Bronfenbrenner finds similar trends in the training of children beyond the age of 2. In the 1930s and 1940s, the middle-class mother was more restrictive of freedom of movement; since then, less so. Also, since World War II, the middle-class mother has become more permissive toward the child's expressed needs and wishes in such diverse areas as oral behavior, toilet accidents, dependency, sex, aggressiveness, and freedom of movement outside the home. At the same time, however, the middle-class mother has higher expectations for the child with respect to independence and achievement.

Methods of discipline were found to differ. Working- and lower-class mothers are more likely to use physical punishment, while the middle-class mothers use more symbolic and manipulative techniques such as reasoning, isolation, and appeals to guilt. But over the 25-year period surveyed, the overall parent-child relationship in the middle class was reported as being more acceptant and egalitarian than in the working class, which is more oriented toward maintaining order and obedience.

THE NATURE OF SOCIAL CLASS DIFFERENCES

The differences in the parent-child relationship between the middle class and the working and lower classes arise from systematically different life experiences that, in turn, lead to differences in basic outlook and lifestyle. Rainwater, Coleman, and Handel (1962) found these important characteristics of the working-class mother: Central to her outlook is her underlying conviction that most significant action originates from the world external to herself rather than from within herself. Further, she sees the

world beyond her doorstep and neighborhood as fairly chaotic and potentially catastrophic. She feels she has little ability to influence events, and
her outlook is shaded by a fairly pervasive anxiety over possible fundamental deprivations. Similarly, she feels it is difficult to influence the behavior of her children. The study found that "the middle-class woman is
more likely to perceive her child's behavior as complex, requiring understanding. The working-class mother is more likely to see her child's behavior as mysterious, beyond understanding. The latter, consequently,
looks for rules or authoritative guidance, which she hopes will work and
take hold on the child." Middle-class mothers want to give their children
"worthwhile experiences" to make them well-rounded; working-class
mothers want their children to grow up to be moral, upright, and
religious-minded.

How can we explain the apparent contradiction resulting from our
finding that working-class mothers want specific rules or authoritative
guidance in dealing with their children and Bronfenbrenner's finding that
middle-class women are more attentive to child-care experts and literature?
Kohn argues—substantially correctly, we believe—that middle-class parents' attentiveness to experts and other sources of relevant information
represents not a search for new values but for better techniques of realizing the values they already have (Kohn, 1969). He believes that middle-
class values have remained substantially the same over the period surveyed by Bronfenbrenner, but that the attentiveness of middle-class
parents to expertise stems from greater readiness to accept innovation in
the service of their unchanging basic goals and from the fact that these parents regard child-rearing as more problematic than do those of the working and lower classes. His interpretation that the middle-class is not only
more receptive to—but also more in search of—innovation than the working classes and lower classes is borne out by much research. However,
the conclusion that basic middle-class values have not changed over 25
years is somewhat more open to question. It does not seem sufficient to
say that earlier middle-class rigidity and more recent middle-class permissiveness are simply two different techniques in the service of the value of
self-direction. Various social analysts have noted, for example, a change
from production-oriented to consumption-oriented values. Insofar as such
a shift in value emphasis has occurred, the increased permissiveness in
child-rearing documented by Bronfenbrenner probably derives from a
more general acceptance of impulsivity in the middle class.

Kohn believes that sociological emphasis on child-rearing techniques
is somewhat misplaced, and he seeks to redirect attention from specific
techniques to the larger question of how the social structure influences
behavior. His analysis takes the following general form: Values (conceptions of the desirable that influence choices) are products of life conditions. Middle-class and working-class parents live under different conditions; they therefore have different values, although they also have some

values in common. The value differences result in differential parental behavior in the different social classes. To understand parental behavior one must know what their values are, particularly those concerned with child-rearing.

Filling in the specifics of his analytic model, Kohn notes that the significant value difference is that working-class and lower-class parents want conformity to external proscriptions while middle-class parents want their children to become self-directing. The life conditions that most directly determine these values are occupational, educational, and economic. Middle-class occupations deal more with manipulation of symbols, ideas, and interpersonal relations; working-class occupations, with manipulation of things. Middle-class occupations are more subject to self-direction, and getting ahead in them depends more on the individual, whereas working-class occupations are more subject to standardization and direct supervision, and getting ahead in them depends more on the collective action of labor unions. The greater income and higher educational preparation of middle-class parents enables them to be more attentive to motives and feelings, including their children's. Thus, in disciplining them, middle-class mothers are more concerned with the child's intent; working-class mothers are more concerned with the overt consequences of the child's act. A more general consequence of the value difference is that middle-class mothers tend to feel a greater obligation to be supportive of their children, whereas working-class and lower-class mothers are more attentive to the parental obligation to impose constraints. In keeping with this, middle-class mothers want their husbands to be supportive of their children, especially the sons, but do not expect them to impose constraints to any great extent. In the working class, the reverse holds: the wives expect their husbands to be more directive and look less to them to give emotional support to the children. However, Kohn finds that while middle-class fathers' own role expectations for themselves accord with what their wives expect, this is not as frequently true in the working class, since the working-class father believes that the most important thing is that the child be taught proper limits, and it doesn't much matter who does the teaching. He would rather not be bothered, and expects his wife to take major responsibility for child care.

A few years ago, after some 10 to 15 years of postwar growth in affluence, there was a growing belief that "now everyone is middle class." This notion proved to have a rather short life, since it was followed by the "rediscovery of poverty." During the interim of popular illusion, however, some research was directed to this question, particularly since it was unmistakable that some working-class families were moving to suburbs and an increasing number of their children were going to college. The fact that suburbanization became a mass phenomenon during the 1950s lent credence to the illusion. Berger, however, studied a new tract suburb settled largely by working-class families and found that the increased level of material comfort had not resulted in any significant shift in outlook or life-style as compared with their life before the move to the new suburb (Berger, 1960). Berger's basic conclusion is that the fact of being of the working class was more influential than the fact of having moved to a suburb. Berger's results are understandable in terms of Kohn's analysis, since the men remained in working-class occupations. At the same time, it should also be said that Berger's study was done only 2½ years after the settling of the new community, perhaps too soon for any suburbanizing effects to become evident. Even so, residence basically follows from oc-cupational level, rather than the other way around, so that the "working classness" of a working-class suburb is likely to remain more consequen-tial than its "suburbanness."

Handel and Rainwater also studied the question of change in the working class and found it useful to distinguish between a traditional and a modern working class. Nonetheless, the basic difference in values be-tween middle class and working class endures, although some changes in outlook occur. For example, the growing working-class interest in a col-lege education for their children is largely focused on their sons, for whom it is seen as a means to a better-paying job rather than as a means of personal inner growth. College education for girls is discouraged unless the girl has a definite vocational objective such as becoming a nurse or a teacher; a year or two of college that does not lead to a definite vocation is seen as wasted (Handel and Rainwater, 1964).

ETHNIC DIFFERENCES IN PARENTHOOD

It was noted earlier that ethnic differences among whites are somewhat less significant than was the case during periods of heavy European im-migration into the United States. However, although increasing intermar-riage leads to a certain amount of blending of the population (Barron, 1972), it is now recognized that the conception of the United States as a "melting pot" is inadequate (Glazer and Moynihan, 1970). Although some of the distinctiveness of earlier immigrant groups has become attenuated, it has not disappeared entirely. Further, new groups have immigrated and retain elements of distinctive identity that affect some aspects of parent-hood. A recent work by Mindel and Habenstein (1976) focused specifi-cally on ethnic differences in family relationships.

It is impossible in a brief space to convey the full range of impacts of ethnic group membership on parenthood. All that can be done is to pre-sent some brief suggestive illustrations. For example, groups differ in the extent to which parents feel obliged to make sacrifices for their children. Two students of the Japanese family in America report that it is common for Japanese immigrant parents to deny their own needs for the sake of their children (Kitano and Kikumura, 1976, p. 51). A different emphasis seems indicated in the French-Canadian working-class family of northern New England; the parents "help their children with emotional concern and support but do not see the wisdom or need for mortgaging their own future to assure that of their offspring" (French, 1976, p. 343).

There appear to be differences among ethnic groups in the distance maintained between adults and children. A study of Chinese-American families reports that:

> . . . Chinese parents take their children with them not only to wedding feasts, funeral breakfasts, and religious celebrations, but also to purely social or business gatherings. A father in business thinks nothing of bringing his boy of six or seven to an executives' conference.
>
> This pattern is still adhered to by the majority of second, third and fourth generation Chinese Americans in Hawaii . . .
>
> This sharing of the world of reality between Chinese children and their parents may be one of the more crucial factors in the process of socialization (Huang, 1976, p. 134).

A contrast with this Chinese-American pattern is discernible among one group of American Irish Catholic middle-class families. A student of this group identifies at least three main types of middle-class American Irish Catholic family. For one of these types she reports, "In these families, the men are likely to be preoccupied with their work. They take little part in the rearing of their children, express most concern when it is time to choose colleges for and with the children, and, having made it themselves, worry little about an improvement in the economic and social welfare of their children" (Biddle, 1976, p. 118).

These brief examples indicate that ethnic traditions may continue to play a significant part in the way that parenthood is carried out. They also indicate two additional points of importance. One is that parents' ethnicity usually needs to be considered in conjunction with their social class, and the observer needs to be on guard against falling victim to simple ethnic stereotypes, favorable or unfavorable. What is true of the Chinese-American father in business may not necessarily be true of the Chinese-American father who is a restaurant waiter. A second point of importance is that even within a social-class level within a particular ethnic group, there are significant variations in family life, including the ways in which parenthood is carried out. Among American Irish Catholics, for example, there are important differences in how families relate to the church, and these differences affect the inner life of the families. Biddle's account is particularly instructive in setting forth these variations in pattern, each of which represents a particular integration of ethnicity, social class, and religion (Biddle, 1976).

FATHER ABSENCE, UNEMPLOYMENT, AND UNDEREMPLOYMENT

Until now, the parental differences we have sketched assume intact families. They assume further that the father is engaged in some kind of gainful work. The presence or absence of the father in the home has significant consequences. The kind of work he does—or his lack of work—is scarcely less consequential. It is therefore useful to indicate here some facts concerning father absence, underemployment, and unemployment, particularly their uneven incidence. Clausen observes that the 1960 U.S. Census reports that 11 percent of all American households with children under 18 had only one parent present; the absent parent was usually the father (Clausen, 1967). Moynihan, in his summary of statistical data pertaining to black families, states that 36 percent of black children live in broken homes at any given time (Moynihan, 1967). In addition, he reports an estimate that only a minority of black children reach the age of 18 having lived all their lives with both parents. More than 20 percent of black households are headed by a female, as compared to 9 percent of white households.[5] Moynihan shows that over a period of years from 1951 to 1963 the number of broken black families rises and falls with black male unemployment. Although both series of statistics show a long-run rising trend, there are numerous fluctuations during the period; an increase in unemployment tends to be followed a year later by an increase in separations, and a decrease in unemployment by a decrease in separations. In 1960, black unemployment was double that of whites; even so, as Moynihan points out, the usual way of reporting unemployment understates the problem. The average monthly black unemployment rate for males in 1964 was 9 percent, but during 1964 some 29 percent of black males were unemployed at one time or other.

The father's occupation is obviously of enormous significance for parenthood. When the father has no sustained gainful occupation, the consequences for the family can be devastating. The discrimination in education and employment directed to the black male plays a significant part in undermining the black (particularly lower-class) family. The destructive effects of unemployment on the family, now most clearly evident among blacks in American society,[6] but also apparent wherever unemployment is pervasive and long-enduring, were epidemic during the

[5] A social psychological analysis of the lower-class female-headed black family is presented by L. Rainwater in his "Crucible of Identity" (Rainwater, 1972).

[6] For a comparable picture among Appalachian whites, see Caudill's *Night Comes to the Cumberlands* (1963). The way in which family relationships are affected by larger social forces has seldom been more effectively traced than in this beautifully written book.

Great Depression (Angell, 1936; Komarovsky, 1940). The amount of evidence accumulated to date is substantial: Long-continued unemployment among males, especially fathers (though also among young unmarried men), is one of the most important causes of pathological conditions within the family, with far-reaching consequences for both parents and children, as well as for the entire society.

A complex picture of the interrelationships among employment, marriage, and fatherhood has emerged from a sensitive study by Liebow (1967) of some two dozen black men who congregate at a particular urban location. These men are all employed irregularly. In terms of the jobs available to them, "the most important fact is that a man who is able and willing to work cannot earn enough money to support himself, his wife, and one or more children. A man's chances for working regularly are good only if he is willing to work for less than he can live on, and sometimes not even then" (pp. 50–51). This fact of occupational life results in a paradoxical pattern of the fathering activity:

> . . . The men who do not live with their own children seem to express more affection for their children and treat them more tenderly than those who do live with them.
>
> Fathers who live with their children, for example, seem to take no pleasure in their children and give them little of their time and attention. They seldom mention their children in casual conversation and are never seen sitting or playing with them on the steps or in the street. The fathers do not take their children to tag along while they lounge on the streetcorner or in the Carry-out. . . .
>
> Compared with fathers who live with their children, separated fathers who remain in touch with their children speak about them more often and show them more warmth when the father and child are together. For separated fathers, the short intermittent contacts with their children are occasions for public display of parental tenderness and affection (Liebow, 1967, pp. 79, 81).

The closest relationships of all are often between a man and the children of a woman he takes up with. The crucial element seems to be the voluntariness of the relationship. Liebow explains his findings in this way: A man who lives with his wife and children is legally obligated to provide for them. Since the man is likely to be failing as a provider, he protects himself against a feeling of failure by minimizing his fatherliness. The father who is separated from his own children can enjoy some modest success as a father with them or with the children of his later woman. "It is as if living with another man's children is, so far as children are concerned, to be in a fail-proof situation: you can win a little or a lot, but, however small your effort or weak your performance, you can almost never lose" (Liebow, 1967, pp. 87–88). Whatever fatherly acts he performs are voluntary—more than expected—and thus to his credit.[7]

STRUCTURED STRAIN IN BECOMING A PARENT

The traditional interest in the study of parenthood, in sociology as in psychiatry and psychology, has been to ascertain the consequences of different kinds of parental performance on the child. It is appropriate to take note of a relatively new line of sociological inquiry that began in the late 1960s, the socially structured strains in becoming a parent, particularly in the middle class and particularly for women. This problem has been addressed most directly by Alice Rossi, who argues that the transition to parenthood is more difficult in American society than either marital or occupational adjustment[8] (Rossi, 1968). She notes Therese Benedek's point that the child's need for mothering is absolute, while the need of an adult woman to mother is relative. Mrs. Rossi then observes: "Yet our family system of isolated households, increasingly distant from kinswomen to assist in mothering, requires that new mothers shoulder total responsibility for the infant precisely for that stage of the child's life when his need for mothering is far in excess of the mother's need for the child." Thus, she continues, what is often interpreted as an individual mother's failure to be adequately maternal "may in fact be a failure of the society to provide institutionalized substitutes for the extended kin to assist in the care of infants and young children." Rossi notes these additional strains in the transition to parenthood: (1) There is great cultural pressure on growing girls and young women to consider maternity necessary for individual fulfillment and adult status. (2) Pregnancy is not always a voluntary decision, but society does not allow the termination of unwanted pregnancies. (3) First pregnancy is now the major transition point in a woman's life, because of the spread of effective contraception. This is a change from the past, when marriage was the major transition and first pregnancy followed closely upon marriage. (4) Parenthood is irrevocable, since society allows one to be rid of wives and jobs but not children, and one consequence of this social fact for women with unwanted children is that "the personal outcome of experience in the parent role is not a higher level of maturation but the negative outcome of a depressed sense of self-worth. . . . The possibility must be faced, and at some point researched, that women lose ground in personal development and self-

---

[7]For other aspects of parenthood among black Americans, see Rainwater (1965; 1970; 1972), Schultz (1969), and Staples (1973).

[8]I wish to express my thanks to my colleague Dr. Betty Yorburg for bringing this article to my attention.

esteem during the early and middle years of adulthood, whereas men gain ground in these respects during the same years.'' (5) American society does not provide adequate preparation and training for the role of mother. (6) The period of pregnancy does not allow adequate training, unlike the period of anticipatory socialization for marriage (i.e., engagement). (7) Finally, the transition from pregnancy to motherhood is abrupt; it does not allow for a gradual taking on of responsibility, as is true in a professional work role.

Thus, Rossi seems to be describing two main kinds of strain: (1) American culture presses many women into maternity who are not very maternal and perhaps should not become mothers and (2) motherhood in America is difficult because the role demands exceed the woman's capacity to meet them adequately and, further, because the social structure provides no built-in surrogates to help the mother, particularly right after delivery but also throughout the rearing of the young.

Rossi's analysis of the strains in the transition to motherhood locates them in the basic structure of American society rather than in any particular segment of it. Some questions arise. Her argument turns to some extent on characterizing our family system as consisting of isolated households that thus deprive the new mother of kinswomen to help in mothering. However, some sociologists have conducted studies that show that the nuclear family is not nearly so isolated as had been commonly supposed. Sussman is most closely identified with this line of inquiry (Sussman, 1974). But while his work shows that there is much more help among kin (including that of parents to their married children and to their minor grandchildren) than had been supposed, the findings are not specific enough to confirm or disconfirm Rossi's specific claim that basic mothering is a solitary task rather than one shared with others, as formerly. Another source of doubt: Perhaps Rossi's analysis holds for the middle class but not for the working class. Numerous studies have shown that working-class married women in several societies retain close ties with their own mothers and other kin. A brief overview will be found in Gans's study of working-class Italians (Gans, 1962). The evidence would seem to suggest that Rossi's analysis may be less tenable for the working class, though again the evidence is not in a form that permits a confident confirmation or disconfirmation of her analysis.

What about the abruptness of full-scale mothering responsibilities in the middle class? Rossi's strongest case would seem to be located here, but numerous questions will have to be laid to rest before it can be accepted. For example, many young newly delivered mothers hire a practical nurse to live in for at least a week after returning home from hospital confinement; others have their own mothers visit to help out. We do not know how widespread such practices are in the middle class. Perhaps this is true in only a small "deviant" group of middle-class mothers. Or perhaps Rossi's mothers constitute the small deviant group rather than the basic pattern to which the middle class is tending. Another informal observation: rooming-in arrangements in maternity hospitals seem to be growing in popularity. If this is a demonstrable fact, how does it fit with Rossi's analysis?

Rossi offers her paper to raise questions and to stimulate rethinking of important issues rather than to provide answers. The largest question she raises is that of the goodness of fit between psychological propensities and the social arrangements that channel wishes, motives, and behavior. This is one of sociology's enduring questions, one that follows close on the heels of the master question: How does society structure wish, motive, and behavior?

SOCIAL CHANGE AND PARENTHOOD

The pace of social change continues to accelerate in our society. This concluding section presents briefly some of the main changes that have been under way in recent years and that affect parenthood.

The Women's Movement

The period of the 1960s gave rise to a markedly heightened awareness of families in the United States (and elsewhere.) This decade was a period of intense social ferment, with many social movements starting up or gathering momentum. The women's liberation movement came to be among the most significant. Under its impact, the rewards and duties of parenthood and family life began to receive a public examination unlike anything that had preceded it in recent memory. The reverberations of this activity are numerous and proceed in many directions, but for the purposes of a brief chapter such as this, the central idea of the movement can be stated quite simply: Anatomy is *not* destiny. In place of a simple taken-for-granted expectation that all women, ideally, are destined for motherhood, the newer ideas stress that motherhood is only one option that a growing girl or mature young woman should consider for herself. Other roads to personal fulfillment are seen as alternatives that merit serious consideration. Further, the new ideology stresses that when motherhood is chosen, it should no longer be regarded as an all-engrossing life commitment. Combining motherhood with productive work is seen as not only a reasonable possibility, but a desirable option and indeed a probable necessity for all except the most wealthy. And still further, the shift from full-time motherhood to a pattern of motherhood-with-work means that fatherhood should become more engrossing for men than it has been heretofore. This is seen as desirable for mother, father, and child alike, since the mother gains help with the burdensome aspects of child-rearing, the father gains added opportunity to have an effect on his child's development, and the child gains a more balanced experience with both parents.

There seems little doubt that the women's movement has had the effect of encouraging women to seek more personalized goals. The age of first marriage for women in the United States has risen between 1956 and 1974 (Carter and Glick, 1976, pp. 406–407). The fact that this trend began before the rise of the women's movement suggests other influences on it as well, though what these are is not clear. It is also not clear what effect the women's movement is having on the actual performance of parenthood, as distinguished from ideas about how parenthood should be carried out.

Working Mothers

One of the most significant social trends that is affecting the way in which the role of mother is performed is the continuing increase in the number of working mothers. In 1890, only 5 percent of *all* married women were employed, and this increased to 12 percent in 1930. (Census figures before 1940 provided no information as to whether employed married women had dependent children.) In 1972, 30 percent of the women with children up to age 5 were in the labor force (i.e., either actually working or actively looking for work); 50 percent of the women with children between the ages of 6 and 17 were in the labor force (Nye, 1974).

This trend has received support in recent years from the women's movement, but the trend began before the movement and is attributable more to demographic and economic changes than to ideology. During and after World War II, the economy was expanding. This followed a period of low birth rates between 1910 and 1945. As the labor force increased from 52 million in 1940 to 80.6 million in 1972, a major part of the increase had to come from women with young children (Nye, 1974, pp. 7–8). The women's movement can be regarded as, in part, a response to changes that had already been under way for some time. One of the goals of the movement can be seen as removing whatever residual stigma still attached to working mothers, in the face of such a clearly changed actuality. A second goal, of course, is to upgrade women's occupational status and compensation so that women would not simply be a source of low-paid labor.

The effects on children of this change have naturally raised curiosity and concern. Research on this question has been begun. Hoffman has reviewed the work done thus far (Hoffman, 1974). She finds some important limitations in the available information, but also some significant and consistent trends. For example, for girls of elementary school age and older, the fact of the mother's working seems to increase self-esteem of the daughter, to stimulate her to develop a wider concept of femininity, and to perceive women as competent and effective, compared to daughters of nonworking mothers. Adolescent daughters of working mothers are more likely than daughters of nonworking mothers to name their mother as the person they most admire.

Studies of effects of maternal employment on boys seem to have been restricted so far to boys from lower-class and working-class families. The results currently available indicate that at these social class levels, sons of working mothers have diminished respect for their fathers, compared with boys from the same levels whose mothers do not work.

The working mother's satisfaction with her work affects her performance as a mother. One study indicates that although working mothers who enjoy their work are not as adequate in parental performance as full-time homemakers who are contented, they are more adequate than full-time homemakers who are discontented with their role. Generally, the impact of a mother's working on her performance as a parent depends on how she feels about her job, and how she and her husband mutually adjust to the multiple competing demands. Studies of two-career families indicate that there are as yet relatively few societal guidelines for dealing with these newly arising problems, and that each family must construct its own solutions (Holmstrom, 1973; Rapoport and Rapoport, 1971).

Marriage, Divorce, and Female-Headed Families

The prevailing conception of "a family" in our society is a group composed of a father, mother, and their biological children. Other societies have other norms of family composition, and other norms prevailed in our own society in earlier times when an unmarried uncle or aunt or a grandparent might often belong to the family that shared a single household. In our own time, however, the nuclear family has been the expected family and the expected household unit.

These expectations require modification in the face of increasingly widespread changes in family composition. These changes are often thought of as part of "the breakup of the family," but such a conception appears unduly simplistic in light of current evidence. It is more accurate to think of many families forming, separating, and then reforming with one or more new members and minus one or more previous members. It will be useful to draw upon demographic statistics to document the trend.

Compared to other industrialized countries, the United States has both a high rate of marriage and a high rate of divorce. Paradoxically, the high divorce rate contributes to the high marriage rate, because a large majority of divorced persons remarry (Carter, 1976, p. 388). Of course, remarriages do not always take place immediately after divorce. The consequence is that the United States has a substantial—and growing—number of female-headed families. This is, in fact, the fastest-growing household type in the country (Ross and Sawhill, 1975, p. 30). The overall situation can be presented compactly in the following list of figures. There were in the United States in 1974 (Ross and Sawhill, 1975, p. 12) about:

70 million households
55 million families
47 million husband-wife families (26 million—56 percent—with children)
6.8 million female-headed families (68 percent with children)
1.5 million male-headed families (36 percent with children)

The percentage of all families with children headed by women had reached 15 percent in 1974, up from 9 percent in 1960; this growth is due primarily to the increasing number of divorced and separated young women with children. (Rising illegitimacy among teen-agers is a less significant factor.) The prospect is for the proportion of female-headed families to increase still more: "The probability of divorcing after, say, 6 to 9 years of marriage has more than doubled in the postwar period, with the result that almost one out of every three marriages among younger couples is predicted to end in divorce" (Ross and Sawhill, 1975, p. 160).

If we look at these changes from the point of view of children's living arrangements, the evidence shows that the proportion of children under age 18 living with two parents declined from 89 percent in 1960 to 81 percent in 1974. The 1974 figure is made up of two disparate components: 87 percent of white children and 51 percent of black children living with two parents (Carter and Glick, 1976, p. 416). All of these figures for two parents combine children living with both natural parents and children living with one natural parent and one stepparent.

Clearly, a great many children—an increasing number—are without a father or surrogate father figure in the home for a portion of their childhood. Accumulating evidence from the work of psychologists indicates that father absence is likely to be deleterious to the developing child's personality; the specific consequences vary for boys and for girls and differ also for middle-class and for lower-class children. The incidence of father absence is much greater in the lower class and some parts of the working class than in the middle class; this means that father absence is often accompanied by poverty, and these two types of deprivation intensify each other (Biller, 1971).

New Family Forms

The increase in number and prominence of the single-parent family is one element in a larger phenomenon: the increasing variegation of family types. Thus, alongside the traditional nuclear family in which the husband-father is provider and the wife-mother the homemaker, there are single-parent families, dual-work families with both parents working, and reconstituted or remarried families with children from three marriages—his, hers, and theirs. While none of these forms is actually new, they are increasingly prevalent and, what is sociologically important, they make claims for recognition as legitimate and honorable forms of family. Added to these types are many types of experimental marriage and family arrangements. One study estimates that 8 percent of the United States population living in families in 1970 live in some form of experimental family (Cogswell and Sussman, 1972, p. 507). The traditional nuclear family is currently expected to remain in the plurality but not in the majority. American society has scarcely begun to recognize, much less integrate, these changes.

Many of these alternative forms of the family are, for their participants, transitory—that is, people move in and out of various family and household arrangements, whether by choice or by force of circumstances. Perhaps the single most important point to be recognized by policy makers, therapists, and all workers in fields concerned with family relations is that contemporary American society no longer has a single, standard family form, whether as ideal or as actuality. The new forms that have been appearing are efforts to solve problems that are perceived as arising from the traditional nuclear family. The increased fluidity of family arrangements is an important fact of contemporary life, and the effort to gain legitimacy for each new form is important for most participants, because they wish to be free of stigma that ordinarily attaches to people whose families and households take deviant forms. (Some persons may take specific satisfaction from living in a family/household form that is denied legitimacy by the larger society. While such a dynamic is undoubtedly one of the contributing factors in the proliferation of new family arrangements, it seems doubtful that this kind of scorn for conventionality is the primary factor. A search for individual fulfillment, however understood, seems to be more widespread, more pervasive, and more fundamental as an explanatory factor.) Whatever the impetus to strike out in a new direction, there may well be some magical thinking in the belief that escaping old norms is in itself a solution to problems. As this writer has pointed out in another context, every family, of whatever composition and no matter by what norms of conduct it seeks to govern itself, faces the task of constructing its own life day by day through interaction around events both chosen and imposed. Norms of family association, whether considered legitimate or not by the larger society, are neither self-fulfilling nor self-enforcing. They merely provide the framework within which interaction takes place (Handel, 1972).

Increased Contraception

The introduction of effective contraceptives also introduced a new conflict into human life—whether reproduction is entirely a matter under the control of God, fate, or nature, or, alternatively, a matter subject to rational human planning. It would appear that efforts to bring reproduction within a framework of planning are increasing. A national study in 1955 found that 70 percent of white married women 18 to 39 years of age reported having used some method of contraception. By 1965, this figure had increased to 84 percent. When adjustments in the figures are made to take account of problems of subfecundity and to include recently married women who plan to use contraception after conceiving, then the use or expected use is virtually universal among these women. "Clearly the norm of fertility control has become universal in contemporary America" (Ryder and Westoff, 1971, p. 107). The proportion of Catholic women conforming to their church's teaching on birth control has been decreasing; by 1965, a majority reported not conforming (Ryder and Westoff, p, 186).

National census data show that the number of children expected by wives 18 to 24 years of age averaged 3.2 in 1955 but only 2.4 in 1971 (Scanzoni, 1975, p. 64). The study of expected family size is a highly technical endeavor, with many conditions having to be considered simultaneously and sequentially. With this caution in mind, it nevertheless seems justifiable to state that Americans are on a continuing trend of having fewer children. This trend is itself made up of two somewhat different trends: (1) Having a large family is an ideal that seems to be losing value among American parents and prospective parents; (2) The birth of unwanted children is being more effectively prevented, both by contraception and by now legal—though not universally accepted—abortion.

In the present context, it is important to note that changes in policy of the United States Government have some effect on parenthood. After long opposition to governmental support of family policy programs, the federal government has become gradually more involved. Only in 1965 was a bill introduced in Congress to repeal the nineteenth-century laws that classified contraceptives as obscene materials and prohibited their mailing and importation, and not until 1971 was this bill actually passed. The amounts of money appropriated for family planning programs remain minuscule (Piotrow, 1973, pp. 119–120).

The Future of Parenthood

Parenthood is a role that is performed in a larger social world. The actions that a person carries out as a mother or a father and the feelings that permeate those actions are influenced by the social world in which mother and father participate, although they are not simply reflections of it. Families are arenas where interactions take place and where choices are made (Handel, 1956, 1972), and the choices are shaped by each member's perceptions of possibilities open in the world beyond the family. Becoming a parent is itself today more a matter of active choice than formerly;

nonparenthood and antinatalism are ideologies that make a claim for serious attention (Bernard, 1974). Economic uncertainty, the population crisis, the threats of war and of environmental damage, the alternative possibilities for women's self-fulfillment, the rise of "the singles' way of life," the possibilities for enjoyment of life in a companionable childless marriage—all of these new developments and more contribute to a climate in which people more frequently ask themselves whether they wish to become parents rather than simply taking for granted that every person "naturally" should become a parent. Indeed, the tradition of self-scrutiny that was initiated by psychoanalysis has led, in a modern-day derivative, to such candid self-interrogations as: Is parenthood the right choice for me?

Yet with all the factors that lead people to pause and question whether they should become parents, the likelihood is that most persons in the United States will marry and most will become parents. They will do so in a society in which various trends are under way that are changing the roles and status relationships of men and women and therefore changing what will be expected of a mother and of a father. As one historian has noted:

> After 1960 the era of tranquil domesticity dissolved into hurly-burly scenes of rebellion. The camera eye swung from the pine-paneled family room to the campuses and streets, where young people chanted the birth of a "new generation." Suddenly the established cultural institutions and values shook under the assault of youth. Racism, capitalism and imperialism, higher education and professionalism, marriage and parenthood and sexual mores—all came into radical question. . . . By the 1970's many Americans were asking, with fresh confusion or exhilaration: "What does it mean to be a (male) (female) person?" (Filene, 1975, p. 202)

The questioning goes on most actively among the educated upper-middle class and proceeds more slowly to segments of society that are less idea-conscious. Nevertheless, there is wide awareness that the world is changing. Parenthood becomes a new kind of challenge—preparing children for a world that parents know will be very different from their own.

REFERENCES

Angell, R. C. *The family encounters the depression.* New York: Scribners, 1936.
Barron, M. *The blending American.* Chicago: Quadrangle, 1972.
Berger, B. M. *Working-class suburb: A study of auto workers in suburbia.* Berkeley, Cal.: University of California Press, 1960.
Bernard, J. *The future of motherhood.* New York: Dial Press, 1974.
Biddle, E. H. *The American Catholic Irish family.* In C. H. Mindel & R. W. Habenstein (Eds.), *Ethnic families in America.* New York: Elsevier, 1976.

Biller, H. B. *Father, child, and sex role*. Lexington, Mass.: Heath, 1971.

Bronfenbrenner, U. Socialization and social class through time and space. In E. E. Maccoby, T. M. Newcomb, & E. L. Hartley (Eds.), *Readings in social psychology* (3d ed.). New York: Holt, Rinehart and Winston, 1958.

Carter, H., & Glick, P. H. *Marriage and divorce: A social and economic study*. (Rev. ed.). Cambridge, Mass.: Harvard University Pres, 1976.

Caudill, H. *Night comes to the Cumberlands*. Boston: Little, Brown, 1963.

Clausen, J. Family structure, socialization and personality. In M. Hoffman (Ed.), *Review of child development research* (Vol. II). New York: Russell Sage, 1967.

Cogswell, B. E., & Sussman, M. B. Changing family and marriage forms: Complications for human service systems. *The Family Coordinator*, 1972, *21*,(4), 505.

Davis, A., & Havighurst, R. J. Social class and color differences in child rearing. *American Sociological Review*, 1946, *11*, 698–710.

Filene, P. G. *Him/her/self. Sex roles in modern America*. New York: Harcourt Brace Jovanovich, 1975.

French, L. The Franco-American working class family. In C. Mindel & R. W. Habenstein (Eds.), *Ethnic families in America*. New York: Elsevier, 1976.

Gans, H. J. *The urban villagers: Group and class in the life of Italian-Americans*. New York: Free Press, 1962.

Glazer, N., & Moynihan, D. P. *Beyond the melting pot: The Negroes, Puerto Ricans, Jews, Italians and Irish of New York City* (2d ed.). Cambridge, Mass.: MIT Press, 1970.

Handel, G. Views of a changing interior. In G. Handel (Ed.), *The psychosocial interior of the family: A sourcebook for the study of whole families* (2d ed.). Chicago: Aldine, 1972.

————, & Hess, R. D. The family as an emotional organization. *Marriage and Family Living*, 1956, *18*(2), 99–101.

————, & Rainwater, L. Persistence and change in working class life style. *Sociology and Social Research*, 1964, *48*, 280–288. Reprinted in A. Shostak & W. Gomberg (Eds.), *Blue-collar world*. Englewood Cliffs, N.J.: Prentice-Hall, 1964.

Hoffman, L. W. Effects on the child. In L. W. Hoffman & F. I. Nye (Eds.), *Working mothers. An evaluative review of the consequences for wife, husband and child*. San Francisco: Jossey-Bass, 1974.

Holmstrom, L. L. *The two-career family*. Cambridge, Mass.: Schenkman, 1973.

Hsu, F. L. K. *American museum science book* (2d ed.). Garden City, N.Y.: Doubleday Natural History Press, 1972. (Cited in Huang.)

Huang, L. J. The Chinese American family. In C. H. Mindel & R. W. Habenstein (Eds.), *Ethnic families in America*. New York: Elsevier, 1976.

Kitano, H. H. L., & Kikumura, A. The Japanese American family. In C. H. Mindel & R. W. Habenstein (Eds.), *Ethnic families in America*. New York: Elsevier, 1976.

Kohn, M. L. *Class and conformity. A study of values*. Homewood, Ill.: Dorsey Press, 1969.

Komarovsky, M. *The unemployed man and his family*. New York: Dryden, 1940.

Lenski, G. *The religious factor: A sociological study of religion's impact on politics, economics and family life* (Rev. ed.). Garden City, N.Y.: Anchor, 1963.

Liebow, E. *Tally's Corner. A study of Negro streetcorner men.* Boston: Little, Brown, 1967.

Mindel, C. H., & Habenstein, R. W. (Eds.) *Ethnic families in America.* New York: Elsevier, 1976.

Moynihan, D. P. The Negro family: The case for national action. Washington: Office of Policy Planning and Research, U.S. Department of Labor, March, 1965. pp. 6, 9. Reprinted in L. Rainwater & W. L. Yancey, *The Moynihan report and the politics of controversy.* Cambridge, Mass.: MIT Press, 1967.

Nye, F. I. Sociocultural context. In L. W. Hoffman & F. I. Nye (Eds.) *Working mothers. An evaluative review of the consequences for wife, husband, and child.* San Francisco: Jossey-Bass, 1974.

Piotrow, P. T. *World population crisis. The United States reponse.* New York: Praeger, 1973.

Rainwater, L. *Behind ghetto walls. Black family life in a federal slum.* Chicago: Aldine, 1970.

————. *Family design: Marital sexuality, family size and contraception.* Chicago: Aldine, 1965.

————. Crucible of identity: The Negro lower class family. *Daedalus,* 1966, *95*(1). Reprinted in G. Handel (Ed.), *The psychosocial interior of the family.* Chicago: Aldine, 1972.

————, Coleman, R., & Handel, G. *Workingman's wife: Her personality, world and life style.* New York: Oceana, 1959; paperback ed., Macfadden, 1962.

Rapoport, R., & Rapoport, R. *Dual-career families.* Harmondsworth, England: Penguin, 1971.

Ross, H. L., & Sawhill, I. V. *Time of transition. The growth of families headed by women.* Washington, D.C.: The Urban Institute, 1975.

Rossi, A. S. Transition to parenthood. *Journal of Marriage and the Family.* 1968, *30,* 26–39.

Ryder, N. B., & Westoff, C. F. *Reproduction in the United States, 1965.* Princeton, N.J.: Princeton University Press, 1971.

Scanzoni, J. H. *Sex roles, life styles, and childbearing.* New York: Free Press, 1975.

Schulz, D. *Coming up black. Patterns of ghetto socialization.* Englewood Cliffs, N.J.: Prentice-Hall, 1969.

Staples, R., *The black woman in America.* Chicago: Nelson-Hall, 1973.

Sussman, M. B. The isolated nuclear family: Fact or fiction? In M. B. Sussman (Ed.), *Sourcebook in marriage and the family.* Boston: Houghton Mifflin, 1974.

Vincent, C. E. Teen-age unwed mothers in American society. *Journal of Sociological Issues,* 1966, *22,* 22–23.

Wolfenstein, M. Trends in infant care. *American Journal of Orthopsychiatry,* 1953, *23,* 120–130.

CHAPTER FOUR

THE AMERICAN FAMILY: AN HISTORICAL PERSPECTIVE

MICHAEL P. FARRELL AND MADELINE H. SCHMITT

INTRODUCTION

In this chapter, we draw on recent findings to present an historical perspective of the American family. This history has only been written in the past decade by a generation of historians determined to write a history of family life. Their theory and methods of sampling and data analysis have become increasingly sophisticated as they attempt to use untapped data sources to describe life outside the political and economic elite. By combing through old parish and state-house records, some researchers are compiling demographic histories of birth rates, illegitimacy rates, marriage rates, household size, death rates, and so on. These variables are interpreted in light of social-historical theories of family development. Other researchers, known as psychohistorians, make use of art, literature, and personal documents to piece together a qualitative picture of family life in past times. A third group carries out a comparative analysis of cultures around the world at various stages of economic development, then draws inferences about how family structure is related to the type of economic structure, and extrapolates these inferences to the development of family structure in Western culture. The findings are still coming in, and it is too soon to build a final composite picture of the history of the family. But, we can bring together some selected findings that seem solid and point out controversial areas where they still exist.

We focus particularly on the changes in four areas: family formation, husband-wife relations, parent-child relations, and extended-kinship relations. Finally, we draw some general implications for family health care based on these changes.

HISTORICAL THEORIES ABOUT CHANGES IN THE FAMILY

It is one thing to build an accurate description in history of the family and it is quite another thing to conceptualize and explain the changes in family structure. As usual in the social sciences, the theory has been far ahead of the data. It is only recently that systematic data has been gathered that enables us to test the many theories about the changes in family structure.

The theories have ranged from being very optimistic to being very pessimistic about the future of the family. Carl Zimmerman (1949) argues that family structure is progressing toward a stage of disintegration that will coincide with the disintegration of the whole culture. He claims that, looking at the changes in family structure in Greek, Roman, and Western society, including the United States, he observes a cyclical pattern. In each case, the society begins with what he calls a trustee family. Under this system, each person is merely the trustee of the name, the property, and blood of the family. Individuation is minimal; the family has the power of life and death over the individual. Divorce in uncommon at this point. The family is the major social unit and most functions of social, economic, political, educational, and religious life occur within the family. The state consists of the confederations of families into a tribal structure. In the next phase of development of societies, the state begins to gain more power and becomes a countervailing force vis-à-vis the family. The family structure during this phase—the domestic family—is an extended family embedded in a larger system with an autonomous political structure. During this period, the concept of individual rights emerges and the state makes provisions to protect individual rights against the demands of familialism. For example, legal separation is allowed within a marriage. It is during this period that the flowering of a culture occurs. It is followed by the atomistic family structure, in which individualism becomes even more valued and the power of family constraints is minimal. Marriage becomes a civil contract and divorce is common. Illegitimate children have full rights protected by the state. Involvement of women in politics and economics increases. A generation gap develops between parents and children and childlessness becomes common. The dominant motive among the society's members becomes fulfillment of the self rather than fulfillment of family responsibilities. This phase is followed by the disintegration of the whole society.

Obviously, Zimmerman saw our society as headed toward or already into the atomistic phase of development. However, his and other pessimistic interpretations of the development of the atomized nuclear family in modern society were challenged by Parsons (1955). Parsons argued that the family, rather than disintegrating in modern industrialized societies was becoming more specialized in its functions. Like other more specialized institutions in the society, it was performing a few functions much better than any other institution in the society and much better than it itself had ever done. Besides providing for physiological needs, he saw the family as specializing in the preparation of children's personalities to fit into modern industrialized systems and in the maintenance of adults' personality systems. He saw the flexibility, and the physical and social mobility of the nuclear family structure, as essential to adaptation in modern industrialized systems.

Both Parsons and Zimmerman have been criticized thoroughly over the past 20 years. Their brand of speculative grand theories has been replaced by more modest attempts to test limited hypotheses with empirical data. However, their theoretical frameworks set the backdrop of questions that guide modern research. How has the family structure changed? How are the changes in family structure related to changes in economic systems? Have relationships within the family become qualitatively better or worse? It is these questions that modern research is attempting to answer. The answers are coming from four types of research: (1) the work of sociologists studying census documents and other reports from this century, (2) the work of a new generation of social historians using quantitative data to trace the history of the family prior to industrialization, (3) the work of comparative anthropologists who attempt to piece together hypotheses about the prehistory of the family by comparing family structures in industrial, agricultural, and preagricultural societies, and (4) the work of psychohistorians who attempt to reconstruct the history of childhood, making use of artistic, literary, and personal documents.

THE ECONOMIC SYSTEM AND FAMILY STRUCTURE

From comparative analyses of anthropological data, it can be inferred that prior to the agricultural era, family structure tended to be nuclear. The basic unit was husband, wife, and children. During this period, people lived in bands of 50 to 200 people and frequently had to cover great distances to hunt and gather food. In such societies, the accumulation of property was minimal, especially property that could not be moved, such as land or houses. There was little division of labor or stratification, with everyone assisting in major tasks. The socialization of children was integrated into the work of the adults, and relations between parents and children and husbands and wives tended to be warm and casual (Stephans, 1963).

Planned cultivation of food permitted the development of more complex societies. Extensive stratification developed, eventually culminating in a ruling class with strata between them and the actual producers. Land became the basis of wealth, and physical mobility was replaced with routine and discipline. The increased food supply permitted the development of some large towns and cities, where the division of labor became more complex.

In this environment, the extended family became more common, though not nearly as extensive as previously assumed. For the wealthier portions of society, marriage became an economic business supervised by parents or professional matchmakers. In our own history, the marriage of the first-born son was particularly important, as it brought to the family a dowry of land or goods that would be the basis of family wealth and provide for the later-born children. The whole family's economic and social standing in the community depended on making a wise transaction at this point.

Contrary to popular myths about the warmth of the extended family, available information now indicates that relations between parents and children and husband and wife tended to be formal and cold. DeMause (1974) argues that abuse of children was common during this period. He argues that, ". . . the further back one goes in history, the less effective parents are in meeting the developing needs of the child" (p. 3). His descriptions of the responses of respected people to their children fit current findings of the treatment of children by child-abusing parents. The children were not treated as separate persons with needs of their own, but rather were seen as projective extensions of the parents' own internal world. Thus, when Cotton Mather's daughter fell into the fireplace and was severely burned, he saw it as a punishment for something he himself had done wrong, and was more sensitive to his own subsequent moral pain than he was to his daughter's suffering (deMause, 1974, p.9). DeMause describes even more dramatic cases where children were brutally whipped or burned for vague reasons that seemed to be based on the parents' projection of their own problematic sexual and aggressive impulses onto the child.

Few children had formal schooling in traditional society. They were sent out as shepherds, apprentices, or servants into the homes of other people as early as 8 to 10 years of age. Children were valued for their contributions to the work of the farm or shop, and they stayed attached to the family because it provided the easiest route to a livelihood and social standing in the community. In other words, there was at least as much greed as affection that held the unit together.

As societies all over the world have become even more complex, the extended family form has become less common (Winch and Blumberg, 1968). Nimkoff and Middleton (1960) argue that the nuclear family reappears in modern times as the predominant form for the same reasons that it appeared in the hunting and gathering societies, ". . . namely, limited need for family labor and physical mobility . . . to achieve economic goals. The hunter is mobile because he pursues the game; the industrial worker because of the job" (p. 225). Thus, there is a curvilinear relationship between family structure and societal complexity, with extended families being more common during the intermediate agricultural era.

Having taken a broad overview of changes in family structure, it is possible now to look in more detail at the changes in family structure, moving from agricultural to industrialized modern societies. First, the traditional family in preindustrial Western societies is discussed. Then, the evidence for a revolution in family structure that began roughly around 1700 to 1750 is examined. Finally, the variations in family processes occurring during the past century in the United States are examined.

TRADITIONAL FAMILY DURING THE AGRICULTURAL ERA

Prior to the eighteenth century, family life was embedded in the community. Most people lived in small villages dominated by a manor house. Generations of dowry exchanges resulted in the farm land being divided into the crazy quilt of irregular strips and patches on the outskirts of the village, with each family's holdings being spread around the general area. The men and boys went off to work in the fields together, and had ample opportunity to become aware of one another's business. Younger boys might be left to tend the sheep and cattle in the communal green. Women and girls stayed nearer the home, preparing food and maintaining the home. Much of their activity involved being with or being visible to nearby neighbors or family. During frequent holiday celebrations, the family became enmeshed in communal celebrations.

That privacy was a rare experience was reflected in the structure of the home. Even in the manor house, most family activities took place in a single room that was simply rearranged like a stage setting for different times of the day. During meal times, the table and hearth were center stage. The folding table may have also been the place where visitors were received and business transacted. Neighbors moved in and out all day long, easily viewing the whole family setting. At night, cots and mats were spread around the floor and the whole family slept within earshot of each other. Most of the functions of life took place within the family. Work, education, recreation, religious worship, health care, business transactions, political activities were all managed by the family, usually under the supervision of the family patriarch.

Among the elite, marriages were formed by arrangement of the family patriarchs. Marriage was a business transaction, too important to be left to children. The marriage of the first-born male was particularly important. For one thing, it often marked the transition of authority from one generation to the next. Upon marriage, the oldest son assumed responsibility for the family land and control over the family work force. The transition was often marked with strain. Greven (1973) reports that early patriarchs in Andover, Massachusetts, were particularly long-lived, and they held on to their authority until they were well into their seventies, maintaining control over their sons until they were well into their forties. Berkner (1973) reports that the protection of the rights of the patriarch had to be maintained with legal contracts, and folk songs portray a theme of strain in father-son relations over control of the land.

Eventually, the transition took place, but under the control of the patriarch. If he did not select the family into which his son would marry, he at least maintained veto power. Upon agreeing to the marriage, the father of the bride would then "walk-off" the land to be given as her dowry, or he would show the shop or tools if he were a craftsman or merchant. These items would be used in the dowry exchange of the first patriarch's daughters, or they could be used to establish his other sons.

Among the poorer serfs and laborers, marriage was less controlled and less stable. They may have relied more on romantic love than economic gain as a guide in selection. But even the landless laborer had to consider the need for a mate with a strong back to carry out the cycle of agricultural work (Shorter, 1971). Husband-wife relations tended to be distant, with the husband maintaining formality and control, as is reflected in the legal code. Women's work and men's work were sharply defined. When the boundaries were crossed and a woman dominated a man, informal ridicule was brought to bear by the community. If things seemed to be going too far in a relationship, the men in the community might appear one night and place the henpecked husband facing backwards on a horse and ride him through town. His position on the horse reflected his misconception of proper husband-wife relations (Shorter, 1971, p. 222).

1700 TO 1850: THE REVOLUTION IN FAMILY STRUCTURE

Revolutionary changes in family relations seems to have begun in the early 1700s. One of the most obvious pieces of evidence of the change is the change of housing architecture. First among the wealthy, then among the poorer people, space in the home began to be parceled off into rooms.

First, sleeping was separated from other activity. Then, husband and wife quarters were separated from children's rooms. Then, beginning in the large towns and later spreading to the country, a separate room was set aside to retire to after dinner and to receive guests. The bell cord appeared in wealthier homes as a means to summon servants. Privacy appears to have become a value.

In the eighteenth century, the family began to hold society at a distance, to push it back beyond a steadily extending zone of private life. The organization of the house altered in conformity with this new desire to keep the world at bay. It became the modern type of house, with rooms that were independent because they opened onto a corridor (Aries, 1962, p. 398).

Around this same period, romantic love began to spread into the upper classes and replace matchmaking as the basis of mate selection. That courtship became less controlled is reflected in the rising rates of illegitimate births and pregnant brides all over Europe (Shorter, 1975) and New England (Smith, 1973). The trend increased as young men became more mobile, with more opportunities opening up in the towns and cities. Shorter refers to this period as the first sexual revolution. Husband and wife relations may have become more tender during this period, if the romantic love pattern persisted after the marriage. The increase in privacy for the couple points in that direction.

The middle class developed a pattern of sentimental feelings toward children. Middle-class women began to breast feed their own children, rather than send them out to a wet nurse. Children often were sent to school to learn to read and write. A drop in infant mortality coincides with this period. Whether the decline in mortality was caused by better treatment or vice versa, parents began to invest more in their children.

1850 TO 1970: THE FAMILY DURING THE PAST CENTURY

As late as 1850, 85 percent of the population in the United States lived in rural areas. Over a 100-year period that pattern was reversed, so that now close to 90 percent live in urban areas. In this section we trace some of the concomitant changes in family relations.

The political and economic changes in Europe in the nineteenth century led to drastic changes in social life. As factories began to grow in the cities, more and more opportunities to make a living appeared outside the small villages. In many places, the increased attractiveness of the cities coincided with overpopulation or disaster in the countryside. For example, in Ireland the population doubled during the 50 years prior to the potato blight that led to mass starvation. In other areas, political changes or reorganization of the land by capitalists undermined the old ways. The combination of forces led to waves of migration, out of the countryside, into the cities of Europe and America.

The loss of an ability to provide for his family and the opening of new opportunities undermined the authority of the family patriarch. However, in many cases familial pressures operated even at a distance. Wages were sent home to help the family, and established urban dwellers were expected to help younger siblings find a place in the city when they arrived. The networks of family ties often resulted in single ethnic groups dominating particular professions or industries or segments of the country—such as the Irish with the police force, and the Jews with the garment industry, and the Swedes with the dairy industry. But adjustments to urbanization and industrialization eventually led to major changes in the family's structure and functions. In adapting to the new setting, the family began to lose a variety of functions to agents in the outside world.

First, economic functions moved out of the home. To support his family the patriarch had to leave his home each day and be out of touch for most of the day. At first, wives and children went to work in factories too and their wages fed into the patriarch's resources. At times, it was easier for children to find work, for they demanded less pay and conformed with less resistance to the routine of the job. A whole generation grew up having learned as children to take for granted the deadening monotony of the factory.

Then, educational functions moved out of the family. To learn the language, skills, and values necessary to do well in the system, children had to be educated in schools by specialists. Soon, many other community functions were being handled by specialists outside the family—recreation, medical care, food processing, political maneuvering, conflict resolutions, and so on. Each day, the family members left the home to carry out their most important activities. They went off to operate in separate worlds, returning at the end of the day to the empty shell of a structure that once provided for everything. This erosion of functions has led some theorists to conceive of the family as an obsolete vestige of a previous era—a structure, like the monarchy, kept alive for sentimental reasons, but performing no really essential functions for its members.

However, many writers still see marital and family relations as very much alive and well and performing more specialized functions in industrialized societies. The family remains the basic unit providing for physical needs and for psychological development and maintenance. There is still no major competitor for the family in the building of the basic groundwork of personalities for children. And, it is in the family that adults can set aside the facades used in their roles in outside institutions and express and resolve unresolved tensions from their past and from dealing with the outside world. At the least, the significant others in the family play a part in the maintenance of defenses and fantasies that compensate for deprivations in other areas of life.

Marital Formation

Romantic love is now accepted as the "natural" basis for mate selection in our culture. The mass media reinforce this notion regularly—with songs, stories, and advertisements providing cues as to how to go about mate selection and what to expect at each phase of the relationship. For many people the emotional storms that occur in this process are reflected and amplified by the popular culture. Perhaps marrying someone with whom you have fallen in love increases the chances of the relationship's providing psychological gratification throughout life—which is supposedly a major function of marriage today. But, our knowledge of the causes and consequences of romantic love are overlaid with myth. Much research is being done and still needs to be done in this area.

In the nineteenth century and early twentieth century, a majority of marriages took place within ethnic boundaries. As assimilation progressed, marriages began to take place outside ethnic boundaries but within religious groups. Thus, an Irish Catholic might marry an Italian Catholic. As assimilation progresses even further, religious barriers are breaking down more, though even now most marriages take place between two persons of the same religion.

There have been significant changes in sexual behavior during courtship over this century. Kinsey (1953) reports that the first sexual revolution of this century took place during the 1920s. Among women born prior to 1910, he finds approximately 25 percent having had sexual relations prior to marriage. Among women born after this period, he finds approximately 50 percent reporting having had sexual intercourse prior to marriage. Religious values seemed to play an important part in this change. For example, among devout Catholics he finds only 24 percent had coitus, whereas among the religiously inactive he finds 55 percent had such experience. Among males, he finds that level of education was an important predictor of sexual behavior. Ninety-eight percent of males who stopped at the grade school level reported premarital coitus. The figures for high school- and college-level males were 84 percent and 67 percent, respectively.

Hunt's (1973) report of current sexual practices is one of the few large-scale attempts to study the changes that have occurred during the 1960s. He reports that the younger the age of his respondents, the greater the percentage reporting premarital sexual relations. For males, the figures range from 84 percent for those age 55 and older to 95 percent for those males under age 25. For females the range is from 31 percent for those over age 55 to 81 percent for those under age 25. However, Hunt (1973) and Reiss (1972) both find that the greatest proportion of this sexual behavior still occurs within an intimate love relation, usually with a person one intends to marry. Impersonal sex is a rare phenomenon, and close to two-thirds of the females report regret and worry afterwards.

In 1890, the median age of first marriage was 26.1 years for males and 22.0 years for females. This figure continued to decline by a few months each decade until 1960, when it reached 22.8 years for males and 20.3 years for females. Since then it has begun to rise again, so that by 1975 it stood close to the 1940 figures—23.5 years for males and 21.1 years for females.

This recent pattern of delaying marriage also shows up in the data on the proportion of people in the population who are married. That proportion had been increasing for every age group until 1970. For example, in 1900, for the age range of 30 to 34 years, the proportions of the population that had ever been married for males was 72 percent, and for females 83 percent. By 1970, those proportions had climbed to 91 percent for males and 94 percent for females. Since 1970, the proportions have begun to decline for the younger age groups, with the 20- to 25-year-old group showing a decrease of 5 percent.

Husband-Wife Relations

Empirical research on the "period of adjustment" immediately after marriage presents a paradox. On the one hand, we hear that it is the period of greatest satisfaction with the relationship (e.g., Rollins and Feldman, 1970), and, on the other, it continues to be the period in the family life cycle when divorce is most likely to occur. Across the family life cycle, the period when divorce is most likely is during the first few years, with 50 percent of all divorces occurring during the first 8 years of marriage (*U.S. Fact Book,* 1977, p. 55).

If nothing else, the indications are that the negotiations of husband-wife relations during this period are characterized by high and low points. These negotiations are usually guided by parental models of male-female relations or images provided by the popular culture. These vague conceptions get expressed in the form of metaphors. In some cases, the appropriate metaphor has gone from the "king and his castle" and the "captain and his ship" to "a democratic friendship" or the "patient and his therapist." In the latter case, the expectation is that the spouse will be able to assess one's deepest needs and help one fulfill one's greatest potential. No wonder there are such highs and lows. The general trend seems to be toward more equality and companionship. Perhaps this trend is reflected in the finding of women marrying someone closer to their own age rather than someone older than themselves. Surprisingly, Lantz, Schultz, and O'Hara (1977) find evidence for this trend toward equality developing force as early as the 1850s. Their content analysis of magazines shows women portrayed as overtly powerful in family relations in 56 percent of the 1338 articles.

Along with the trend toward companionship is a trend toward the de-differentiation of roles. Women are more likely to take on some of the bread-winning functions; and men may be more likely to take on house-keeping functions. In 1920, only 23 percent of all women aged 20 to 60 were in the labor force. Today almost half (45 percent) of the women in the age range 18 to 64 are working. The life cycle stage affects this pattern. As Suelzle (1973) reports: In 1920, female participation in the labor force dropped off at age 25, decreased steadily with age, and by the time women were age 45 to 54 only 18 percent were working. In contrast, female participation in the labor force today drops off at age 25, but rises again at 35 to a second peak of 54 percent at age 45 to 54. The trend, then, is toward more and more families juggling two work schedules, especially after all the children have been established in school. At home, this pattern is associated with more egalitarian relationships both in the distribution of power and in the division of labor.

The pattern of dual careers is likely to become more common in the future. In the previous century, most couples could expect that one or the other would be dead before the last child had left the home. With smaller families and increased life spans, the more common pattern now is for the couple to have a prolonged period during which the children are raised and both remain healthy enough to continue working for years. We do not yet have a name for this period. We refer to it in negatives such as "post-parental," "pre-retirement," or "empty nest." This period is likely to continue to lengthen in the future, and, as the postwar baby-boom cohort goes through this phase, a greater percentage of the population will be facing this period of life. If conditions are created that enable the bulk of this group to gain a sense of "generativity" rather than "stagnation" (Erikson, 1950), the society will have an abundant source of resources for constructive services.

Divorce Rates

Divorce rates have been climbing throughout this century, but with some interesting fluctuations. First, there was a slight decline during the first years of the Depression, with a level in 1929 of 1.7 per 1000 population not being recovered until 1935 (see Figure 4-1). The marriage rate dropped during these same years. After 1935, it continued to rise, picking up tempo

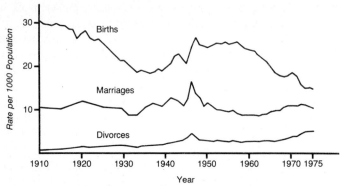

Figure 4-1 Changes in the rate of births, marriages, and divorces per 100 population between 1910 and 1975. (From *The U.S. Fact Book, The Statistical Abstract of the U.S.*, U.S. Bureau of the Census, 1977, Grosset and Dunlap, New York, and *A Statistical History of the United States from Colonial Times to the Present*, U.S. Bureau of the Census, 1977.)

during the war years, until by 1944 it had reached 2.0 per 1000. Then, as soldiers returned and people attempted to put their lives together, the rate hit a peak that was not to be topped until 1973. In 1945, it rose to 3.5; in 1946, it peaked at 4.3; then, in 1947, it began to recede to 3.4 per 1000. It finally leveled off at an average of 2.3 through the 1950s and early sixties. But by 1964 it began to climb again. In 1970, it reached 3.5; and, by 1973, it had broken through the previous ceiling, reaching 4.7 per 1000 population by 1975.

Parent-Child Relations

In general, the quality of parent-child relations seems to be improving (deMause, 1974). A number of factors contribute to this trend. The first factor is the continued decline of infant mortality and death due to childhood disease. The increased likelihood of children remaining alive certainly encourages more investment in them. Another factor is probably the increased awareness of the importance of parental behavior in the molding of personality.

Another factor that probably will contribute to improvement of parent-child relations is the trend toward smaller family size. In 1910, the crude birth rate (per 1000 population) was 30.1 (Figure 4-1). This rate dropped steadily through the first quarter of the century, reaching a low of 18.4 during the Depression year of 1936. It began to climb gradually after that, reaching 22.7 during the war year of 1943. Then it surged in 1946 to 24.1, peaking in 1947 at 26.6, and stayed relatively high during the 1950s, roughly 25 per 1000 population. However, through the 1960s and 1970s it has dropped steadily, reaching 18.4 in 1970 and 14.8 in 1975. This decline in the birth rate is reflected in the decrease in the average number of children per family, going from 4 in 1960 to 1.8 in 1975.[1]

Extended Family Relations

We have seen the reports of comparative studies of family structure that indicate the prevalence of extended family forms declined as societies became more complex. Textbooks on the family often assert that, in our own history, the growth of urbanization and industrialization has coincided with the decline of the extended family. However, in the past, this paradigm has never been tested through careful historical research. Rather, it has been inferred on the basis of a few literary reports and, perhaps, a nostalgic myth that somehow family life was better in the good old days. This paradigm has been shattered by recent research. In reviewing the literature, one gets the sense that some patterns exist, but they do not seem to be interpretable within the old grand theories nor within the paradigm developed through comparative analysis of contemporary societies.

At this point, numerous historical studies of the proportion of households containing extended families indicate that the proportion of extended families living in one household have not declined with industrialization. Laslett (1972, p. 51) traces the change in proportion of extended families in samples of English communities from the late 1600s to the late 1800s. In the preindustrial period, he finds an average of only 6 percent extended family households. As if this small number is not enough to call in question the old myth of extended families living together in rural togetherness, he finds an *increase* in the number of extended families as England moved through the period of industrialization, reaching an average of around 16 percent during the period of 1850 to 1880. Anderson's findings (1973), in his study of Preston during the period of the growth of industrialization, supports this finding. Housing shortages plus the economic gains that came from having an older relative care for children while the mother worked seem to have led to the extended family's being a feasible pattern for a minority of the population during this period. Thus, extended families living in a single household never were common in our history, and, if anything, they became slightly more common during the early period of industrialization.

---

[1] This decline in the crude birth rate should not be interpreted as the end of the population explosion problem. A huge wave of women are now in the age range of greatest fertility (15 to 34 years); thus a net increase in the number of births seems inevitable. In order to curb the explosion, each family would have to limit their average size to 1.2 children per family, and the birth rate would have to equal a death rate of approximately 9.4 per 1000 population (Frejka, 1968).

Furthermore, the mean size of household in England remained nearly constant during the whole period of industrialization. From the late sixteenth to the early twentieth century, it stayed roughly at a level of 4.75 persons per household (Laslett, 1973, p. 22). The data for American families are different, showing a decline from an average of 5.8 per household in 1790 to 4.75 by 1900. However, the larger size of households was due to a prodigious birth rate rather than the presence of relatives in the home. Berkner (1973) questions Laslett's interpretation of his findings. He argues that the extended family living together was common in traditional societies, but only occurred at the beginning or end of the family life cycle, when the patriarch stepped down and turned the farm or business over to his son.

Though these quantitative findings call into question the old myths about the extended family living together, they tell us little about the relationships between family members living near each other. As Greven (1973) points out, a patriarch might still maintain firm control over his sons by virtue of his control over the family land, even if they lived in separate households. In seventeenth-century Andover, he found that fathers maintained control over sons by retaining legal control of their son's land even after the son had married and moved away from the homestead. The strength of extended family controls at a distance in traditional society is amply described in other settings also (e.g., Arensberg and Kimball, 1948). It is the decline of these kinds of control networks that probably coincided with the rise of industrialization and urbanization. When a new husband and wife did not need to depend on the familial network for their economic and social status, the old order began to erode.

However, recent research in urban settings shows that the network has not completely disintegrated. For example, Sussman (1959) and Litwak (1960) find that the majority of families in their studies maintain extensive ties with their extended families. Through the exchange of services, gifts, and help during crises the network is kept very much alive. Gathering the family together at holidays and maintaining communication is still important to a great many people. The difference between traditional and modern extended family ties is that they have become less necessary and more voluntary. Like husband-wife relations they now serve more social-emotional than instrumental needs.

SOME IMPLICATIONS FOR FAMILY HEALTH CARE

As with other family functions, the management of physical and emotional illness was a responsibility contained largely within the confines of the traditional family. Folk knowledge of how to treat common illnesses was passed on from one generation to the next. Only the indigent received care for illness in institutions as the result of the charity of religious orders. These institutions were perceived as death houses by the society as a whole. During the period 1700 to 1850, separate occupations devoted to treatment of various kinds of ills emerged outside the family structure, so that, by 1850, families shared the task of caring for the ill with several emerging occupations, e.g., medicine, osteopathy, chiropractic, and naturopathy. However, it is only in the most recent era of family change that the science of medicine has become sufficiently developed as to clearly usurp the major role of the family in knowledge about treatment of disease. Thus, the management of physical and emotional illness, like so many other family functions, has moved out of the family into an increasingly complex and specialized institution we have come to know as the "health care system."

Part of Rodgers' paradigm (1973) is useful for looking at the situation the modern family finds itself in, with so many of the old family functions moved into complex institutions in the larger society. He points to the task of the family as one of "transaction" with the many complex institutions in order to meet the needs of family members. He points to the fact that, although much work has been done on transactions between the family and the political system, the family and the educational system, the family and the religious system, and so forth, few studies have focused on transactions between the family and the health care system. With what paradigm do we understand these transactions? Only a few are available that utilize a family rather than or in addition to an individual focus (Anderson, 1968; Suchman, 1964, 1965, 1966; Geertsen et al., 1975). The need for such transactions obviously puts a large burden on the family system to know what is available in health care, how to gain access to it, and how to work in cooperation with it. How do health professionals assess families' capabilities for transaction with the health care system and assist families to further develop these transaction skills? One wonders whether the current, renewed interest by some families in "natural" treatments reflects a wish for a return to a simpler time, when knowledge and management of illness called primarily for resources contained within the family system.

Beyond the general implication for family health care of the need for assessment and assistance in families' transactions with the health care system are the myriad of specific implications of societal and family change for assistance in specific areas of health care. To point to a few examples:

1. Houses are much more complex structures as the result of long-term trends in privatization, individuation, and technology. This creates

demands for awareness by families of environmental hazards that have simply never existed before.

2. The availability of a complex food technology makes providing for basic nutritional needs a more difficult endeavor.
3. Establishing regular cycles of sleep, eating, work, and recreation is complicated by family members going in many different directions on a daily basis.
4. The discovery of the importance of childhood experiences in personality formation has made the complex responsibilities of parenthood apparent and creates the demand for parents to assimilate a growing quantity of information and advice.
5. The change in the relations between the sexes has created a need for sexual counseling for purposes of genetic counseling, fertility counseling, facilitating mutually satisfying sexual relations, and preparing for parenthood experiences.
6. Management of illness among family members requires use of sophisticated medical regimens and, in some instances such as organized home care, a complex cooperative effort with multiple representatives of the health care system.

SUMMARY

In this chapter, we have traced the history of the family and how its structure and function have changed as the economic forces in society have changed. Discussion has centered particularly on family formation, husband-wife relations, parent-child relations, and extended-kinship relations. General implications for family health care were drawn.

It is important to remember that the historical research providing the basis for the review in this chapter is recent and that some of the research is contradictory. Much additional work remains to be done. Though some general implications for family health care can be and have been drawn from this recent research, none of it deals explicitly with the family's past functioning in relation to health and illness. This remains as an area to be explored in future work.

REFERENCES

Anderson, M. Family, household, and the industrial revolution. In M. Gorden (Ed.), *The American family in social-historical perspective.* New York: St. Martin's Press, 1973.

Anderson, R. *A behavioral model of families' use of health services.* Chicago: University of Chicago, Center for Health Administration Studies, 1968.

Arensberg, C. M., & Kimball, S. T. *Family and community in Ireland*. Cambridge, Mass.: Harvard University Press, 1948.

Aries, P. *Centuries of childhood*. New York: Vintage Books, 1962.

Berkner, L. K. The stem family and the developmental cycle of peasant household: An 18th century Austrian example. In M. Gorden (Ed.), *The American family in social-historical perspective*. New York: St. Martin's Press, 1973.

deMause, L. The evolution of childhood. In L. deMause (Ed.), *The history of childhood*, New York: Harper & Row, 1974.

Erikson, E. H. *Childhood and society*. New York: W. W. Norton, 1950.

Frejka, T. Reflections on the demographic conditions needed to establish a United States stationary population growth. *Population Studies*, 1968, *22*, 379–397.

Geertsen, R., Klauber, M. R., Rindflesh, M., Kane, R. L., & Gray, R. A reexamination of Suchman's view on social factors in health care utilization. *Journal of Health and Social Behavior*, 1975, *16*, 226–237.

Greven, P. J., Jr. Family structure in seventeenth century Andover, Massachusetts. In M. Gorden (Ed.), *The American family in social-historical perspective*. New York: St. Martin's Press, 1973.

Hunt, M. Sexual behavior in the 1970's. Part II: Premarital sex. *Playboy*, 1973, *11*, 74.

Kinsey, A., & Gebhard, P. *Sexual behavior in the human female*. Philadelphia: W. B. Saunders, 1953.

Lantz, H., Schultz, M., & O'Hara, M. The changing American family from the preindustrial to the industrial period: A final report. *American Sociological Review*, 1977, *42*, 406–421.

Laslett, P. Introduction: The history of the family. In P. Laslett (Ed.), *Household and family in past time*. Cambridge, Mass.: Harvard University Press, 1972.

———. The comparative history of household and family. In M. Gorden (Ed.), *The American family in social-historical perspective*. New York: St. Martin's Press, 1973.

Litwak, E. Occupational mobility and extended family cohesion. *American Sociological Review*, 1960, *25*, 9–21.

Nimkoff, M. F., and Middleton, R. Types of family and types of economy. *American Journal of Sociology*, 1960, *66*, 215–225.

Parsons, T. The American family: Its relations to personality and the social structure. In T. Parsons & R. F. Bales (Eds.), *Family, socialization and interaction process*, Glencoe, Ill.: Free Press, 1955.

Reiss, I. L. Premarital sexuality: Past, present and future. In I. L. Reiss (Ed.), *Readings on the family system*. New York: Holt, Rinehart and Winston, 1972.

Rodgers, R. H. *Family interaction and transaction: A developmental approach*. Englewood Cliffs, N.J.: Prentice-Hall, 1973.

Rollins, B. C., and Feldman, H. Marital satisfaction over the family life cycle. *Journal of Marriage and the Family*, 1970, *32*, 20–28.

Shorter, E. Illegitimacy, sexual revolution, and social change in modern Europe. In T. K. Rabb & R. J. Rotberg (Eds.), *The family in history*. New York: Harper Torchbooks, 1971.

———. *The making of the modern family*. New York: Basic Books, 1975.

Smith, D. S. The dating of the American sexual revolution: Evidence and interpretation. In M. Gorden (Ed.), *The American family in social-historical perspective*. New York: St. Martin's Press, 1973.

Stephans, W. N. *The family in cross-cultural perspective*. New York: Holt, Rinehart and Winston, 1963.

Suchman, E. A. Health orientation and medical care. *American Journal of Public Health*, 1966, *56*(1), 97–105.

————. Social patterns of illness and medical care. *Journal of Health and Human Behavior*, 1965, *6*, 2–16.

————. Sociomedical variations among ethnic groups. *American Journal of Sociology*, 1964, *10*, 319–331.

Suelzle, M. Women in labor. In H. Z Lopata (Ed.), *Marriages and families*. New York: D. Van Nostrand, 1973.

Sussman, M. The isolated nuclear family: Fact or fiction? *Social Problems*, 1959, *6*, 333–340.

Winch, R. F., & Blumberg, R. L. Societal complexity and familial reorganization. In R. F. Winch & L. W. Goodman, (Eds.), *Selected studies in marriage and the family* (3d ed.). New York: Holt, Rinehart and Winston, 1968.

Zimmerman, C. C. *The family of tomorrow: The cultural crisis and the way out*. New York: Harper & Row, 1949.

CHAPTER FIVE

THEORIES OF FAMILY CRISIS

CAROLYN BROSE

Increased interest has been focused in the last few years on crisis and crisis intervention. Much attention has been given to psychological and mental health crises, since the consequences of crisis management often have significant and long-lasting effects on the level of a person's mental functioning (Bloom, 1963, p. 498). Crisis theorists have shown that crisis situations have predictable outcomes and that timely intervention will greatly influence the predicted result. Not only can intervention affect the outcome of the actual crisis, but also it can influence the adaptation or maladaptation that the person will continue to make to the situation. For some people, the changes wrought by crisis may mean increased health and maturity, while for others the changes may be the beginning of incapacity to deal effectively with life's problems.

From the physiological point of view, crisis intervention may entail life-and-death situations. Death from trauma, especially in our age of increasing power and speed potential, added to acute, life-threatening medical emergencies such as myocardial infarctions, accentuates the need for crisis intervention. Despite the movement of the medical health systems in the direction of preventive medicine versus acute, episodic care, one cannot negate the need for a functional crisis-oriented system to provide life support for the physiological crisis. Immediate action must be taken in the true physiological crisis if the organism is to survive. The biggest problem seems to be one of a gap between knowledge and its application.

CRISIS DEFINITIONS

Today, *crisis* is almost a household word. We hear of the political crisis, the international crisis, the economic crisis, and the drug crisis, to mention only a few. Often we hear *crisis* used interchangeably with *stress* (Selye, 1956) because both terms imply actual or potential disruption of the stable state of those involved.

A leading crisis theorist, Gerald Caplan, and his colleagues have described crisis as an "upset in the steady state" (Caplan, 1964, p. 40; Parad, 1965). They believe a crisis is produced when a person finds the usual methods of problem solving ineffective when coping with an obstacle to important life goals. Fink defines crisis as "an event in which the individual's normal coping abilities are inadequate to meet the demands of the situation" (1967, p. 592). Miller and Iscoe present crisis as "the experiencing of an acute situation where one's repertoire of coping responses is inadequate in effecting a resolution of the stress" (1963, p. 196). Bloom states that crisis will vary in severity as determined by the degree of reorganization required to cope with the situation and that a crisis represents a turning point in one's life. The crisis, therefore, necessitates a reorganization of some of the important aspects of the individual's structure (Bloom, 1963, p. 498).

McHugh (1960, p. 227) describes a crisis as an event that disturbs the equilibrium of social relationships in a situation. Erikson (1965) expands the definition by classifying crises as *developmental* (maturational) or *situational* (accidental). A situational crisis is an external event or stress, such as illness or death of a loved one. Developmental, or maturational, crisis is a normal and expected occurrence in the process of one's psychosocial development. Puberty, courtship, marriage, pregnancy, and menopause are examples of developmental times of increased susceptibility to crisis. Developmental and situational crises may occur simultaneously, as in the case of the adolescent facing hospitalization. It appears evident that crisis may assume different forms to different persons or even to the same person at different times. Although these definitions vary, we might generalize to say that crisis involves a threat, either real or implied, to the person or persons involved, even though the threat may take different forms.

RESPONSE TO A CRISIS SITUATION: THE BYSTANDER

It is important that the nurse have an understanding of the actions and reactions that may occur in a crisis. The nurse who understands possible response mechanisms, their causes and meanings, is better equipped to cope with a personal response as well as those of the victim, family and bystanders. The nurse may also better understand the effect of crisis on the victim and the victim's ability or inability to make decisions or use other resources available.

To fully appreciate crisis responses, we should look at both the bystander's and the victim's points of view. A great deal of the bystander's behavior can be explained by listing the characteristics of an emergency situation (Latanè and Darley, 1969). Threat is inherent in an emergency, perhaps to one's well-being, life, or property. Rewards for successful intervention in an emergency, such as self-satisfaction, public recognition, or even financial reward, are possible but may be difficult to assess in value. On the other hand, one must consider that the rescuer often must enter into a dangerous situation to aid the victim. A man standing at the water's edge, hearing the call for help from a drowning man, must decide within himself the potential cost. Will he take the risk of losing his own life in an attempt to save another's? Does he consider the possibility of endangering his own family's support if he is drowned in the attempt? At the scene of an auto accident, will he attempt to give care to the injured, even though he may be sued for his well-intentioned actions? Witnessing a mugging, will he go to the aid of the victim and perhaps be required to appear in court as a witness against the assailant? How much time, effort, and funds will such follow-up activities take? Would it be easier to not get involved? Is he prepared in the first place to intervene?

An emergency is a rare event. Statisticians have presented evidence that truly critical medical emergencies may occur only once or twice to a person during a lifetime. Other statistics indicate that, on the average, a person may encounter fewer than six serious emergencies of all types in a lifetime. It becomes obvious that the individual is poorly prepared to meet these emergencies. Human beings, used to adapting to new situations by recalling previous situations, will find they have limited reference experience to guide them in a new crisis. They are much like the actor who is thrust onto the stage to perform a new role without the benefit of rehearsal.

Another basic characteristic of emergencies is that they differ in type and character. Problems presented to the rescuer of the drowning man and those presented to the rescuer of a potential suicide victim are vastly different. The nurse faced with a patient on a bad LSD trip finds different problems than the nurse caring for a patient who has been severely burned. Just as the situations are different, so are the actions to be taken.

Emergencies are unforeseen events that arrive suddenly, with little or no warning. Time to think through feasible courses of action and alternatives is denied. Immediate action is a necessity. Time to consult with others of greater knowledge and experience cannot usually be taken. The individual *must* act if the condition is to be rectified. Stress will begin to bear influence. How then will one perform? Will the effect of the stress spur one to greater action, or will the stress level be of such a degree that one will become immobile under its influence? This depends a great deal on the individual's personality and previous exposure and manner (coping mechanisms) in being able to function under other stresses.

Another important element in the understanding of reactions to crisis is the decision-making processes that are inherent in each situation. Before a person can intervene in a crisis situation, the fact that a crisis exists must be recognized. That is, the person must be aware that an event is taking place and must also decide if something is awry.

As you hurry down a busy street crowded with shoppers, do you notice the young man leaning in the doorway of a building, clutching his abdomen and moaning? Or, is your mind crowded with the pressures of the day so that the young man goes unnoticed in the crowd? Let us assume that you have seen him. You must now decide if there is something wrong. In our culture, we are hesitant to be too observing of others, especially strangers. For example, have you ever felt the flush of unexplained embarrassment when you realize that you are unwittingly caught staring at another, or vice versa? It is not polite to stare or gape at another person. It is not proper to examine another, especially a stranger. Another factor that may influence your decision is the young man's mode of dress. Is he clean-shaven and neatly dressed in a suit; or is he a hippie with beard, beads, and long hair? Maybe he is on dope or on a "bad trip." Maybe he is pretending to be ill to lure a victim to him, whom he will then assault. Even if you have decided that something is wrong, will you next make the decision to take on the responsibility of action? If you do, you must next decide what form of aid is needed and how its implementation will be carried out. Finally, you must decide where your responsibility for the young man ends.

As has just been demonstrated, a series of decisions must be made if one is to intervene in a crisis. A logical sequence of decisions is rarely made. The bystander may overlook some decisions, or may simultaneously make several decisions and vacillate between possible actions and outcomes before actually initiating intervention. The bystander, therefore, is not an objective observer, but is caught up in the crisis, with an emotional level that is probably high.

Social determinants also will strongly affect the decision-making process and, therefore, the intervention or lack of intervention that occurs. An individual will be strongly influenced by the decisions others are perceived to be making. Let us return to the young man in the street. If, while he leans against the building and moans, people hurry by him with only side glances and indicate by their behavior that nothing is out of the ordinary, you are apt to follow suit. This behavior is demonstrated by one who goes to a very formal dinner with copious quantities of silverware on the table, and watches the behavior of others—what spoon or fork is picked up first and used in what manner. In strange situations, we check others for cues to how we are expected to perform. As a result, in our case of the young man, the inaction of other passersby may present the situation as less serious than perhaps you would determine if you were alone.

Not only will the perceived decisions that others are making influence your actions, but also the knowledge that others are watching your behavior will affect your decision. To be a "good nurse" you must remain calm and poised in the face of crisis. To show emotion or undue concern would possibly open the door to ridicule and weaken your professional image. In the hospital setting, emotion or undue concern may be equated with inexperience or lack of knowledge. Therefore, it is very possible, even in the hospital, to misjudge the seriousness of a crisis when behavioral cues alone are taken. One needs to remain calm and collected to function effectively, but too much calm can be calamitous for the patient.

There is safety in numbers, or is there? Research has shown that when faced with a stressful situation, most people do seem less afraid when they are in the presence of others than if they are alone (Latanè and Darley, 1969, p. 226; Latanè, 1969, pp. 61–69; Latanè, 1968, pp. 142–146). Who does not find comfort in the fact that there are many others moving about the street on a dark, misty night? What nurse has not found comfort in the knowledge that supervisor and peers from other units can come if help is called for? We may feel our chances for assistance are greater with a greater number of people around us. Research has disproven this (Latanè and Darley, 1969, p. 249; Darley and Latanè, 1968; Latanè and Darley, 1968).

Take, for example, the reports in the newspapers in 1963 of a young woman in New York City coming home from work in the early hours of the morning and being attacked by a maniac. Her cries for help attracted a total of thirty-eight neighbors and witnesses, surely enough people to overpower her attacker and rescue the victim. These people watched for over half an hour while the maniac slowly killed his victim. Such incidents have spurred research into bystander apathy. These studies have shown that the greater the number of people who witness a crisis situation, the less likley the victim is to receive aid. This information has also filtered into the lay literature (Blank, 1970, p. 73).

We have already presented some of the possible causes of the reluctance to offer aid in the presence of others. Real or potential threat to one's own life, fear of litigation for the efforts made, unwillingness to "appear against" the wrongdoer, and the inaction of others can encourage a person not to become involved. However, other factors should also be considered. In a large crowd of onlookers, who has the responsibility of stepping forward and taking charge? Should the bystander in a crowd rush to a phone to summon an ambulance or the police, or has someone already called for help? Are one's efforts necessary or will they be wasted? While responsibility can be delegated to an individual—for example, to the surgical resident in the emergency room who is responsible for the management of all cases of serious trauma—who is responsible when the designated person is absent? No one, everyone, or someone else?

The sins of omission and commission are equally important in the action that a person takes in face of an emergency. This is still a persistent concern to physicians and nurses despite the Good Samaritan Laws that have been passed in many states (Chayet, 1969, pp. 275–294). A person who witnesses an emergency situation alone bears the total responsibility for subsequent action or inaction. But, if there are others who also witness the emergency, the blame is diffused and not focused on any one person. Courts may decide such cases on the basis of what was "wise and prudent" for the person of such training and experience to have done. A nurse, who has been trained to give care, is held more responsible for providing such care than a person without such training. A nurse may have been off duty at the time of the emergency, but is, nevertheless, a nurse, on duty or off.

Research has shown that people are more willing to take the chance of exposure and action when in the presence of friends than when in the presence of strangers (Latanè and Darley, 1969, p. 263). If the emergency is witnessed by a group of friends rather than by a group of total strangers, the victim will be somewhat more apt to receive aid. In view of the decisions that one must make and the forces that impinge upon the decision-making process in the face of a crisis situation, it becomes almost a miracle that intervention ever occurs.

RESPONSE TO CRISIS FROM THE VICTIM'S POINT OF VIEW

Fink (1967, p. 592) has presented a theoretical model of changes that he feels occur in the person who is experiencing a crisis situation. This model is a useful one, for it provides the profesional with a systematic organization of events that otherwise appear chaotic and incomprehensible. As such, this model offers information on what behavior the rescuer might expect from the victim, as well as the type of aid that would best be given and its timing.

The model consists of four sequential phases: (1) shock, (2) defensive retreat, (3) acknowledgment, (4) adaptation. Each of these phases is described in terms of self-experience, reality perception, emotional experience, and cognitive structure (see Table 5-1).

The shock phase represents the individual's first moments of encounter with the crisis situation. This phase may last only a few minutes or may extend over a period of hours.

Table 5-1 Psychologic phases of crisis

Phase	Self-experience	Reality perception	Emotional experience	Cognitive structure	Physical parallels	Social parallels
Shock (impact)	Depersonalization	Sharp; clear; "objective"	None; possible euphoria; indifference	Organized; automatic functioning	Shock; emergency reactions	Individual centering; associality; docility
Realization	Collapse of existing structure	Reality seems overwhelming	Panic; high anxiety; helplessness	Inability to plan, reason, or understand situation	Objective somatic damage requiring immediate care	Breakdown of ordinary social controls; chaos
Defensive retreat	Attempt to reestablish previous identity	Avoidance of reality; wishful thinking; denial	Indifference or euphoria except when challenged, in which case, anger	Progressive rigidity; situation-bound thinking; resistance to change	Recovery from acute phase; rapid improvement. Treatment plans solidify.	Authoritarian control; tightening of structure; use or organized force
Acknowledgment	Disintegration; self-depreciation	Reality "imposes itself"	Depression; apathy, agitation, or bitterness. If overwhelming, suicide	Disorganization; reorganization in accord with altered reality perceptions	Physical plateau. Rate of improvement slows	Recognition of inadequacies in old system; reevaluation of structure; plan for change
Adaptation; change	New identity appears; new sense of personal worth	Reality testing; mastery efforts	Anxiety decreases; satisfaction increases	Stabilization of reorganization; integration with earlier structure	"Functional improvement" with no change in actual disability status	Repatterning of behavior and environment to cope with or avoid future similar crises

Shontz (1964) has divided the shock phase into two periods. The first period is the *impact phase,* in which the person understands that "something is wrong." For example, a mill worker reaches full realization that his hand has just been severed by his machine, yet he may not panic or express overwhelming anguish at what has just happened. Rather, he appears to become emotionally numb. He clearly understands that he has just lost his hand, but is unable to formulate a plan of action to cope with the situation. He is at a prime stage for help and will be submissive to the will of others. Depersonalization will begin, and he will not see himself as the one who has just lost the hand. It is obvious that the victim should not be required or expected to make decisions regarding his care or well-being. Someone else must formulate a plan of action and communicate this plan to the victim, if the sitaution is to be managed efficiently.

The second period of the shock phase, as reported by Shontz, is *realization,* when panic begins to set in. At this point, the victim may be overwhelmed by what has happened to him, because the situation may appear totally hopeless. His anxieties may soar. Although he may begin to feel the need to plan a course of action, he is unable to do so because of his clouded perceptions and high level of anxiety. At this stage, he will usually be very open to suggestions. Help might need to be presented to him in a very firm and decisive manner in order for him to control his own behavior and cooperate with the rescuer's efforts. During this stage, attention is focused upon the damage and its repair. It is during this stage that the victim is usually first seen by the nurse or physician. The total phase of realization may last for weeks or be reasonably brief.

The next stage into which the individual will move is that of *defensive retreat.* This stage can be compared with the "fight or flight" behavior exhibited by an organism under attack. The victim will seek ways in which to lower the stress felt at the moment. Reality will become an element which he will attempt to avoid. He may express anger, and denial may begin.

Denial should be considered in the victim's response to a crisis as it is very much a part of one's reaction to the stressful event. Denial becomes a useful tool, which the victim uses in attempting to maintain some degree of equilibrium during a period of disorganization. As such, denial becomes a normal and inevitable response to a crisis. Just as a crisis event will vary in severity, so will the degree of denial that may be exhibited.

With a serious crisis, however, denial cannot be maintained. According to Shontz, a person has three alternatives: (1) withdraw entirely from the situation, (2) express anger or despair, or (3) yield, or succumb, to the disorganization and disruption imposed by the situation. If the victim withdraws, he then must find gratifications and his being in a fantasy world. If he expresses anger or despair, he will have resorted to destructive emotions; and a constructive solution to the situation will not be forthcoming. If the victim yields, he has at least broached upon the vital element of realism.

It is during the response of yielding that many medically trained persons lose grasp of what is happening to the victim. If the victim "yields" by hysterical outbursts of crying, the physician or nurse may see this as unacceptable and annoying behavior. This behavior is, in fact, acceptable for the victim at that particular time. The victim, by yielding, has let reality overwhelm him. The passive, very quiet, stoic patient might be completely denying and avoiding all contact with reality. This reaction is obviously not healthful and should not be allowed to continue. The nurse and/or physician must try to see the crisis from the patient's point of view, rather than viewing it in coldly objective reality.

Take, for example, a young woman who is brought into the emergency room after sustaining facial lacerations in an auto accident. Despite reassurances that her injuries are not serious, she continues to cry hysterically. The emergency room staff becomes increasingly annoyed with the patient, because she is not responding correctly as gauged by the reality of the situation. Unknown to the staff, however, this young woman is a model, and she equates the facial lacerations with scarring and potential loss of her livelihood. She is overwhelmed and cannot think in rational terms, such as plastic revision of any scarring.

Unless the victim totally maladapts, he or she will not be able to forever suppress reality, and will, finally, move into the stage of *acknowledgment*. This becomes a period of increased stress, for the victim not only *recognizes* reality but also is forced to *accept* reality. This phase is a gradual one, which may last a period of years, and perhaps the rest of the victim's life.

The final phase is that of *adaptation*. Shontz emphasizes that adaptation necessitates a change, not a resumption, of preexisting structure. A reorganization, a restructuring, and a new approach to management of life's demands constitute adaptation to a crisis situation.

GENERALIZATIONS

If one were to combine the previously mentioned observations of crisis theory and intervention with other related studies, four major generalizations might be made. The first is that whether a person emerges stronger or weaker as a result of crisis experience is not based so much on previous character makeup as on the kind of help received during the actual crisis (Caplan, 1964, p. 53). This fact places great responsibility upon the nurse who is faced with the patient and/or family in a crisis situation. The nurse must recognize that a crisis exists, attempt to understand its impact on the family, and must render "crisis care" or call upon others to assist with the patient and/or family. It is important to realize that there may be others, for example, a social worker, a physician, or minister, who may be more effective as the "crisis manager." This utilization of others should not be a mode of escape, however, for the nurse who would rather evade responsibility for crisis management.

The second generalization is that people become more amenable to suggestions and open to help during the actual crisis (Brandon, 1970, p. 631; Robischon, 1967, p. 29; Caplan, 1964, p. 53). In the hospital setting, this fact means that the responsibility for dealing with the crisis is assumed by the emergency room nurse, by the intensive care nurse, and by the floor nurse. As time passes, even the community health nurse should assume some of the intervention role. The ideal opportunity and time to render aid is now.

Family support is also very important. The person who is in crisis needs the support and encouragement of those most close. The family can help the person by acknowledging the trouble and indicating their concern (Caplan, 1964, pp. 44–47). It must be emphasized that the family may need support from the nurse or others in order to recognize this need and to cope with it effectively. The basic strength of the family must also be considered. If the family is crisis prone, consistently passing from one crisis to another, resolution and opportunity for growth and maturation may never be realized. Maladaptive behavior may be encouraged by this type of family, because they have not yet learned effective ways of coping with the stress of life. Cultural factors are also relevant. The person's cultural heritage may be responsible for some ability to deal with the more complex problems (Brandon, 1970, p. 628).

The need for the nurse to be keenly aware of the family and to assess the family as well as the individual patient should be self-evident if optimum crisis care is to be realized. Take, for example, the family of a 16-year-old boy who was brought to the emergency room by the police after he was apprehended during an armed robbery attempt on a bank. The staff's primary concern was quickly directed to physical care, since the youth had sustained a gunshot wound resulting in a sucking chest wound. After the physical crisis was stabilized, attention could then be diverted to the psychosocial crisis, considered from both developmental and situational crisis standpoints. Here was an adolescent (developmental crisis-prone time) facing a life-threatening physical crisis as well as a situational crisis, a felony charge. The family situation was assessed as malignant. The mother came into the emergency room, where she was first detained and questioned by FBI agents. When she was allowed to see her son, she stood at a distance from the cart for several minutes in stony silence. Her only comment was, "Who was in this with you?" The boy stared at the ceiling and yelled, "No one!" At this point, the mother left the room and refused to accompany her son to the hospital unit. Brief assessment of the family from an interview with the mother yielded the following information. This was a crisis-prone family. Their life was a long series of one crisis followed by another, none of which appeared to result in maturation or growth for the family. The family was of a lower-socioeconomic level and daily faced crucial financial problems of providing the essentials of living. There had been no stable father figure in the home. All the children over 14 years of age had dropped out of school. One older son was in prison, convicted of assault with a deadly weapon. It is obvious that this family will most likely be unable to cope with the new crisis in an acceptable manner. The addition of the act of crime, subsequently resulting in the injury, further isolated the victim from some type of family support. The identical injury, if it had been sustained accidentally, might have mobilized greater support.

The nurse in the emergency room will not be able to deal with all the problems involved, but should be aware of their presence and base professional involvement upon an assessment of the patient and family. The nurse should then convey this information, along with the need for additional information, to the floor nurse and others needed to cope with the crisis resolution. The crisis for this family will not be resolved in a short period of time. It may take many weeks, months, or years, and many people assisting the family and boy to adjust. Hopefully, the emergency room nurse will start the intervention to help this family learn to better cope with the crisis and emerge as a more healthy entity.

A third generalization is that with the onset of a crisis situation, old memories of past crises may be evoked. If maladaptive behavior was used to deal with previous situations, the same type of behavior may be repeated in the face of the new crisis. Another example of this behavior was reported by Hiatt and Spurlock (1970, p. 53) as what they term *geographical flight*. This behavior is a "pattern of travel wherein motionless and geographical fleeing has become a chronically episodic way of coping—characteristic of a way of life or life style." The onset of the flight coping mechanism appears to begin in childhood, for example, in the runaway child.

A fourth generalization is that the only way to survive a crisis is to be aware of its existence. This generalization is reinforced by the work done by Lindemann on the Coconut Grove fire and the process of grieving (1965, pp. 7–21). He concluded that people who adjusted stoically to their loss (denied the loss to a degree) were, in the long run, the ones who suffered the most, as evidenced by the decline in their mental health in the following years. Lindemann pointed out the need to face the fact of death and to go through a grieving process.

Related to the preceding generalizations, Cadden (1964, pp. 288–296) has listed seven ways she feels a person can help another who is in crisis:

1. Help the victim to confront reality, to speak of unspoken fears, and to cry.
2. Help the victim to confront reality in manageable doses. Rest is important, but do not misgive drugs to induce excessive sleep when the person needs assistance to look at reality.
3. Help the victim to find the facts. Fantasy is always much worse than fact. The nurse can assist greatly in this area by being truthful with the patient and the family as well as promoting communications between doctor and family.
4. Do not give false reassurances.
5. Do not encourage the victim or family to blame others.
6. Help the victim to accept help.
7. Help the victim and family with the everyday tasks of living until resolution or stabilization is attained.

CONCLUSION

The intricate blend of the psychological and physiological factors makes it impractical, if not impossible, to consider the patient on only a physiological basis. The psychological crisis involving the realization of an injury and the impending medical care, its costs, and the potential loss of income and rearrangement of family structure, even on a temporary basis, may well overwhelm the patient with even a minor illness or injury. The professional nurse, therefore, needs to consider the patient as a whole being rather than "the fracture in room nine" or "the stroke in the medical room." Perhaps the nurses who should be most aware of these problems, by nature of their work in acute episodic care areas, are the least sensitive to the more subtle crisis that the patient and the family may feel. With an understanding of the many factors that may influence the patient's response and reactions to crisis, the professional nurse will, it is hoped, take the additional step in providing more comprehensive crisis care.

REFERENCES

Aquilera, D. C., & Messick, J. M. *Crisis intervention and methodology* (2d ed.). St. Louis: C. V. Mosby, 1974.
———, ———, & Farrell, M. S. *Crisis intervention: Theory and methodology,* St. Louis: C. V. Mosby, 1970.
Barrell, L. M. Crisis intervention—Partnership in problem solving. *Nursing Clinics of North America,* 1974, *9,* 5–16.
Blank, J. P. "Rescue on the freeway," *Reader's Digest,* 97:73–80, 1970.
Bloom, B. L. Definitional aspects of the crisis concept. *Journal of Consulting Psychology,* 1963, *27,* 498–502.

Brandon, S. Crisis theory and possibilities of therapeutic intervention. *British Journal of Psychiatry,* 1970, *117,* 627–633.

Cadden, V. Crisis in the family. In G. Caplan (Ed.), *Principles of preventive psychiatry.* New York: Basic Books, 1964.

Caplan. G. *Principles of preventive psychiatry.* New York: Basic Books, 1964.

Chayet, N. L. *Legal implications of emergency care.* New York: Appleton-Century-Crofts, 1969.

Darley, J., & Latanè, B. Bystander intervention in emergencies: Diffusion of responsibility. *Journal of Personality and Social Psychology,* 1968, *8,* 377–383.

Eastham, K., Coates, D., & Allodi, F. The concept of crisis. *Canadian Psychiatric Association Journal,* 1970, *15,* 463–472.

Erikson, E. H. *Childhood and society.* New York: Penguin Books, 1965.

Fink, S. L. Crisis and motivation: A theoretical model. *Archives of Physical Medicine and Rehabilitation,* 1967, *48,* 592–597.

Hiatt, C. C., & Spurlock, R. E. Geographical flight and its relation to crisis theory. *American Journal of Orthopsychiatry,* 1970, *40,* 53–57.

Latanè, B. Gregariousness and fear in laboratory rats. *Journal of Experimental Social Psychology,* 1969, *5,* 61–69.

――――, & Darley, J. Bystander apathy. *American Scientist,* 1969, *57,* 244–268.

――――, & ――――. Group inhibition by bystander intervention in emergencies. *Journal of Personality and Social Psychology,* 1968, *10,* 215–221.

――――, & Glass, D. C. Social and non-social attraction in rats. *Journal of Personality and Social Psychology,* 1968, *9,* 142–146.

Lindemann, E. Symptomatology and management of acute grief. In H. J. Parad (Ed.), *Crisis intervention: Selected readings.* New York: Family Service Association of America, 1965.

McHugh, M. The management of crisis in human situations. *The Canadian Nurse,* 1960, *56,* 227–229.

Miller, K. The concept of crisis: Current status and mental health implications. *Human Organizations,* 1963, *22,* 195–201.

Parad, H. J. (Ed.) *Crisis intervention: Selected readings.* New York: Family Service Association of America, 1965.

Robischon, P. The challenge of crisis theory for nursing. *Nursing Outlook,* 1967, *15,* 28–32.

Selye, H. *The stress of life.* New York: McGraw-Hill, 1956.

Shontz, F. C. Reactions to crisis. Paper presented at Speech and Hearing Workshop, Kansas City: University of Kansas Medical Center, May 14, 1964.

Smith. L. L. A general model of crisis intervention. *Clinical Social Work Journal,* 1976, *4,* 162–171.

CHAPTER SIX

THE DEVELOPMENT OF FAMILY NURSING

LORETTA C. FORD

Tracing the development of family nursing in the emergence of professional nursing preparation and practice is a frustrating endeavor. Factors and forces within the profession, in related disciplines, and in the context of social evolution, make the identification and analysis complex and multidimensional. Time and relationships of movements and events overlap, lack sequential evolvement, and, for all intents and purposes, appear unplanned. In one sense, family nursing has grown in response to the zephyrs and hurricanes of change within nursing as well as in external forces.

In another sense, the elusive quality of "becoming" rather than "being" characterizes the state of the art and science of family nursing today. To capture a composite picture of this growth, four major dimensions are explored: advances in nursing and nursing education, contributions of professional organizations, theory development in nursing and related disciplines, and changes in needs, demands, and aspirations of society. Recent and long-term trend data from epidemiological and sociological sources on population and families give rise to questions about future directions for nursing practice. A preliminary review of the history of nursing education and practice serves as a point of departure.

The concept of family nursing has always been with us. Some arenas of practice, notably public health nursing, have claimed more interest, expertise, opportunities, and responsibilities for family care than others in nursing practice. Delivering service in the patient's home fostered the nurse's insights about the family as a resource in the maintenance or disruption of health and also afforded opportunities to view holistically the problems and progress of patients and families.

Public health nursing in its initial stages began by providing care to the sick poor; it later emerged as a force in augmenting preventive health services and family care. As society grew and developed by grouping people in schools, industries, and communities, specialized nursing practices evolved. Public health nurses struggled with the problems of specialization and finally laid claim to a practice known as *generalized nursing services,* or *family nursing.* Essentially it meant nursing care of the sick and health counseling and teaching for all members of the family under the sponsorship of governmental or voluntary health agencies. Some agency programs, of course, while directing their efforts toward specific disease eradication or other specialized goals, used family service as their basic philosophical orientation. Notable among these was the tuberculosis control program sponsored by the federal government in the forties.

Early in the growth of public health nursing practice, nurses recognized that their preparation in hospital schools was inadequate to serve families. Demands for advanced preparation in institutions of higher education were met first in 1910 by Columbia University. The movement of nursing education programs into collegiate settings began. Braving the resistance to change, many courageous nursing leaders introduced concepts of family care in the basic nursing curricula (Committee on Education, 1919; Committee on Grading, 1934; Report of the Committee, 1923).

Admittedly, the theoretical orientations often were lacking; however, the operational aspects that gave recognition to the family as a unit of service and study were identified as principles. No effort will be made to recount this very early history verbatim. It exists and is well documented in the literature of the field (Gardner, 1936; National Association for Public Health Nursing, 1939).

It suffices to say that the history of public health nursing practice is replete with undulating curves of crises and plateaus reflecting the changes and stresses in society. Unfortunately, despite these early advantages to promote family nursing care, often agency policies and procedures controlled nursing practice, unconsciously undermining the basic stated philosophy of family care. Referral policies, established daytime hours of duty, health insurance coverage limitations, reimbursement policies from government sources, mechanized recording, and the demands for certain types of disease-identification statistics all required operationalizing the nursing service given by public health nurses to an individually oriented care system. As Freeman (1967) points out, some record systems organized for the collation, storage, and retrieval of data were devised for care of an individual, not a family unit.

Other factors mitigated against delivering family nursing care. Nurses themselves played a large part in giving lip service to family care concepts and in actuality practiced nursing as they had basically learned it in hospital settings. Nursing care plans frequently revealed that service was rendered to individual patients, rather than to the family. Though the National Organization for Public Health Nursing enunciated a cardinal principle in 1932 that identified the family as the basic unit of service, as Freeman points out, "practice does not always follow precept" (1970, p. 109). Influxes into the public health nursing field of ill-prepared nurses at certain times in history, such as in pre- and post-World Wars I and II, undoubtedly accounted for the widening gap between promise and performance in the delivery of family care.

Following World War II, changes in undergraduate and graduate collegiate nursing education influenced positively the development of family nursing. Content from the social sciences was explored and selected for its applicability to nursing curricula. Introductory courses in sociology and advanced courses on the study of the family as a basic social group and an institution in society were included in many programs. In special certificate programs, public health nursing courses offered extended study of the family and the community.

As the scope and nature of nursing came under scrutiny by nursing educators, an intensive examination of educational processes was begun. Collegiate schools introduced a new field teaching pattern that made public health nursing faculty members primarily responsible for the student's education during clinical experiences in the community. When the National League for Nursing Accrediting Service required that public health nursing courses be integrated into all generic baccalaureate educational programs by 1963, emphasis on the family in patient care became an integral component of every professional nurse's education. All faculties were required to have basic public health nursing preparation. Nursing itself was fast being professionalized. As nurses began to formulate basic conceptualizations about nursing, there was movement away from the medical model, disease-oriented, largely technical programs. Many nursing school faculties engaged in all-out efforts to create curricula based on a philosophy and goals commensurate with nursing's commitment to care for people. Debates about nursing's goals and identification of the client were heard in national and local arenas. The search for the body of nursing knowledge began.

The emphasis on research, the recognition of the care concept as a philosophical commitment, the efforts to redirect nursing potential to clinical rather than managerial responsibilities in the health care system, the desire for autonomy in clinical practice, and the demands for rigorous scientific and theoretical bases for changing and developing nursing practice all contributed to the growth of an increasingly sophisticated knowledgeable group of professionals.

Conceptual frameworks were created. Nursing was introduced as an integrated subject matter; clinical resources were expanded; and the student's clinical study was balanced with general education courses. Some programs quickly launched into extensive use of ambulatory care settings for learning experiences. Preventive and promotional aspects of nursing and health care were emphasized. As new basic curricula evolved, advanced preparation for leaders in nursing received increasing attention. Certainly, psychiatric nursing with its early financial support from the federal Mental Health Act led the field in the expansion of graduate programs and in the preparation of clinicians (Peplau, 1959). The patterns of operation for the distribution of those original grant funds, the mid-fifties National Institutes of Health study on families of schizophrenics, the increasing interest and research in family therapy in psychiatry, the federal government's later commitment to community mental health programs influenced greatly the contributions that psychiatric nurses have made and are making to the growth of family nursing as a field of study (Joint Commission on Mental Illness and Health, 1961).

Psychiatric nurses entered the community from a relatively stagnant position in hospital care to find the dynamic, exciting world of families and the community ready and willing for their specialized psychotherapeutic skills. Early hospital discharge of the mentally ill forced public health nurses to examine their abilities to cope with family problems in this relocation effort and seek consultation from psychiatric nurse clinicians and others in the mental health field. Emphasis on health counseling of the family group, team delivery of mental health care, and the reduction of the mystique of psychiatric diagnosis to behaviorally describable terms all added appreciably to the development of understanding among nurses and helped immeasurably toward working constructively with families.

Other nursing specialists, notably those in maternal and child care, have demonstrated extended interest in family care, focusing initially on the mother-child dyad and later on parenting. Historically, midwifery used a family-centered approach, particularly in home delivery services when family resources were explored and activated in preparation for care of the mother and newborn in the home setting. Leading the way for parents' classes, nurses in such well-known agencies as the Maternity Center Association of New York and the Child Study Association in association with the Children's Bureau also promoted the development, over time, of nursing care of the family (Auerbach and Taylor, 1960; Corbin, 1960).

Philosophically, the uniqueness of this approach in group education was to meet expressed needs and concerns of parents through the nurse's group leadership role, and not through a preplanned course of instruction.

Probably the decision to prepare nurse clinicians at the graduate level was a major step in redirecting the educational endeavors of the profession. Certainly, professional organizations played a major part in this, and their influence in the development of family nursing can be traced throughout history.

Early, the National Organization for Public Health Nursing championed the cause of family nursing practice; later the National League for Nursing assumed leadership through its community commitments and its influence in nursing education. Only a few specific details can be mentioned here. The NLN's Committee on Perspectives began agitating for expanding nursing's role and serving families and communities through improved patterns of health care delivery (National League for Nursing, 1967). Changes in the National League for Nursing accreditation criteria also played a part in emphasizing care of the family and the community. Efforts of the 1967 Records Committee NLN-PHS committee are also worthy of mention (National League for Nursing, 1970). The product of their labors, the family record system, focused on assessment and intervention using the locus of the family. The American Nurses' Association also gave direction for nursing practice and nursing education. The *Position Paper* (1965) was followed by a *Statement on Graduate Education in Nursing* by the ANA's Commission on Nursing Education (1969). The latter helped identify as the major purpose of graduate programs the preparation of clinical specialists for leadership responsibilities. The commission's charge to the profession was to advance the science of nursing through research. The ANA organizational restructuring, which provided for Divisions on Practice, a Congress for Nursing Practice, and an Academy of Nursing, called national attention to a core value in nursing—the direct care of people. Statements on the standards of practice have been formulated by the Congress for Nursing Practice as charged by the ANA board of directors.

In 1967, the following definition was approved by the Division on Community Health Nursing Practice:

> Community Health Nursing Practice is a field of nursing practice for which there exists a body of knowledge and related skills which is applied in meeting the health needs of communities and of individuals and families in their normal environment, such as the home, the school, and the place of work. It is an area of practice which lies primarily outside the therapeutic institutions (ANA, 1967).

Other divisions struggled with definitions, some of which included family concern. Attempts to prevent duplication and overlapping now are in progress with the eventual goal of establishing standards of nursing care. In addition to the American Nurses' Association's and the National League for Nursing's activities, the Western Council for Higher Education for Nursing's actions deserve recognition. In 1958, the graduate seminar of the Western Council on Higher Education for Nursing

(WICHEN) of the Western Interstate Commission on Higher Education published *Guidelines for Developing Master's Degree Programs in the West* (1958). These guidelines publicly announced the belief of Western deans and some graduate faculty that clinical nursing should be an integral part of graduate education in nursing. Further, the graduate seminar sought action. It applied for and was granted project funds from the United States Public Health Service for graduate faculty in Western schools to clarify and delineate clinical content appropriate to the four major nursing areas: maternal and child nursing, psychiatric nursing, medical-surgical nursing, and public health nursing, later called community health nursing. Reports on this project were published in 1967 (*Defining Clinical Content*, 1967). The impact of these reports on the total nursing community has never been researched. However, Western faculty members involved in the years of collaborative effort attest to the great insights they gained from this rare learning experience. The Public Health Nursing Section of the American Public Health Association, initially through a special joint ad hoc committee, with the American Nurses' Association formulated a statement on the nursing specialist in public health nursing (Public Health Nursing Statement, 1967). This statement emphasized expertise in family and community nursing practice.

Probably no force has been so potent or recent as that provided by theorists and researchers in the social and behavioral sciences. In describing the development of the family as a field of study, Christensen (1964) identifies four time spans and phases: (1) preresearch—activities until the mid-nineteenth century; (2) social Darwinism—from the end of the preresearch period to the twentieth century's beginning; (3) emerging science—the first 50 years of the twentieth century; and (4) systematic theory building—from 1950 to the present and into the future. Obvious strides in theory building were made in the sixties. Efforts to theorize and conduct research about families as a social phenomenon brought together many disciplines, and, to a great extent, encouraged cooperation and collaboration in the study of this complex social entity—the family. These multidisciplinary contributions derived from collaborative studies of the family have greatly motivated many teachers and scholars of nursing to seek advanced preparation and conduct research about families.

Identification and categorization of conceptual frameworks by Hill and Hansen (1960) afforded the field of family study a tremendous growth spurt. They also served to attract community health nurses whose longstanding interest in the family served as a primary motivator. Christensen's 1964 *Handbook of Marriage and the Family* provided a comprehensive overview of the field of family study and brought together many eminent authors and researchers. In a compilation of conceptual frameworks for family analysis, Nye and Berardo (1966) presented eleven frameworks in an effort to advance theory building by introducing "orderliness into research processes and findings" (p. 6). Many nursing teachers in graduate programs, particularly in community health nursing, found these published works on family helpful resources for the newly organized clinical nursing courses. Some students used the conceptual frameworks for the development of assessment tools and for testing nursing intervention techniques. Clinical studies in nursing evolved from the theories and research of these behavioral scientists—particularly in the sixties.

Recently, as the decade ended, historical perspectives and future projections were in order. The *Journal of Marriage and the Family* gave public recognition of this point in history by publishing decade reviews in three parts. In one of these reviews, a comprehensive and astutely analytical article by Broderick (1971) traced a decade of development of family theory.

Essentially the development of family theory in the sixties advanced the field of family nursing appreciably from a relative static, philosophical concept to a dynamic, operational testing ground. Social scientists' contributions to systematic theory building have had a great influence in altering circumstances, identifying conceptual frameworks for testing and analysis, and providing direction and substance to the field. Emphasis on the scientific approaches through research about family life has encouraged scholars in nursing to view these aspects of family nursing. Though few erudite studies have been published to date, current explorations offer much potential.

Perhaps most significantly, nursing is joining with other disciplines from related fields whose basic interests and competencies in the family may someday ensure team approaches in family care, in multidisciplinary educational programs, and in research. In projecting future directions, Broderick (1971, p. 153) suggests three new strategies for future research: (1) systematic theory building, which would in Hill's suggestion provide an organized research effort in "systematically abstracting general principles from empirical generalizations"; (2) multiple perspective strategies, which promote the integration of specific social processes related to family life using the established conceptual frameworks; and (3) modern systems analysis, which uses complex, simulated computer programming for cognitive mapping and information networks.

This latter strategy requires extended periods of time for data collection and skilled analysis. The continuity of care responsibilities and the new emerging community and statewide health information systems that Glasser (1971) describes in a recent article may make modern systems analysis particularly fruitful for research in family nursing.

Efforts in theory construction in nursing are recorded by King in her publication, *Toward a Theory for Nursing* (1971). The contributions of Rogers, Quint, Brown, Gunther, Orlando, Abdellah, McCain, and others, while not specifically directed toward family nursing, deserve recognition for lending force and direction to the total field of nursing (King, 1971).

Within their focus on nursing practice, one finds concepts and constructs particularly applicable to family nursing.

But the growth of family nursing as a field of study and practice in large measure is dependent upon powerful, dynamic, societal forces. The expanding knowledge base about man and technology, the evolving philosophies of equality and humanism, the changing value system, the concern for population growth and the environment all have their impact. One of the most remarkable influences today is the demand to activate the long-enunciated democratic philosophical concept of equality for all—including health care. The implications of this are not only for the development of quality health services, but also for health care to be comprehensive and primarily oriented toward the promotion of health and the prevention of disease. Many health service organizations today are restating their goals in terms of high-level wellness, which Dunn (1961, p. 3) defines as:

> An integrated method of functioning which is oriented toward maximizing the potential of which the individual is capable within the environment where he is functioning.

Dunn applies his concept to individuals, families, and communities in an ecological framework. Though the terms *health, wellness,* and *illness* are difficult to define, often highly subjective and culturally determined, and impossible to measure precisely, society is beginning to recognize positive health as a value, a goal, and a right. Society's demands, needs, and aspirations are making rapid changes in all health arenas—including nursing practice and educational programs. Tired of fragmentation in service, high costs, barriers, and the inertia and unresponsiveness of the health care system, consumers are taking action.

With this powerful movement in society, health professionals find themselves in the center of a revolution in the health care system. One such outcome of consumer input affecting family care is the emerging neighborhood health center phenomenon, encouraged and supported by the Economic Opportunity Act of 1964 (Curry, 1971).

Efforts to make health care accessible, adequate, available, and acceptable to deprived populations required ecological and creative approaches. It meant serving families in their neighborhoods, using patterns of health care delivery that were not conducive to the highly specialized, infinitely technical, and controlled professional practice arenas. Health care in these centers tends to be holistic, humanized, and informal. Cutting the red tape rituals of the formalized health care system became necessary if groups of deprived people were to be brought into the mainstream of our society through the health care system. Health then becomes a mechanism for social progress as well as a social goal and a right. Individual rights extend to family and community rights—giving the consumer of health care decision-making power. Consumers of health services assume major responsibility in planning, developing, and managing their own health centers. Health professionals become learners and followers in certain aspects of the neighborhood health programs.

From the consumer groups, the indigenous family health worker came into existence. Functioning as case finder, interpreter, and liaison personnel between the consumers and providers of care, the family health worker introduced a new element in health care delivery patterns. Articulating roles for the team delivery of care became a necessity—and the transition was not always smooth and efficient. Nor is the concept of neighborhood health centers totally new. Rosen's historical review (1971) documents the rise and fall of early neighborhood health centers. The need for a national health policy is glaringly apparent throughout history.

Only recently, a national health policy directed toward developing a comprehensive health strategy for health maintenance was announced. This strategy employs health maintenance organizations and area health education centers (U.S. Department of Health, Education, and Welfare, 1971). The mechanism of family health insurance plans using the public and private sectors is proposed to provide competitive, capitalistic, and pluralistic components of the nation's political economy. This is the new health care system look for the 1970s. Will nursing, and more particularly, the family nursing proponents be ready? Perhaps.

In the late sixties, society's needs and demands for primary care fostered the development of new health workers. Family nurse practitioner programs have become increasingly visible (AJN, "Editorial," 1971). Their first appearance is recorded at the annual meeting of the American Public Health Association in October 1964, when Dr. Duncan E. Reid of the Harvard Medical School introduced his concept of a family nurse practitioner. Primarily, Reid's practitioner would provide the major portion of health care for normal expectant mothers and for newborn care in satellite community health clinics. In discussing Dr. Reid's proposal, Weidenbach (1965) astutely analyzes some of its shortcomings and adds the professional nursing perspective, promoting comprehensive maternal and child care through advanced preparation for collaborative physician-nurse relationships in practice. Just prior to this, Siegel et al. (1963) had reported successful work in expanding the role of the nurse in well child care in California.

By this time, national concern for the crisis in health care, and more particularly the horrendous problems of preparation and utilization of the country's health manpower, began to be heard in medical circles. Physicians and others realized that doctors were not meeting total health care needs of people; indeed they should not and could not be expected to do this. The dwindling supply of general medical practitioners, the lack of responsiveness of the health care system to meet people's needs, the health manpower crisis, and the insistent demands of society for quality and comprehensive health care all contributed to experimenting with new roles for nurses and other health personnel. Siegel's work was followed by other projects that were designed to tap nursing's potential for expansion. The Pediatric Nurse Practitioner Project at the University of Colorado and the studies at Montefiore, Massachusetts General, and the University of Kansas Medical Center are excellent demonstrations of the time and directions that pioneered nursing's future (Ford and Silver, 1967; Ford et al., 1966; Stoeckle, 1963; Lewis and Resnik, 1967). All these projects developed a clinically oriented, independent nursing role with collaborative, interdependent functioning with physicians in the ambulatory health care systems.

The heavy work loads of physicians created an opportunity to take a new look at current, available manpower resources and encouraged cooperative arrangements among health professionals to work together for a common goal—to provide quality health care to people. Further, it forced nurses to take a hard look at their role and its articulation with fellow team members.

The advent of the expanded role of the nurse for specific age groups and conditions was a phasing-in of the current interest and direction for the development in the late sixties of a *family nurse practitioner*. There are as many definitions of this term as there are programs, projects, and interested people.

Conant (1970–1971, p. 5) describes one such project and illuminates the model with the following framework:

> The family nurse practitioner is a practitioner who is prepared to make independent judgments and to assume principal responsibility for primary health care of individuals and families in organized services. She assumes major professional responsibility for decision making in relation to health needs. She works collaboratively with physicians and other members of the health team in the delivery of health services to individuals and families. Her practice is community oriented, related to needs, concerns, and priorities of the consumers.
>
> The family nurse practitioner will have responsibility for the following:

I Wellness
  A Health maintenance of all age groups—provision of continuing care to assist the patient and/or family to function at their individual optimum level of wellness
  B Prevention
    1 Instituting known procedures to prevent illness

    2 Screening procedures for purpose of early detection, primary prevention, health counseling, and appropriate referral

    3 Health teaching and counseling of patients and families related to need and interest

    4 Periodic examination of well infants, children, and adults

II Illness

  A An initial assessment and evaluation of the health status of the patient with needed diagnostic procedures to enable the family nurse practitioner to make one of three decisions for the care of the patient:

    1 Immediate intervention with or without medical consultation

    2 Arrangement for emergency care

    3 Referral of the patient to the physician

  B Provision of on-going health maintenance and clinical management of stable chronically ill patients

  C Identify the impact of the health status on the individual and family in order to:

    1 Help the patient and/or family cope with the situation

    2 Plan for continuity of care

The nurses who completed the initial course for family nurse practitioners say that what they learned is the link that has been missing previously in their nursing practice. No longer do they have to stop when someone presents symptoms of illness, instead they can evaluate and make plans in relation to their assessment of the patient's condition.

Some people view the family nurse practitioner as one who not only serves as the primary care specialist for individual members, but also is qualified to serve the family as a unit. This nurse relates to the family in an interactional relationship offering continuous coordinated health care to the total family as a group. Few of the programs articulate the more sophisticated definition of family nursing, where the practice of nursing is defined in terms of concepts of family care and sophisticated nursing practice, e.g., working on a contractual basis with the family as the unit of service, making complex multidimensional assessments of the family group's resources and "cope-abilities," applying therapeutic interventions from autonomous interpretations of family interactional patterns, and employing prediction models for future family development. A current major problem is the variety of programs and models, the level of educational preparation of the candidates, and the eventual certification of the nursing practitioner. The words "practitioner" and "clinician" have variant meanings and do not always differentiate types and levels of preparation. In the early models of practitioner programs, the basic preparation was the baccalaureate degree in nursing. Not all later models demanded this educational base. In the minds of nurse educators, the nurse clinician is clearly a product of graduate education.

Concepts of the nurse's role in primary care are now under exploration by nursing leaders. A statement by the Western Council of Higher Education in Nursing boldly directs nurses toward exciting new roles as primary care takers (*Western Interstate Commission on Higher Education,* 1971).

In discussing the past, present, and future development of family specialists without identifying any specific discipline, Mace (1971) lists two criteria for the contemporary family specialist giving direction and substance for the future: (1) The family specialist's primary function is to deal exclusively with the family itself. (2) The family specialist is prepared from a scientific base and with specialized skills.

Nursing has not yet articulated such criteria to give direction for the development of programs in family nursing at the graduate level. Currently the state of the art is understandably fuzzy. Family nurse practitioners and community health nurses, maternal and child nursing specialists, and psychiatric nursing clinicians all promote their own territorial claims. In the meantime, families in the community are seeking comprehensive health care that will assure them the quality of life they have been promised and deserve. Today the horrendous crisis in the health care system is causing nurses to take a new look at their roles and goals. There appears to be a decided shift to search out nursing's professional role in health maintenance as a primary care agent, emphasizing the delivery of family services. Recommendations of the National Commission for the Study of Nursing and Nursing Education include developing the science and art of nursing through research, expanding role articulations in the delivery of health care, creating statewide planning committees for nursing education, and increasing governmental support for education and research (Lysaught, 1970). Pointing toward the current fallacies in the organization of the health care system, which unselectively lumps the well with the sick, Garfield (1971) suggests a four-pronged approach that separates the well from the sick and the worried well from the early sick. Norris (1970) adds her influence with her insightful article about the nurse's role as one of the gatekeepers of the health care system. Ideas such as those presented by the National Commission on Nursing and Nursing Eduation, Garfield, Norris, and others have evolved from the acute and astute concerns about the inability of the present health care system to meet even minimum standards of quality health care. The continuing misutilization and maldistribution of health manpower resources, the escalating costs of health care, and the potential for society's consumers to erupt into violent action have catapulted health professionals into action—finally. In terms of delivering family care, it may be later than we think, particularly if the assumption is that the family of the future will be the same as it is today or was yesterday.

THE NEXT DECADE

In 1970, Toffler predicted accurately that families of the future would be quite different in structure, organization, and function. New families, childless couples, homosexual unions, foster parents, and unmarried elderly couples have come to public attention. Some of the new relationships have caused political embarrassments and problems for protocol officers and presidents alike. Recently, President Carter insisted that male members of his staff either marry the women with whom they were living or not accept a position of public service.

Social mores are also influenced by demographic shifts. Epidemiological evidence indicates that adult male and female populations are experiencing recent and long-term declines in death rates. Though women still have a longer life expectancy at birth (76.4 years) than men (68.5 years), gains in both sexes, particularly in white populations, are impressive indeed. The undulating, though generally reduced birth rate, and paradoxically the alarming epidemic of teenage pregnancies, the increasing emphasis on no-growth population policies, the altered composition of the population in age, sex ratio, and health status, and the changing social values and concerns reflecting new rights and relationships offer unusual opportunities for the practice of nursing, particularly for nurses with broad preparation and interest in family care.

The family in the seventies is as diverse as Toffler predicted it would be. Despite the economic slump and concern for the distribution of resources, there is continuing concern for the quality of life. Families are taking a much more assertive role in decision making about matters of living and dying. Demanding full disclosure of risks and benefits, knowledgeable consumers and families are becoming full-fledged members of the health team.

In some instances, notably the prepaid insurance plans offered by the growing number of health maintenance organizations, families are partners with the health professionals. All share in the benefits of maintaining health, because illness, disability, and death are costly. Everyone loses if a partner becomes ill and requires expensive, sophisticated medical treatment. Incentives and rewards to maintain wellness, while still in their infancy as concepts in health care plans, are expanding in number and kind. Negotiations over health benefits in labor contracts require more knowledge and effort these days than do the discussions about wages and nonhealth-related benefits. Soon, management and labor will find themselves collaborators in developing healthful work environments, preventive and promotional health services, and family health insurance that focuses on the worker and family life-styles. Attention given to environmental safety in the work environment in the sixties will expand the

current federal legislation (OSHA) to psychosocial and physical maintenance of well worker populations.

Increasingly, nurses in almost every area of specialty services from
occupational health to the traditional public health nurse of an earlier era
will require extensive preparation in family care, because of the
broadened definition and diversity found in the so-called family.

Professional nursing curriculums, created from philosophical statements and conceptual frameworks on nursing and health care, have im-
pacted on nursing practice. New patterns of delivering care through primary nursing care and primary health care have been introduced relatively
recently. Primary nursing, a patient-centered concept with identified accountability, autonomy, and authority for nursing functions, is replacing
team nursing in many in-patient settings (Marram, Schlegal, and Bevis,
1974).

In ambulatory care, professional nurses are assuming roles as providers of primary care. Often in collaboration with physicians, nurses are
helping patients and their families to gain direct access to health care services, provide continuous comprehensive care, including prevention and
promotion of health and coordination of health services to accomplish
nursing's goal to "help people attain, regain and retain health" (Schlotfeldt, 1972).

Understanding the changing social phenomenon known as the family
will require professional nurses to become more theoretically and clinically competent to address the needs and demands of the future family.
Nurse clinicians, prepared at the graduate level today in various specialties, will need to broaden their preparation and perspectives to deal with
the stresses of the family that are exhibited in deviant behaviors such as
child abuse, wife beating, rape and incest, marriages of mental retardates,
cohabitation of the elderly, and a host of other unique and growing social
phenomena.

As the social codes are altered, changes in the laws, as a form of
social control, will be forthcoming. Individuals and families are seeking
extensive control over their own lives. Legal, ethical, and moral issues
about abortion and euthanasia are discussed publicly. Supreme Court rul-
ings and legislation seem to emphasize individual and family choice and
the quality of life. Bio-ethics and the control of research in creating new
forms of life have great implications for the preparation and practice of all
health professionals and scientists. On these, public debate abounds. No
longer can important decisions about research and clinical matters be the
sole province of the health care provider. Legally, morally, and ethically,
the consumer has rights and responsibilities to which institutions must be
responsive. The messages of consumer dissatisfaction with health services cannot be ignored either. Women have taken the lead in expressing
their displeasure by organizing their own clinics, publishing self-care lit-

erature, and demanding legislation that promotes the rights of women (Proceedings, 1975; Lytle, 1977). Assertiveness training and action by women are altering their relationship to men, children, and others, with a resultant role blurring, growing equality and parity, and new expectations and, it is hoped, extending freedom for men and rights for children.

Health care delivery patterns involving women and families are showing some responsiveness to new demands and understanding about people. The concept of attachment, which emphasizes immediate family participation in the birth process, has created demands for home deliveries, the establishment of birthing rooms in institutions, and the provision of midwifery services along with traditional medical practices. Family crisis centers, services for rape victims, and lifeline phone resources are also community service innovations. With changing roles between and among family members, there are new demands for the health practitioners to humanize their care, to teach and counsel families for self-care, and expand the accessibility and availability of health services.

A recent interesting visual experience in family life was provided to the American public over a national television network with the televising of Haley's poignant accounts from his book *Roots* (Haley, 1976). National interest was aroused and many people were moved to seek their own roots through investigations into public records, familial historical documents, and accounts from aging relatives. It will be interesting to observe how long this renewed appreciation and activity on the family survives.

One hopes that imaginative nurse-researchers and investigators from other disciplines will use this current interest in the family to encourage studies of physiological and psychological responses to states of health and illness and thereby increase the body of knowledge upon which nursing curricula and professional practice are built. The effective domain of nursing will continue to expand only as long as it finds its basis in scientific development and humane goals.

The family in the decade ahead and those professionals who attempt to serve it will need to adopt a philosophy of becoming to accommodate the inevitable changes. The professional nurses who serve best will be those who have researched well the problem of daily living and dying that families face and can help families find innovative and creative ways to deal with the internal and external stresses and strains of complex, multidimensional relationships of the difficult to define family within contemporary society.

How well will nursing be able to cope with the problems of preparing future practitioners for family nursing? Developmentally, family nursing of the type families need, demand, and desire is in its infancy. It is a time of searching and thoughtful becoming. Now is the time to take advantage of these growing years.

THE DEVELOPMENT OF FAMILY NURSING

REFERENCES

American Nurses' Association. *Division of Community Health Nursing Practice*. New York, April 1967 (mimeographed).

American Nurses' Association. *A position paper: Educational preparation for nurse practitioners and assistants to nurses*. New York, 1965.

American Nurses' Association. *Statement on graduate education in nursing*. New York, 1969.

Auerbach, A. B., & Taylor, R. G. An experiment in training nurses for leadership. *The bulletin for maternal and infant health, a symposium: Education for parenthood*. American Association for Maternal and Infant Health, Inc., 1960.

Broderick, C. B. Beyond the five conceptual frameworks: A decade of development in family theory. *Journal of Marriage and the Family*, 1971, *33*, 139–159.

Christensen, H. T. (Ed.). *Handbook of marriage and the family*. Chicago: Rand McNally, 1964.

Committee on Education of the National League for Nursing Education. *Standard curriculum for schools of nursing*. New York: National Nursing Association, 1919.

Committee on the Grading of Nursing Schools. *Nursing schools today and tomorrow*. New York, 1964.

Conant, L. B. The nature of nursing tomorrow. *Image: Sigma Theta Tau National Honor Society of Nursing*, *4*, 1970–1971.

Corbin, H. Development of parent classes in the United States. *The bulletin for maternal and child health, a symposium: Education for parenthood*, American Association for Maternal and Infant Health, Inc., 1960.

Curry, F. J. Neighborhood health centers, planned, developed, and managed by neighborhood groups, should be a top priority in bringing tomorrow's medicine today. *California's Health*, 1971.

Dunn, H. L. *High level wellness*. Arlington, Va.: R. W. Beatty, 1961.

Editorial. *American Journal of Nursing*, 1971, *71*, 489.

Ford, L. C., & Silver, H. K. The expanded role of the nurse in child care. *Nursing Outlook*, 1967, *15*, 43–45.

Ford, P. A., Seacat, M. S., & Silver, G. A. The relative roles of the public health nurse and the physician in prenatal and infant supervision. *American Journal of Public Health*, 1966, *56*, 1097–1103.

Freeman, R. B. *Community health nursing practice*. Philadelphia: W. B. Saunders, 1970.

———. The criterion of relevance. *American Journal of Public Health*, 1967, *57*, 1522–1531.

Gardner, M. S. *Public health nursing*. New York: Macmillan, 1936.

Garfield, S. R. Prevention of dissipation of health services resources. *American Journal of Public Health*, 1971, *61*, 1499–1506.

Glasser, J. H. Health information systems: A crisis or just more of the usual? *American Journal of Public Health*, 1971, *61*, 1524–1530.

Haley, A. *Roots*. Garden City, N.Y.: Doubleday, 1976.

Hill, R., & Hansen, D. A. The identification of conceptual frameworks utilized in family study. *Marriage and Family Living*, 1960, *22*, 299–311.

Joint Commission on Mental Illness and Health. *Action for mental health*. New York: Basic Books, 1961.

King, I. M. *Toward a theory for nursing: General concepts of human behavior*. New York: John Wiley and Sons, 1971, pp. 2–6.

Lewis, C. E., & Resnik, B. A. Nurse clinics and progressive ambulatory patient care. *New England Journal of Medicine*, 1967, *277*, 1236–1241.

Lysaught, J. P. *An abstract for action*. New York: McGraw-Hill, 1970.

Lytle, N. A. (Ed.). *Nursing of women in the age of liberation*. Dubuque, Iowa: Wm. C. Brown, 1977.

Mace, D. R. The family specialist, past, present, and future. *Family Coordinator*, 1971, *21*, 291–294.

Marram, G. D., Schlegel, M. W., & Bevis, E. M. *Primary nursing: A model for individualized care*. St. Louis: C. V. Mosby, 1974.

National Association for Public Health Nursing. *Manual for public health nursing*. New York: Macmillan, 1939.

National League for Nursing. *Record system guide for a community health service*. New York, 1970.

National League for Nursing Committee on Perspectives. *Change, collaboration and community involvement*. New York: National League for Nursing, 1970.

Norris, C. M. Direct access to the patient. *American Journal of Nursing*, 1970, *70*, 1006–1010.

Nye, I., & Berardo, F. *Conceptual frameworks for the study of the family*. New York: Macmillan, 1966.

Peplau, H. E. Principles of psychiatric nursing. In S. Arieti (Ed.), *American Handbook of Psychiatry* (Vol. II). New York: Basic Books, 1959.

Proceedings for the 1975 Conference on Women and Health. Boston, Massachusetts, April 4–7, 1975.

Report on the Committee for the Study of Nursing Education. *Nursing and nursing education in the United States*. New York: Macmillan, 1923.

Report of Joint Ad Hoc Committee of A.N.A.–A.P.H.A. *Public health nursing specialist*, 1967 (mimeographed).

Rosen, G. Public health: Then and now—the first neighborhood health center movement—its rise and fall. *American Journal of Public Health*, 1971, *61*, 1620–1637.

Schlotfeldt, R. M. This I believe . . . nursing is health care. *Nursing Outlook*, 1972, *4*, 245.

Siegel, E., & Bryson, S. L. Redefinition of the role of the public health nurse in child health definition. *American Journal of Public Health*, 1963, *53*, 1015–1024.

Siegel, E., Dillehay, R., & Fitzgerald, C. J. Role changes within the child health conference: Attitudes and professional preparedness of public health nurses and physicians. *American Journal of Health*, 1965, *55*, 832–841.

Stoeckle, J. D., Noonan, B., Farrisey, R. M., & Sweatt, A. Medical nursing clinic for chronically ill. *American Journal of Nursing*, 1963, *63*, 87–89.

Toffler, A. *Future Shock*. New York: Bantam Books, 1970.

U.S. Department of Health, Education, and Welfare. *Toward a comprehensive health policy for the 1970's: A white paper.* Washington, D.C., 1971.

Western Interstate Commission on Higher Education. *Defining clinical content, graduate nursing programs: Community health nursing.* Boulder, Colorado, 1967.

Western Interstate Commission on Higher Education. *Defining clinical content, graduate nursing programs: Maternal and child nursing.* Boulder, Colorado, 1967.

Western Interstate Commission on Higher Education. *Defining clinical content, graduate nursing programs: Medical surgical nursing.* Boulder, Colorado, 1967.

Western Interstate Commission on Higher Education. *Defining clinical content, graduate nursing programs: Psychiatric nursing,* Boulder, Colorado, 1967.

Western Interstate Commission on Higher Education. *Guidelines for developing master's degree programs in the West.* Western Council on Higher Education for Nursing. Boulder, Colorado, 1958.

Western Interstate Commission on Higher Education. *Statement on primary care in progress.* Western Council on Higher Education for Nursing. Boulder, Colorado, 1971.

Wiedenbach, E. Family nurse practitioner for maternal and child care. *Nursing Outlook,* 1965, *13,* 50–52.

PART TWO

FACTORS AFFECTING THE FAMILY

This section presents some of the numerous variables that affect family development and interaction. Because there are so many factors affecting the family, and, consequently, the delivery of health services, it is not possible to adequately cover all variables. Consequently, we have selected those that present the reader with a broad perspective of these factors, all of which have implications for the delivery of health care services.

In Chapter 7, *Law and the Family,* we are introduced to several common legal problems faced by families in America. Legal issues related to marriage, divorce, child custody, adoption, child abuse, juvenile delinquency, incompetent persons, and death are included. The individual and collective family decision-making behaviors regarding goods and services and the distribution of income among family members are the topics covered in Chapter 8, *Economics and the Family.* The next two chapters offer the reader an opportunity to examine the influence of culture on individual and family behavior. Because there is wide range of sociocultural backgrounds and life-styles that nurses are likely to encounter in their professional roles, we have in Chapter 9, *Cultural Barriers: An Anthropological Perspective,* included an introductory chapter with a broad anthropological view of cultural variations. The Mexican American family (Chapters 10 and 11) and the low-income family (Chapter 12) were selected as examples to illustrate the way these sociocultural differences may become barriers to the delivery of effective health care. Chapter 13,

Urban Family Health Care, dicusses health problems and the needs of urban family dwellers and provides insights into the challenges presented to our health care delivery system if we are to meet the needs of these people.

Chapter 14, *Changing Nutritional Styles within the Context of the Modern Family,* reveals the significant changes in individual and family eating patterns wrought by social, cultural, political, and technological developments. In Chapter 15, *Dental Health and the Family,* the author gives us an overview of the common preventable dental diseases of which we need to be aware. A section is also devoted to discussion of oral cancer and its treatment. The final chapter of this section, *The Family with a Career Mother,* deals with one of the prevalent changes in our society: the increased number of mothers entering the labor force. Insights regarding the impact of this change on individuals and families are provided as well as suggestions for parental guidance.

CHAPTER SEVEN

LAW AND THE FAMILY

JED B. MAEBIUS, JR.

The purpose of this chapter is to acquaint the reader with several common legal problems that are faced by families of all socioeconomic levels. Whether working in a hospital, a doctor's office, or the community, health care workers are bound to encounter families with some of these problems. A basic introduction to such problems will help them better understand how the family unit functions. In giving nursing care to a patient, professional assessment of the patient's family situation should reflect the family's legal problems.

The laws dealing with family problems emanate primarily from court decisions and state statutes. As such, these laws vary from state to state. Therefore, a general statement of the law will be given, with occasional references to specific statutes. The reader should keep in mind that in any particular state the law may be different from statements made in this chapter.

The scope of this chapter will be limited to a discussion of family legal problems. There will be no discussion of the legal aspects of nursing, although the bibliography at the end of this chapter supplies helpful references in this area and this topic is covered in Chapter 25 of this volume.

LEGAL ASPECTS AND PROBLEMS OF THE FAMILY

Marriage

The couple, composed of husband and wife, or the group, composed of husband, wife, and children, constitutes the family. The relationship begins with the marriage; this can be accomplished by a ceremony performed upon the issuance of a marriage permit after certain legal prerequisites have been met. The marriage relationship, with all its legal implications, can also exist without formal entry into a marriage contract according to law. Certain marriages are prohibited according to laws of the various states. A person may not marry any close blood relative. A person may not marry if he or she has not dissolved a prior marriage. There are also minimum age requirements in all states for males and females; the age requirement is usually lower for females.

Many centuries ago husband and wife legally became "one person" by marriage, and the entire legal status of the woman was completely incorporated into that of the husband. However, the evolution of the law has seen the emergence of the separate legal existence of the wife and her property. The relationship of husband and wife imposes on each of them certain legal marital rights and duties. Each spouse has a right to the support, company, affection, and service of the other. If either party fails to live up to these obligations of the marriage contract to the extent that the purpose of the marriage is defeated, the law will allow the innocent party to dissolve the marriage contract.

In addition to divorce, the family relationship is terminated by the death of one spouse if there are no children or by annulment. The family unit continues after death if there are children and after the divorce for the spouse who retains legal custody of the children. All states have laws prescribing grounds for having a marriage annulled. Typical of these is the situation where one party was under the influence of drugs or alcohol at the time of the marriage and has not voluntarily cohabited with the other party since the marriage; impotency of either party; marriage by inducement by fraud, duress, or force; mental incompetency of one party; and others.

A parent is under an obligation to furnish support for his or her infant children. If the parent neglects that duty, any person who supplies items such as food and clothing is deemed to have an implied promise to pay on the part of the parent. The reasoning behind this rule is the inability of the child to maintain self care and the public policy of not leaving such care in the hands of the state, except as a last resort.

Divorce

The state statutes providing for divorce specify the grounds for which a divorce can be granted, and include such grounds as cruelty, adultery, conviction of the other spouse of a felony, abandonment, etc. Traditionally, divorce has been handled as any other lawsuit is handled in our adversary system. Our adversary system of justice operates on the premise that if each side to a lawsuit has an attorney and prepares its case in the best possible way to promote that side's "best interests," the judge or jury will be able to choose the better of the two sides. In this way, a just decision can be reached.

A divorce suit is instituted in the following manner. One party files a petition for divorce, in the name of John Smith versus Mary Smith, alleging that the other party has been cruel or alleging any other legal basis for the divorce that may exist. The other party may or may not hire an attorney to contest the divorce.

Many state statutes have a mandatory waiting period after the petition is filed for the divorce hearing, such as 60 days. The theory behind this waiting period is that the two parties will have time to think about what they are doing and perhaps reconsider. The setup of our system usually results in a court having to find one of the parties to blame for the failure of the marriage. The other party is then granted the divorce.

In addition to granting the divorce, the court must also divide the parties' property equitably between them. In many, but not all, states, the court must prescribe alimony payments for the husband to make to the wife. All states provide for child support, and the husband is usually required to make support payments for the children who are in the wife's custody.

It is interesting to note that the evolving legal approach to problem solving with the family is inverse to the contemporary health care approach. At a time when the health care professions stress the consideration of the family as a whole in assessing a patient's problem, in some respects, the law has evolved from the concept of the family entity and is emphasizing the rights of individual members of that family. For example, as was previously mentioned, in providing care to an individual patient, the task of assessment now considers the entire family unit and not just the individual patient. The law, however, stresses the individual's rights more and more, rather than the family unit as a whole. This is best illustrated by the law dealing with credit. On October 28, 1975, the Equal Credit Opportunity Act was passed by the United States Congress.[1] The primary purpose of the act is to provide more individual attention and equal treatment for women. The act gives married persons the right to have credit information included in credit reports at banks or department stores in the name of both the wife and husband if both use or are responsible for the account. This right was created, in part, to insure that credit histories will be available to women who become divorced or widowed. Generally the act prohibits credit discrimination on the basis of race, color, religion, natural origin, sex, marital status, and age. In addition, a person may not be discriminated against because all or part of his or her income derives from a public assistance program. If an account at a bank or a department store is one that both the husband and the wife sign for or is an account that is used by one who did not sign, each is entitled to have

---

[1] Title V, P.L. 93-495, §§ 501 et seq., 15 U.S.C. 1691.

credit information reported in his or her own name. The point is that each partner of the marriage is being treated equally and an attempt is being made to give women, who have been discriminated against in the past, an equal legal identity with men. Therefore, a woman's legal identity is becoming less dependent upon that of her husband.

In fashion with the increasing focus on the individual's legal rights, children's rights are receiving more recognition by legislatures and courts. No longer is there a blind presumption that the family "by birth" is the best home for the child. Increasing emphasis on the "best interest" of the child has led the legal sector to treat children as individuals rather than as chattels of their parents.

A New Bill of Rights for Children[2]

1. Any and every child has a right to a family who wants him or her—the child's *own* family, if possible.
2. Any child has a right to the kind of physical safety and health care that ensures the best growth and development before and after birth.
3. Any child has a right to the basics of life itself; enough *good* food and water, clothing, shelter and love.
4. Any child has a *right to learn* (to be educated) about himself or herself, the human race, the world—in order to find ways for self-protection, self-support, and ways to live with others.
5. Any child has a right to enjoyment, a right to play, a right to laugh.
6. Any child has a right to a community that cares for him and his family in ways that help his or her life and growth.
7. Any child has a right to professional help for himself and for his or her family, to enable the family to stay (and grow) together.
8. Any child has a right to a government that protects him or her from neglect, cruelty, and exploitation of any kind, and yet recognizes a child's need for independence, as well as dependence.
9. Any child has a right to the same constitutional protections (federal or state or local) that anyone else is entitled to.
10. Any child, whatever his or her condition, has a right to understanding, tolerance, and acceptance on the part of all adults.
11. Any child has a right to adult models who demonstrate consideration for others, integrity in living, a desire to work out problems, a sense of ethical values, and most especially, compassion and empathy.
12. Any child has a right to a peaceful, non-racist world where violence and massacres and wars are considered obsolete.
13. Any child has a right to his or her own identity as an individual.
14. Any baby, any child born alive has the right to live.

[2]A New "Bill of Rights for Children" was written by Mrs. Shirley Soman and appeared in her recent book *Let's Stop Destroying Our Children*, Hawthorn Books, New York, 1974. Reprinted by permission.

Child Custody

It is the general rule that, if for any reason a husband and wife have divorced or legally separated, the court has the power to determine which parent shall have the custody of the children. It is the court's duty in such cases to place the best interests of the children above the rights of either parent and to make provisions for their care and custody as will best serve their welfare.

It is within a court's power in making such a determination to award custody to neither parent, but rather to a third person, if the best interests of the child so dictate. A parent who is not awarded custody still has the right of reasonable visitation with such child, and some divorce decrees will enumerate specific times at which the parent can visit with the child, such as every other weekend from Saturday morning until Sunday evening and one month each summer. Many times divorce decrees provide simply for "reasonable visitation" by the parent who does not have custody. Such language can lead to a conflict between the parents over the meaning of "reasonable."

An additional problem that must be solved at the time custody of the children is awarded to one or the other of the parents is that of child support. There is no set schedule or formula for reaching an equitable amount of child support. The problem to be dealt with is one of striking a balance between the needs of the children living with the custodial parent and the future life of the noncustodial parent, who is making child support payments to the custodial parent for the benefit of the children. Implicit in such an arrangement is continual struggle, both in court and out of court, between the custodial and noncustodial parent until such time as the youngest child reaches the required age for legal independence. Perhaps this one problem creates more emotional drain on single parents with children than any other, after the divorce. In recent years, attempts have been made to arrive at some sort of preset schedule that judges could use as a guideline in awarding child support. This would avoid arbitrary and capricious awards by judges, and would allow the parents notice of what to expect. For example, in Texas, a schedule has been developed by Judge Harold A. Thomas, of the Domestic Relations Court in Nueces County, which provides a specific amount for a specific salary less deductions for a number of children ranging in age from 1 to 5 years. In Texas, the State Welfare Department and its various local agencies have been using this schedule for the making of informal agreements for the payment of child support by welfare parents. The military services have been using such a schedule in attempting to work out agreements between divorcing spouses. [State Bar of Texas, State Bar Section Report-Family Law, Volume 77-1, March, 1977, "Using a Formula to Set Child Support," John J. Sampson (p. 29)].

An additional problem that has become more profound in recent years is that of "child-napping" by the noncustodial parent. Typically, the parent not having custody who lives out of state, makes the arrangements exercising visitation rights with the child, for the period of time during which the child comes to visit with the noncustodial parent. At the end of the appointed time, the noncustodial parent refuses to return the child to the custodial parent. The custodial parent is then left with serious problems in legally having the child returned. The state court having jurisdiction of domestic disputes in which the custodial parent lives does not have jurisdiction over the noncustodial parent living in a separate state. Therefore, legislation has been proposed and enacted in several states to minimize the problem. A recent California statute provides that a noncustodial parent who wrongfully denies the return of the child to the custodial parent shall be punished by imprisonment for a period of no more than 10 years, a fine of not more than $10,000, or both (Cal. Laws 1976, Chapter 1399, effective January 1, 1977).

Adoption

The family unit can be legally expanded by adoption of a child as well as by the birth of one. However, adoption poses questions relating to the legal status of the child and the new adoptive parents as well as that of the child and the natural parents. Generally the adopted child and the new parents take on the same legal relationship of a natural child and the parents. The legal relationship between the adopted child and the natural parents is severed.

The law has not always been this way, and adopted children were often denied the rights of natural-born children in many situations, such as not being given the right to inherit from their adoptive parents. Most courts and state legislatures have attempted to give the child the rights and obligations that a natural child has. Some states have enacted statutes that allow an adopted child to inherit through adoptive parents as well as from them. [A recent Wyoming statute provides that an adopted person can inherit from all relatives of the new parents, just as a natural child, and all of the parents' relatives can inherit from the adopted person (Wyoming Laws of 1969, Chapter 74).] Many states, however, still have statutes that do not allow a child to inherit from relatives of adoptive parents. For example, if a grandparent in such a state leaves property in a will to "grandchildren," only natural-born grandchildren would inherit. In order for an adopted grandchild to inherit, the will would have to specifically mention the adopted grandchild.

The adoptive process generally takes 1 to 2 months from the time the petition for adoption is filed. Many states have statutes requiring a specified waiting period before the court can hear the adoption. During this time the child may live with the prospective parents. Also during this period, many states require that a social worker be appointed by the court to make an investigation of the family and of the child's background to see if they are suitable for each other. The social worker then recommends to the court whether or not the adoption should take place.

The Abused Child

One of the most difficult family problems to deal with from a legal standpoint, as well as medical and sociological standpoints, is that of the abused child. State statutes require child abuse cases to be reported by health care workers to public agencies or law enforcement agencies. The statutes are designed to prevent further abuse to children. In addition, statutes provide criminal penalties for parents who are convicted of inflicting physical injury on their children.

The responsibility of parenthood carries with it the duty to train and educate children. Involved in the execution of these duties is the right of the parent to exercise reasonable control over the child in the form of discipline. The right to discipline children is based on the premise that a certain amount of discipline is in the best interests of the child. The limits of reasonable discipline are determined according to standards that foster the best interests of the child. A parent is allowed to inflict such punishment and to use such force as is reasonable under the circumstances. The circumstances that determine what is reasonable are age, sex, physical condition, and other characteristics of the child.

The legal machinery presently existing to deal with the problem is inadequate in many areas. The statutes requiring reports of child abuse are lacking in many particulars. One problem is that the only requirement is that a report be made, and, once the report is made, there is little assurance of a follow-up. In many areas, there is also no centralized reporting. This means that a parent who has been guilty of child abuse more than one time can go to a different hospital in the city each time and avoid discovery of previous incidents (Grumet, 1970, p. 306).

Criminal prosecution of the parents has proved to be ineffective. In the first place, it is very difficult to obtain convictions. Even if a conviction is obtained and a sentence is imposed, the problem itself is not being solved. Often criminal prosecution destroys the possibility of being able to work with the parents (Grumet, 1970, p. 307). Some courts have taken custody of children away from parents in these circumstances, and it appears to be necessary in many cases.

Even in the most extreme cases, it is difficult to obtain convictions. An example is the case of *State v. England* [349 P. 2d 668 (Ore. Sup. 1960)]. The defendant was charged with involuntary manslaughter of his 12-year-old son. The father was accused of striking his son about the head and face with such force and violence that the injuries eventually caused his son's death. The manslaughter statute of Oregon contained a provision that stated that the killing of a human being is excusable when it is committed by accident or misfortune when lawfully correcting a child or in doing any other lawful act, by lawful means with usual and ordinary caution and without any unlawful intent. In this case, the father was not convicted, because the court held that the evidence showed that the death resulted from the negligence of the father while he was correcting the child.

It would seem that health care workers, lawyers, law enforcement officials, and social workers will all have to work together to bring about the best possible solutions for child abuse cases, for both the parent and the child. It is obvious that a family with such a problem is undergoing a volatile and stressful period.

Juvenile Courts

There are many definitions of the term "juvenile delinquency," but, generally, it can be said to mean conduct of a child that would be considered criminal in an adult. Many states have established juvenile courts by statute to administer the problems of juvenile delinquents. Such courts can also be empowered to handle dependent, neglected, and abandoned children.

These are special courts designed to deal only with the problems of juveniles. The justification for such courts is that a juvenile delinquent should not be considered as or treated as a criminal, but rather handled as a person requiring care, education, and protection.

Incompetent Persons

All states have laws providing for the care, treatment, and commitment to institutions of persons (either adults or minors) who are mentally ill or mentally retarded.[3] Legal proceedings for the commitment of such a person can be instituted by the state upon motion or information filed by an adult stating that the person in question should be committed. Often an affidavit from a family member is filed stating that it would be in the best interest of such a person to be committed. Traditionally, these legal proceedings have been adversary in nature, with the state attempting to show that the person should be committed by means of medical testimony from

[3]For a thorough treatment of the laws relating to and the legal problems of mentally ill and mentally retarded persons, see Allen, Ferster, and Weihofen, *Mental Impairment and Legal Incompetency,* Prentice-Hall, Inc., Report of the Mental Competency Study: An Empirical Research Project Conducted by the George Washington University Institute of Law, Psychiatry and Criminology (1968).

one or two doctors. The person who is the subject of the commitment proceedings can have an attorney, and in many states the court is required to appoint such an attorney to undertake a defense. In actual practice, it is doubtful that such a system results in serving the best interests of the person who is the subject of the commitment proceedings in all cases.

Traditionally, the only alternatives open at such a hearing are either total commitment or total freedom. Often a statute requires commitment for a temporary period before there can be an indefinite commitment. There are likewise statutory provisions for commitment of habitual drunkards and sexual psychopaths.

Death

In addition to being a very emotionally upsetting experience for the family unit, death of a family member has several immediate legal implications for the family. The most immediate legal problem facing the family unit is disposal of the body. The disposal of the dead has such a relation to public health that the state has the power to regulate such disposal, as an incident of its power to provide for the public health of the people. There may be laws and regulations providing for cemetery locations, burial permits, and many other necessities. Most cities have ordinances stating that there can be no burial of a body within the city limits until a permit has been issued by the proper city authority. Generally, on the death of a husband or wife, the surviving spouse is the person in charge of making the necessary legal arrangements for burial. Otherwise the next of kin has the duty and right.

Additional laws that come into immediate effect at the death of a family member are those relating to the disposition of property. If the deceased person has written a valid will in accordance with the law, the property passes under the terms of the will, but only after the will has been admitted to probate in the particular state where the deceased resided.

If there is no will, state statutes contain rules of descent and distribution and designate the persons who are to take the deceased's property; it is usually on the basis of closest relatives first, such as spouse and children, parents and grandchildren, brothers and sisters, etc.

A person's debts must be paid at the time of death, and the property is subject to being sold to satisfy all such debts and taxes. If the debts of a decedent are not paid before the property passes to surviving heirs, or devisees, creditors may sue the heirs in order to be paid upon a valid claim. Whatever remains after debts have been paid is distributed to the heirs, or devisees.

The rules governing who should take a decedent's property become complicated in certain situations. If a person lives in Iowa, owns land in

Iowa and Minnesota, and dies without a will, which state laws control how the land is divided? Iowa law might provide that the land should go to a surviving spouse. Minnesota law might provide that the land should go to the surviving children. It is the general rule that the state where the land is located has the paramount interest in having its laws regulate land in that state. Therefore, in the above example, the surviving spouse would inherit the Iowa land, and the children would inherit the Minnesota land.

Even if a person dies without having executed a will, there can be an administration of the estate in the probate court if the necessity exists. In such a situation, the court would appoint some person or some institution as administrator to take charge of the assets and to administer the decedent's estate. Sometimes, if the deceased had no debts and no substantial assets, there will not be a necessity to have an administration of any kind. It may be necessary to prepare an affidavit, however, to indicate the heirs. Such an affidavit would be filed in the county records to show the "chain of title" of any property the decedent did have.

An additional problem affecting the family unit with children at death is that of the necessity of appointing a guardian for the estate of the children. If a deceased person dies leaving property to children while they are minors and did not make special provision for the care of that property, the laws of most states require that a guardian be appointed. This property is called a minor's estate, and the guardian serves until the minor reaches maturity. Court supervision over a minor's estate is felt to be necessary in order to protect minors from family members or others who might take advantage of them. Of course, the surviving parent or other family member of age can apply to be appointed guardian for the minor children's property, but he or she must account to the court for all actions taken with regard to such property. Ordinarily a guardian must post a bond, guaranteeing the faithful performance of duties.

A NEW APPROACH TO SOLVING FAMILY LEGAL PROBLEMS

The above outline of some of the legal aspects and problems of the family is intended to give the nurse an idea of the effect that such legal aspects and problems of the family have on the well-being of the family unit. It can be seen that when the family unit faces a problem such as divorce, death, or possible commitment of one of its members, a great amount of emotional stress can result. Perhaps the adversary process of solving such problems as divorce and commitment adds to the trauma facing the family unit. In recent years, new legislation and court opinions have reflected a different attitude of our society to the solution of such problems. The examples of divorce and commitment will be discussed as illustrations.

When a husband and wife are having marital problems, and one of them has reached the point of filing a suit for divorce, the adversary process requires that the husband and wife be pitted against each other in a "legal battle." Much harm to the family, especially to the children, can result from these battles (Hawke, 1970).

In 1969, the Texas legislature passed the Texas Family Code, which establishes a new direction for handling divorce. A divorce petition in Texas is not now entitled Mr. Smith versus Mrs. Smith, but rather the petition is entitled "In the Matter of the Marriage of Mr. & Mrs. Smith" (*Texas Family Code Annals,* 1969). Although the traditional grounds for divorce, such as cruelty, adultery, abandonment, or conviction of a felony exist under this new code, an important new ground has been added. On the petition of either party to a marriage, a divorce may be granted without regard to fault if the marriage has become "insupportable" because of discord or conflict of personalities that destroys the legitimate ends of the marriage relationship and prevents any reasonable expectation of reconciliation (*Texas Family Code Annals,* 1969).

The importance of the new grounds of "insupportability" for divorce is that the statute makes legal the reasons that are actually the basis for most divorce suits. In most divorce situations, there is simply not one party who is the sole blame for the divorce. Prior to the new code, it was necessary to allege cruelty in most divorce cases in order to get the divorce granted. If there was any chance of reconciliation, such allegations would certainly not help the possibility. In many cases, there were simply not facts supporting cruelty, and the parties were forced to exaggerate and say things that were not necessarily true in order to get a divorce.

Another section of the statute provides that after a petition for divorce is filed, the court may, in its discretion, direct the parties to counsel with a person or persons named by the court who shall submit a written report to the court stating an opinion as to whether there exists a reasonable expectation of reconciliation, and, if so, whether further counseling would be beneficial (*Texas Family Code Annals,* 1969).

Other states have also adopted such statutes. Some states have established family clinics in an attempt to provide counseling service for persons with marital problems (Hawke, 1970). The importance of these changes is an attempt to provide a basis for the solution of a problem without directly pitting the husband and wife against each other.

It has been reported that the District of Columbia has passed a new divorce law. The residence requirement has been reduced from 1 year to 6 months. All grounds for divorce based upon fault of one party or the other have been eliminated. The only possible grounds available now for divorce are voluntary and continued separation of the parties for a period of 6 months and involuntary and continued separation of the parties for 1 year (American Bar Association, 1977).

Another area of the law in which a change of direction can be seen is in the commitment of mentally ill or retarded persons. As stated previously, the courts traditionally have approached the solution to the problem as being one of either total commitment or total freedom. In a recent case, the United States Court of Appeals for the District of Columbia illustrated a new approach to this problem [*Lake v. Cameron,* 364 F. 2d 657 (Dist. Col. Cir. 1966) *cert. denied,* 382 U.S. 863 (1966)]. The court in this case recognized that there are other alternatives to commitment and freedom. These people are not criminals, and the primary purposes of any type of commitment should be treatment and rehabilitation. The court stated in its opinion as follows:

> Proceedings involving the care and treatment of the mentally ill are not strictly adversary proceedings. . . . The Court may consider, e.g., whether the appellant and the public would be sufficiently protected if she were required to carry an identification card on her person so that the police or others could take her home if she should wander, or whether she should be required to accept public health and day care services, foster care, home help aid services or whether available welfare payments might finance adequate private care. Every effort should be made to find the course of treatment which appellant might be willing to accept.

The court has recognized not only that the state has the burden of showing whether the person is mentally ill or mentally retarded, but also that it has the burden of finding what the best solution is for the problem. Neither total commitment nor total freedom may be the best answer in a particular case. This decision recognizes the fact that family problems such as possible commitment should be treated differently from an ordinary civil lawsuit or criminal lawsuit. The opinion recognizes the fact that an interdisciplinary approach to solutions of such a problem may be in the best interest of both the individual involved and the society.

SUMMARY AND OBSERVATIONS

It is hoped that this chapter has provided the nurse with some small insight into the vast area of legal aspects and problems of the family. The well-being of the family is greatly affected when it faces emotionally upsetting and stressful situations such as divorce, commitment, or death. Perhaps the traditional legal approach to the solution of these problems adds to the trauma of the family. Changes in the approach of legislatures and courts to solutions of these problems, such as were discussed, should help to reduce the trauma of these problems. A basic understanding of the legal aspects and problems of the family unit and the legal approaches to solutions should help the nurse make a more meaningful assessment of the patient and his family.

REFERENCES

Allen, R., Ferster, E., Weihofen, H. *Mental impairment and legal incompetency.* Englewood Cliffs, N.J.: Prentice-Hall. Report of the Mental Competency Study: An Empirical Research Project Conducted by the George Washington University Institute of Law, Psychiatry and Criminology, 1968.

American Bar Association, Section of Family Law. *Family Law Newsletter,* 1977, *17*(3), 11.

Anderson, B. Orderly transfer of procedural responsibilities from medical to nursing practice, *Nursing Clinics of North America,* 1970, *5*(2), 311–319.

Creighton, H *Law every nurse should know* (2d ed.). Philadelphia: W. B. Saunders, 1970.

Curran, W. Public health and the law. *American Journal of Public Health,* 1970, *60*, 2400–2401.

Grumet, R. The plaintive plaintiffs: Victims of the battered child syndrome. *Family Law Quarterly,* Section of Family Law, American Bar Association, 1970, *4*(3), 296.

Hawke, L. Divorce procedure: A fraud on children, spouses and society. *Family Law Quarterly,* 1969, *3*, 240–253.

Kempe C., Silverman, F., Steele, B., Droegemueller, W., & Silver, H. The battered child syndrome. *Journal of the American Medical Association,* 1962, *181*, 17–24.

Parker, S. Lake v. Cameron: Involuntary civil commitment storm warnings, *Family Law Quarterly,* Section of Family Law, American Bar Association, 1970, *4*(1), 81–89.

Sadusk, J. Legal implications of changing patterns of practice. *Journal of the American Medical Association,* 1964, *190*, 1135–1136.

Springer, E. *Nursing and the law.* Pittsburgh: Health Law Center, Aspen Systems Corporation, 1970.

State v. England, 349 P. 2d 668 (Ore. Sup. 1960).

Texas Family Code Annals, 1969.

Willig, S. *The nurse's guide to the law,* New York: McGraw-Hill, 1970.

Wyoming Laws of 1969, chapter 74.

CHAPTER EIGHT

ECONOMICS AND THE FAMILY

MICHAEL A. VIREN

The word "economics," like the word "engineering," has been so commonly misused that its true meaning has become lost. From the economist's view, economics is a very general science that yields implications about many specific areas such as the stock market, finance, government spending, taxes, money, income, consumption, and so on that have become synonymous with the term "economics." This chapter addresses the more general and theoretical aspects of economics and the family, leaving to others the more specific aspects of family finances, income, and consumption.

Economics, to simplify, is involved with the concept of supply and demand. This concept holds that there is, at some price, a point of equilibrium where the demander will demand exactly the same amount of a certain good or service that the supplier will supply. However, this view of economics is too simplistic and yields too few fruitful implications. Thus what this chapter attempts to accomplish is to develop economics in a manner more complex than simply supply and demand and then see what implications it might have for the family.

The available literature on the economics of the family is discussed primarily in terms of financial aspects of family behavior. In addition, most literature on the subject tends to treat the family as some kind of whole. This macroscopic view, along with limiting the analysis to only the financial aspects of the economic behavior of the family, has tended to create in the literature gross generalization and value judgments—thus resulting in very few fruitful implications about family economic behavior. This chapter hopes to overcome this problem by viewing the family in the microscopic view, i.e., as a collection of individuals. Viewing the family at the micro level yields two sets of implications. The first set pertains to individual and collective decision making by the family, and the second pertains to the distribution of income among family members.

Before proceeding, it might be important to explain why implications of family economic behavior are important to health professionals involved in a helping relationship with families. The reason is simple and straightforward. Decisions of families and members of families may seem irrational when viewed by an outsider. However, when the set of assumptions upon which a family makes a decision is known to the outsider, the seemingly irrational decision often becomes logical. Hopefully, the economics developed below will allow the health professional to more clearly understand the process by which individuals and families make decisions.

INDIVIDUAL BEHAVIOR

Economics assumes that the world is made up of agents. An agent is either an individual, a productive organization (i.e., a company, corporation, farm, store, or business), or a government. Each agent performs two activities: (1) consumption and (2) production. All agents, whether they be individuals or large corporations, consume; and they all produce. An individual produces a supply of labor and uses the proceeds of this labor for consumption. The productive organization (and government) consumes labor and other inputs (like land, capital, and raw materials) and produces the goods and services that are consumed by the individuals. Thus all the individuals in a society, in their efforts to consume, generate a *demand* that is fulfilled by the *supply* of goods and services that were produced through the use of labor and other inputs supplied by the individuals in society. This dual behavior of all agents is the essential basis of an economic system.

To further complicate the matter, goods and services are a large bundle consisting of commodities, services, experiences, happenings, and so on. For example, a boat trip down the Green River in Utah is considered a good or service, so also is a picnic in the park, even though it may not cost anything to visit the park. The point being made here is that the concept of goods and services is an all-encompassing one used to describe all possible items that an agent may want to demand or supply. To complicate the matter still further, agents of an economy must choose among not only a large variety of goods and services, but also the quantity of each good and service to be produced and consumed.

Individual agents make these decisions with the guidance of a utility or preference function. (Other agents in the economy have different methods for making decisions. For example, corporations have the profit motive to guide their decision making. However, since we are only concerned with the family, which is made up of individual agents, we will simply assume that other agents exist but will not be discussed.) This function is a system of values that allows individual agents to rank all possible bundles of goods and services they could possibly produce or consume. For example, suppose an individual has three bundles, each with the same three kinds of goods, but in varying amounts (i.e., bundle one contains two cans of beer, one sandwich, and three boiled eggs; bundle two contains one can of beer, two sandwiches, and two boiled eggs; and bundle three contains three cans of beer, three sandwiches, and one boiled egg). It would seem reasonable that it would be possible to rank the bundles as to which was preferred the most, the next best, and the least. However, we still do not have sufficient information to make a decision as to which of the three bundles to consume. As stated above, each individual must produce as well as consume; i.e., the individual most likely produces labor, working or selling skills from which an income is derived. Now, combining the fact of the existence of a preference function and the existence of an income gives sufficient information for an individual to make a decision. The decision would be to choose the most preferred bundle the individual can afford. In other words, individuals will choose a bundle of goods and services that has the highest preference ranking subject to the constraint that the bundle does not cost more than their income.

We can now introduce slightly more complexity by acknowledging the fact that income is not the only constraint that may keep an individual from choosing the highest rank bundle. This can be understood by considering that the act of consumption also requires the use of time and energy. Thus the price of each good or service in a bundle has three components: the money price, the time price, and the energy price. This implies that it might not be possible for a person to purchase the most preferred bundle of goods and services; i.e., there may be sufficient income, but in fact a less preferred bundle is chosen because the most preferred requires the use of too much time or energy.

We now have sufficient information to draw some implications about individual economic behavior. This can be done by keeping in mind that all individuals are not equally endowed with talent, intelligence, physical stamina, and emotional stability. These inequitable endowments imply that individuals have different endowments of the resources of income, time, and energy. Thus each individual goes about choosing the most preferred bundle of goods and services subject to different constraint levels. These different constraint levels can be used to draw implications about the behavior of individuals.

Health Care: Want Versus Need

The idea that there is a difference in understanding between the economist and the health professional over the meaning of demand was first suggested by Boulding (1966). He introduced the idea that demand was a collection of wants and needs. He stated that the behavior of individuals toward their wants could be explained by economic reasoning but that needs were more basic and were beyond economic reasoning. As could be expected this idea was well received among health professionals and not so well received by economists. In order to maintain economics as a useful tool in the solution of health problems, Jeffers et al. (1971) pointed out that need was a technically defined concept. That is, the amount of goods and services that are needed for the maintenance of health is defined by the health professional. The amount of health goods and services that an individual will consume depends upon resources and income; time and energy; and the price of health goods and services in terms of money, time, and energy. The amount of goods and services supplied depends upon the amount of revenue derived from selling the goods and services. This is to say, the higher the monetary price of goods and services, the greater the supply of health goods and services. Since there is no relationship between the technically defined quantity of health care and the quantity demanded and supplied, the actual quantity of health care goods and services delivered would equal the amount *needed* only by accident. If, somehow, individuals changed their demand for health goods and services as they became more educated, the economic mechanism would bring about an equilibrium between what is demanded, what is supplied, and what is needed. However, if the technology base the health professional uses to define need is expanding faster than the education of health consumers, equilibrium will not be reached. There is considerable evidence to indicate that this is the case.

A better understanding of why consumers do not consume what they *need* can be obtained by referring back to the individual, preference functions, and resource constraints. Note that the preference function is a value system that allows an individual to rank all choices available. The goods and services that are *needed* to maintain health are in a sense competing with other goods and services. Assume that an individual has sufficient resources to purchase the needed amount of health care. Let the other goods and services in the consumption bundle be classified as *wants*. If the individual consumes less health goods and services than are *needed* the individual's resources are also sufficient to purchase the goods and services *wanted*, and if the *wants* are valued sufficiently high by the individual's preference function, the individual will trade off *needed* health goods and services for the goods and services *wanted*.

This seemingly irrational behavior is observed with great regularity. The classic example is the poor family that has barely sufficient funds to buy food, yet purchases a color TV set. However, when viewed from the perspective of the individual's value system, i.e., preference function, the choice made is perfectly logical.

Present versus Future Consumption

Before concluding the discussion of the behavior of individuals, the relationship between present versus future consumption should be highlighted. Just as the individual's value system allows trade-off between wants and needs, it is possible to make trade-offs between present and future consumption. This is particularly easy in the United States economy with its large system of retail credit and savings institutions.

Basic to the relationship between present and future consumption is that for two identical goods or services the one consumed now is valued higher than the one consumed in the future. A second devaluation of future consumption occurs when there exists a lack of knowledge as to the benefits from the consumption of goods and services. The reverse is true, of course, for goods and services that are detrimental to the individual.

The effect on individual behavior is even more pronounced when considering the consumption of health promotional goods and services. Individuals tend to undervalue the benefits of health promotional goods and services not only because of the two reasons cited above, but also because resources must be expended now in order to receive the benefits (i.e., the value of the consumption of health promotional goods and services) in the future. Take, for example, the decision-making process that a pregnant woman uses in deciding to expend resources in order to obtain a program of prenatal care. The benefits from the program are mostly in the future, and therefore, the benefits to her now are some discounted value of her future benefits. Secondly, since she lacks perfect knowledge as to exactly what the benefits of prenatal care are, she may tend to underestimate the future benefits. This does not deny the possibility that out of ignorance and optimism she could overestimate the future benefits of prenatal care. Finally, since the value of the consumption of prenatal services is separated in time from the expenditure of her resources on the purchase of prenatal services, she must also forgo the consumption of some other goods and services while waiting for the value of prenatal care to be received in the future.

The last point to be made about individual behavior pertains to an economic explanation of a statement that poor health creates poverty and that poverty creates poor health. The definition of the level of consumption of health goods and services that is *needed* to maintain an individual at some minimum level of health is independent of endowment of resources. That is, if a person *needs* 2,000 calories per day to keep in health, that amount would not change if the person became wealthier.

This in general causes poor individuals to spend a higher proportion of their income in just meeting needs. Further, this causes a consumption of wants in the present over future consumption of wants and needs to be valued more highly than the same comparison made at higher levels of endowed resources. A person on a $3000 income values the consumption of wants in the present at a higher level than the person who earns $10,000. This phenomenon manifests itself in the inverse relationship that exists between the interest rate individuals will pay in order to consume a product. Individuals from poor urban communities are willing to borrow from "loan sharks" and finance companies at high interest rates; and high- and middle-income individuals will borrow on their life insurance policy at low interest rates. Thus, when faced with a choice of either purchasing health promotion services or consuming *wants* in the present, the individual with a low endowment of resources chooses to sacrifice health goods and services, which may result in declining health. A reduced level of health in turn impairs the individual's earning capacity. The cycle again repeats itself with individuals choosing to meet present needs over future health promotional goods and services.

It is important to note that these conclusions do not depend upon rich and poor individuals having different value systems, but simply on having different levels of endowed resources.

COLLECTIVE BEHAVIOR

Up until this point we have been discussing the individual's economic behavior. We now develop the economic behavior of the family. Again, it must be remembered that we are discussing the economics, not the finances, of the family. The family behavior will be based on the same general theory of value that guided the individual in their decision-making processes.

In order to view the family in perspective with the individual, it is important to visualize a hierarchy along a continuum. At the beginning of this continuum is the individual, who must make the decision as to what and how much of a good or service to consume, given a knowledge of the price of that good or service. The goods consumed by individuals are called *private goods*. All the decisions are single-person decisions. This constitutes the first level of the hierarchy.

With the next level of the hierarchy we enter the world of public goods. That is, at this level a collective of two individuals must make the decision of how much and what kinds of goods and services will be consumed at the prevailing price. All decisions at the second level of the hierarchy are *two-person public goods*. (Using this terminology consistently, a private good should be called a *one-person public good*.) The third level of consumption is that of the three-person public goods. The hierarchy continues in increasing numbers of persons forming collectives in order to make consumption decisions about higher-level public goods. As the number of individuals increases, we see the formations of neighborhoods, communities, towns, cities, counties, states, and nations.

The family is a collective formed to make consumption decisions about two-person and larger public goods. Please note that we are discussing the economic basis of family behavior; there clearly are other social and physical reasons for forming the family. In this respect there is nothing special about the family. It is not the foundation of a society. In this framework the individual is the foundation. As will be discussed below, the family is the first step in the hierarchy of collective decision making. All the problems of decision making at the national level can also be found at the family level of the hierarchy.

Public Goods and Services

Before proceeding, we must be sure that the concept of public goods is understood. The family must make a collective decision as to the amount and kind of good or service they wish to consume. This implies that in making the decision to consume a five-bedroom house, or a 17-inch TV set, each member of the family must consume the same amount of the public good. That is, if the family's collective decision is to buy a 17-inch TV, then all members must watch the same size TV set. Whereas, if the same decisions were made by all members of the family as individuals, then each member could purchase the size of television that would be consistent with a personal preference function and the endowment of resources. It is clearly more economical to consume a television as a public good as opposed to a private good provided a collective decision can be made. The making of the collective decision is much more difficult than the making of an individual decision. The problems of such a decision-making process will be developed below.

A second aspect of public goods and services is derived from the fact that the consumption by one individual in the collective does not prohibit another individual from also consuming the public good. For example, a show being watched on a 17-inch TV set by one individual does not interfere with another individual's watching the same show, whereas an individual eating an apple precludes another individual from eating the same apple. Private goods, like apples, have the property of exclusion, whereas public goods are only exclusive between the collective groups. That is, one family may view their TV set as a public good but exclude their neighbors from using it. In like manner two families may view the streetlight in front of their houses as a two-family or neighborhood public good.

But because of the distance, the neighbors down the street are excluded from use of it.

It is hoped that the above discussion of public goods and services has added another dimension to the concept of a good or service. Originally, when there were only individuals who had to make decisions about consumptions, the only dimension we were concerned with was quantity. As we introduced the collective nature of society, we added a *publicness* dimension to the nature of good and service. A TV set might be described as having a quantity measure of 17 inches and have a publicness measure of being a family public good. An apple might weigh 13 ounces and be a one-person public (private) good. The classic example of a nation-level public good is national defense. The quantity dimensions of national defense might be measured by the 2.7-million man army, and its publicness dimensions might be described as a 200-million-person (national) public good.

Collective (Family) Decision Making

One of the distinguishing aspects of public goods is that the quantity consumed by each member must be the same. Yet a family is made up of individuals with individualistic preference functions, i.e., different value systems. It seems reasonable to ask whether family consumption decisions can be made on the same rational, nonconflicting basis that individuals use. To answer this question, we find that conflict is a natural phenomenon in family decision making, and it can only be avoided by establishing rigid family structures that minimize the degree of democracy and freedom of the individuals within the family (or for that matter individuals of higher-order collectives, i.e., the city, state, or nation).

To help support this conclusion, let us return for a moment to a society of only individuals. If we assume that this society is free of monopolies, then certain other assumptions hold. (These assumptions are not important to the present discussion, but those more interested may consult any intermediate microeconomic text, such as Ferguson, 1969.) Then each individual, with an initial endowment of resources (wealth) and guided by preference function (value system), will engage in a decision process that will allocate the initial resource bundle in such a way that the final consumption bundle will be the best choice and that society as a whole cannot be made better off by any other allocation of original endowments. When such a phenomenon occurs, it is referred to by economists as the *Pareto optimal state* of the economy. Any attempt to improve the position of one individual in society would result in someone else being made worse off. It should be noted that it is possible for a society to reach many different Pareto optimal states, depending on the original allocation of wealth to each member of society. The important point here is that it is theoretically possible for a society made up of only individuals who consume only private goods to reach the Pareto optimal state.

Now, as we expand the definition of goods and services by adding a publicness dimension to them, we find in general that it is not theoretically possible for just any initial endowment of wealth to reach a Pareto optimal state. In order to achieve a Pareto optimal state, the most desired state of all possible Pareto states must be selected, and the initial endowment of resources must be allocated in such a way as to ensure that the desired Pareto optimal state will be achieved. The process of selecting the best of all Pareto optimal states develops the majority of fruitful implications about family economic behavior.

Professor Kenneth Arrow presented in *Social Choice and Individual Values* (1963) several conditions that must exist in order for the selection of the best of all Pareto optimal points to somehow reflect the values of all individuals in a society (or a family). Arrow found that there existed no way to select the best state and still have it reflect individual values. However, if those conditions were weakened sufficiently, they would allow for the existence of (1) social customs and religious dogma, (2) a dictatorial decision maker, or (3) a special case of item (2) in which individuals, through conflict, inform others of the strength of the value they place on certain states of the world (or family) and in turn, through conflict, are receptive to the strengths of the value that others place on alternative states of the world (or the family).

A casual tracing of the historic changes in family style will show that all three of these above exceptions to Arrow's conditions were used in directing individuals toward the Pareto optimal state (of their family).

To see this, let us break the dynamics of family decision making into three discrete periods. The first period involved the family in a struggle for survival against predators. Examples of this period occurred many times in the history of man, i.e., the Dark Ages, settlement of the New World, times of war.

The second period involved the family in a struggle for physical survival. During these periods the families' objectives were to ensure an adequate supply of food and shelter. Examples of such periods in Western civilization were the Renaissance and the first half of the twentieth century.

The third period might be described as the modern period of the family. It is the time when the struggle against predators and for physical survival was no longer necessary.

During the first period, the sheer struggle against predators required the family to have a head, a dictator, usually a man, who imposed his value system on the rest of the family. He made the ethical decision as to which Pareto optimal state was best for the family. He then allocated the family resources in such a way as to achieve the desired state of the family.

As mankind mastered the predators, attention was turned to physical needs. This lessened the need for the family to have a dictator to make their ethical decisions. As the dictator rule faded, it was replaced by strong social customs and religious dogmas. These dogmas defined for the family the Pareto optimal state it *should* obtain. The family then allocated their wealth in such a way that the desired state was obtained.

In the third period, succeeding in the struggle against predators and the achieving of physical security also ended the role of man as a dictator of the family and ended the influence of social customs and religous dogma in the decision-making process of the family. Herein lies the final and maybe the most important economic implication for the modern family behavior. We are now only left with conflict if we wish to reach a Pareto optimal state.

This period has also seen the woman's role in the family change and her role in society become more significant. Along with this there has come an increasing amount of conflict within the family structure. This conflict has been interpreted by others to mean the signaling of the end of the family as an institution within society. This author, however, places a different interpretation on this sign. It seems more reasonable to view the increasing conflict as a natural process of weighting individual values within the family such that the best Pareto optimal state can be decided upon.

Having lost the basis for assuming dictatorial power over his family, man has had to accept the competition of the woman in her desire to make decisions that would improve her state of being. In addition, they have both been freed of the strong religious dogma and social customs that had previously dictated the ethical decisions. Thus, both individuals in the family (a man and a woman) must select the Pareto optimal state of their family with equal representation of both of their value systems. The use of the word "equal" does not mean the resources, or the goods and services, that are produced will be divided equally, but instead that the values of individuals have equal weight in the process used to select the Pareto optimal state of each family.

Herein lies the naturalness of conflict as a process of deciding on the Pareto optimal state. When two (or more) individuals consider themselves equals, the expression of their values about various states of nature (or the family) can result in conflict. This conflict allows the expression of the strengths of each individual's value system. The strength of each individual's value system *equally* considered could then lead to a Pareto optimal state.

It is still possible to argue that this conflict will divide the family. This is particularly true when one individual is trying to find the Pareto optimal state through a dictatorial decision or religious dogma and the other individual considers her (or his) value system of lesser importance.

Opposing the pressure to divide the family is the economics of consuming public goods. Also, the increasing awareness of the fact that we live on a finite planet might begin to lay the economic foundation for the explanation of the increasing occurrence of group marriages and multinuclear families. In addition, in a society such as ours with its ever-increasing use of public goods as opposed to private goods, the collective nature of the family might have to be expanded, not contracted, to allow for collections of families in order that decisions can be made about higher-level public goods.

CONCLUSIONS

The important conclusions of this paper can be summarized in the following statements. (1) Individuals, through the guidance of their preference functions and by their constraints of limited resources, are willing to make trade-offs between their wants and their needs. On the surface these trade-offs may appear to outsiders as being irrational, but when viewed within an economic framework, these decisions are founded in logic. (2) Families cannot, by the independent action of their individual members, reach the optimal state of well-being; and in our modern society conflict may be a very rational process by which individuals within a collective arrangement, i.e., a family, can decide upon the optimal state.

REFERENCES

Arrow, K. J. *Social choice and individual values* (2d ed.). New York: John Wiley and Sons, 1963.

Boulding, K. E. The concept of need for health services. *Milbank Memorial Fund Quarterly*, 1966, *44*, 202–223.

Ferguson, G. E. *Microeconomic theory* (2d ed.). Homewood, Ill.: Richard D. Irwin, 1969.

Jeffers, J. R., Bognanno, M. F., & Bartlett, J. C. On the demand versus need for medical services and the concept of shortage. *American Journal of Public Health*, 1971, *61*, 46–63.

CHAPTER NINE

CULTURAL BARRIERS: AN ANTHROPOLOGICAL PERSPECTIVE

CAROL TAYLOR

The anthropologist can help the nurse, or any other person in a helping profession, to recognize cultural barriers and to work around them rather than against them. In this chapter this author will show how the nurse can use anthropological information to improve nursing practice.

But first an exotic example: Some years ago a nurse from Australia described a unique nursing problem. Apparently an acute and chronic problem in bush hospitals is keeping the aborigine in hospital beds. In their natural habitat these nomadic people sleep clustered in groups on the ground. During the rainy season they build shelters with branches and leaves, and in the cold season they sleep in circles around fires. The nurse said, "They leave a nice, clean hospital bed and you (the nurse) spend half the night with a torch (flashlight) in the bush looking for them." She also talked about the difficulties of getting aborigine patients to take proper nourishment.

It seemed that patients accustomed to sleeping in clusters on the ground might not feel safe and comfortable in nice, clean hospital beds. When the author discovered that the proper nourishment provided was Australian rather than aborigine, it was suspected that an alien diet might be a factor contributing to the proper nourishment problem. And I suggested, as tactfully as possible, that something might be done about beds and diets. The nurse raised her eyebrows, pursed her lips, and said, "The proper place for patients is hospital beds."

Possibly because these suggestions would not be used to change the nursing practice in bush hospitals the author began to use this example of two cultural barriers that seemed to interfere with nursing care when lecturing to nursing students. Some years after this particular story was no longer used to explain how anthropological findings might be useful to nurses, a nurse approached me with the following report.

She had spent several years nursing for the military in foreign countries; and, during this stint of duty, she had been assigned to a hospital that, in addition to caring for base personnel and their families, cared for sick natives. Ten to twelve beds routinely were occupied by members of the indigenous population. She said:

> I remembered the aborigines and hospital beds. Fortunately for me an anthropologist was studying the tribe out of which our patients came and he described their way of life to me. Between us we decided on three changes.
> 1. To get patients from his tribe off beds onto floor mats, their way of sleeping.
> 2. To provide them with the diet to which they were accustomed.
> 3. To see to it that minimum communication, in the native tongue, was established between these patients and staff members.
>
> Target number three was simple. With the aid of an interpreter I learned to ask and understand the answers to basic questions—Do you hurt? Where? And so forth. Then I translated this set of questions and possible answers into a phonetic version of the native tongue, which I then translated into English. The how-to-say-it what-does-it-mean approach. This communication system was painted onto the wall of the ward reserved for native patients. Beds and diet were changed in a less straightforward fashion.
>
> The head of the hospital agreed with my rationale for requesting change and admitted that the changes suggested would be desirable. But he said, "My hands are tied by army regulations." He suggested that I talk matters over with the supply officer and the head of dietary. And he dismissed me by saying, "I'd go to the supply officer first."
>
> The supply officer said, "Good thinking. The problem is that as long as we have enough beds to go round everyone, including natives, must be put into beds. That is what we have to do something about: enough beds to go 'round." Systematically, and over a relatively short period of time, the maintenance crew, armed with sledge hammers, saw to it that the supply of usable beds was sufficiently decreased to permit native-style sleeping.
>
> The head of dietary couldn't see the sense of providing a special cuisine for natives. He said, "Much better off on a balanced diet." But, when it was pointed out to him that the patients didn't even appreciate the expensive and superior diet they were offered, he said, "Then they don't deserve anything better than they're used to." And he arranged to feed them native style.

Anthropologists are best known for their work on small preliterate societies and, as the account above suggests, anthropological information can be put to productive use by a nurse working with exotic peoples whose cultures differ so dramatically from the culture in which the nurse grew up and became a nurse. The question is: Has the anthropologist anything to offer the United States nurse caring for her fellow countryman? The answer to this question is two yeses. The first yes concerns ethnic pockets in our population—groups of people who, for one reason or another, are not being assimilated rapidly into the mainstream of our society. These groups have been studied in considerable detail by anthropologists, and the anthropological information about them should be useful to nurses intending to practice on Indian reservations, in Spanish-American communities, and in other ethnic pockets. The second yes has to do with the various subcultures that, on the surface at least, seem to be melting into what most of us think of as the American way of life. Here again anthropologists have provided information that can be used by the nurse. Esther Lucille Brown (1964) had the nurse in mind when she provided thumbnail sketches of Italian, Chinese, Mexican, and other ethnic subcultures in our society. And in the author's book for students in all health-related professions, a subculture, the "Cracker" (a disparaging term for poor whites), not included by Brown, was used in order to add to the literature information that would be pertinent to nurses who might not realize that there are significant cultural differences among people who consider themselves everyday Americans (Taylor, 1970).

In this author's opinion the anthropologist can most help the nurse when he or she turns an anthropological eye on America's mainstream-related subcultures. In part because culturally conditioned biases and blindnesses in the nurse are most acute when dealing with the cultural mainstream and its fringe elements, and in part because the anthropologist's holistic approach to culture yields detailed information about everyday life-styles. A culture is how people eat, sleep, work, play, and relate to their mothers-in-law, as well as their values, beliefs, and superstitions. Down-to-earth information of this sort can be most useful to the nurse. Here is an example of how the anthropological eye can be used to make nursing everyday Americans more productive.

Some years ago a public health nurse had a problem. She was working with white, lower socioeconomic families. The nurse had succeeded in teaching her notions of proper infant care to about half her mothers. The other half could not seem to understand that smothering infants in oil was bad for them. And she had come to the conclusion that these mothers were more stupid than the mothers who learned about oil. To an anthropologist this conclusion does not make sense. If all mothers were capable of learning everything about infant care except the proper use of oil, an anthropologist would wonder why only some of the mothers refused to change their infant oiling patterns, particularly when the person demanding this change had the authority to remove infants she considered unsatisfactorily cared for from their homes.

In this case it was found that coating the skin of young infants was part of the folk tradition in all families. This fact suggested that the refusal of some mothers to abandon this practice might be tied in with their belief systems. On investigation it was discovered that all the refusing mothers attended the same church and that the complying mothers either attended other churches or did not go to church. The minister of the offending church was cooperative. He said, "The Bible teaches that anointing with oil is efficacious. Your problem is that this practice has got out of hand. I will preach on the subject and, in the future, anointing will be limited to a drop of oil on the head."

Some weeks later the nurse reported that her problem had been solved by the preacher and that she had identified other oil-related problems that had also been solved by him. A woman with an infected leg was not responding to treatment, and the nurse was puzzled by this lack of response. Suddenly and rapidly the leg began to mend. The woman said, "I stopped rubbing it (the wound) with oil. Preacher said it was sinful to do so." And the lady's 10–year-old son said, "The thing God gets behind is a reverent drop on the forehead. More than that is a waste of oil and makes God mad."

A hospital nurse said, "I'm doing my best but in three days I cannot give her the help she needs. That's what's so frustrating about this place [the hospital]; we get lots of cases like this." Cases like this were: unmarried mothers who rejected their infants, refused to allow them to be adopted, and forced their grandmothers to care for them. When an anthropological eye was turned onto this problem, it was discovered that the nurse was nursing a problem that did not exist. It also was discovered that society was creating a problem for itself.

The nurse had been culturally conditioned in a subculture where the mobile nuclear family—mother, father, and offspring—was considered normal and where grandmothers were mothers-in-law who should not be allowed to interfere with the rearing of their grandchildren. In this particular subculture unwed mothers customarily delivered their young secretly and arranged for them to be adopted by strangers. In the case of legitimate births the custom was to begin the name-choosing ritual well in advance of birth.

The patients in question came out of a subculture in which the child of an unmarried woman is not stigmatized and in which it is customary for the young to be reared by the mother's mother. In this particular subculture the mother does not name her child. The mother selects a female relative of her own mother's generation as namer of her child. The namer names the infant during a feast to which the entire extended family and close friends are invited. The namer assumes specific responsibilities for the child she names; she becomes a combination of godparent and backup grandmother. For economic reasons birth and funeral feasts frequently are combined. When a child is named at a dual-purpose feast, one of the given names, as distinct from the family name, of the dead person is given to the child even when the dead person and the young infant are of different sexes.

This subculture is matrifocal, one in which the adult male tends to be an in-and-out member of the family. The adult male is expected to contribute to the support of the matriarchy of his origin—his grandmother, his namer, his mother, his sisters, and their children—as much as, if not more than, to the support of his own offspring and their mother. In this particular subculture stable common-law marriages are the rule rather than the exception, and it is common practice to legalize, from the point of view of the larger society, these unions when the children are grown and a marriage feast can be afforded. In short, the couple waits until it can do for itself what the parents of the bride are expected to do in the subculture from which the frustrated nurse came.

The nurse had identified a problem that, under similar circumstances, would have occurred in her own subculture. A member of the nurse's subculture would have felt ashamed and guilty at having a baby out of wedlock. If she planned to keep her child, she would have concocted a cover-up story to protect both the infant and herself, and she would have entered the hospital with both male and female names already selected. Culturally conditioned to think in this fashion, the nurse knew that her patients were in serious trouble. They had what she called denial symptoms. They did not express guilt and shame, and they made no attempt to keep their birth-giving a secret. From her point of view the patients were denying the reality of the situation by not responding to it in the way she herself would have responded to a similar set of circumstances. In addition to denial symptoms, these patients also had proved to the nurse that they had rejected their young. This fact was attested to not only because they had come to the hospital to give birth unprovided with names for the child about to be delivered, but also because they expected the infant to be reared by their own mothers as if they were producing siblings rather than children. The nurse said, "Just think about the havoc that can be wreaked by this sort of burden in the subconscious." When the cultural context within which her patients would view their situations was explained, she said, "If you're right there's nothing to worry about." However, she did not seem entirely satisfied and although she did not say so I suspect she thought that I did not know what I was talking about.

The name-choosing practices of the subculture from which this nurse's patients come must make it difficult for the society to identify at least some of its members. In our society births must be registered; and the registration document demands a first, or Christian, name for the child. Unless they were stillborn, infants may not leave hospitals without names, and in most cases the nurse is expected to secure a name. As this particular nurse said, "With these patients there is no guarantee that they'll even remember the name they agreed to. Probably a lot of the kids grow up with names different from those they were born with." Observations support this conclusion.

The family structure in the subculture described above is characteristically found at lower socioeconomic levels in our society. And, because nurses frequently work with families structured in this fashion, let us look at traditional health care, which has been designed by middle- and upper-middle-class WASPs, and see what can happen when these health practices are imposed on the members of matrifocal families.

According to WASP tradition, the person caring for the infant and young child is its mother, and the health of young children can be improved by teaching mothers to do a better job of child-rearing. In dominant segments of our society, teaching mothers works because mothers rear their own young. In a matrifocal family the outcome is somewhat different. In most cases this is what happens. The grandmother is not taught child-rearing techniques because she should not, according to WASP tradition, be rearing the young. The mother is taught how to rear her young according to the latest child-rearing formula, and she is put under pressure not only to rear her own infants and young children, but also to see to it that her own mother does not interfere in this process. Under these circumstances the nurse tends to become a social reformer. The nurse's need to shape up the mother so that she, the child's mother, fits a WASP stereotype can be both strong and stubborn. In extreme cases, documented by the author, children have been removed from their homes and placed in foster homes not because of failure to thrive, but because the child's mother refused to shape up.

When a child from a matrifocal family is hospitalized, a similar problem may arise. Hospitals and those who work in them expect parents to care for and be responsible for their children. The doctor talks to the mother and in some cases the father, and it does not occur to him that it might be more productive to talk to the child's maternal grandparent. The nurse cares for the child and, if it is necessary to do so, instructs the mother about caring for the child after the return home. The nurse rarely thinks to ask who will be caring for the patient at home. If the hospital considers it desirable for parents to stay with their hospitalized children, the mother of the child is expected to want to do so. If the grandmother who routinely cares for the child volunteers to stay during hospitalization, she is considered an unsatisfactory substitute. In this situation the rapid turnover of hospital patients does not allow time for social reform. As one hospital nurse said, "We don't have time to work on mothers who won't look after their own kids."

During labor and delivery the matrifocal family may produce a more complex problem. In some hospitals fathers are expected, or permitted, to stay with the mothers during labor. The theory is that the fathers support the mothers during this particular crisis. In a number of matrifocal communities, any male, including the father of the child, would be contaminated by being physically present in the labor room. In some of the communities the author studied, the father supports the mother but in a somewhat different fashion. His knife is placed under the mattress to cut pain and his hat is placed on the mother's abdomen to give her strength. In the traditional situation, which in the case of most of our matrifocal subcultures was birth at home with a midwife in attendance, the mother of the woman delivering, or a female relative of that generation, was present both to support the birthing woman and to assist the midwife. Mothers from these subcultures do not expect the fathers of their children to sit with them during labor, but they would welcome and receive support from the presence of their own mothers or from suitable substitutes. My own observations suggest not only that hospitals do not permit the presence of this natural source of support, the patient's mother, but also that the conscientious nurse sometimes substitutes for support attempts to solve problems that may not exist. One nurse said, "If we're not busy, I work on their psychosocial problems during labor. Believe me, they really have them (presumably this sort of a problem), particularly the unweds."

Another area in which the anthropological eye might be useful to the nurse is in identifying and characterizing the natural clustering behavior of families from different subcultures during sickness, dying, and death. Hospital visiting rules are designed for nuclear families, who consider it reasonable and satisfactory to visit the sick and dying in small groups (no more than two at a time). In many of our subcultures, visiting the sick and dying in a pattern reminiscent of Noah leading the animals onto the Ark is most unsatisfactory both to the patient and to the family and friends. As one nurse said about the visiting behavior of people from nonnuclear subcultures, "They don't even know how to behave in hospitals; visitors pour in by the carload." Another nurse said, "They won't even let them die in peace; as soon as your back is turned, they sneak back in. I've seen as many as sixteen people in the room with a terminal [dying patient]. That's no way to die." According to conversations with those guilty of this sort of behavior, some people do consider a crowd around the bed the right way to die. One man put it bluntly, "Dad is too far gone for the nurses to take it out on him because they're mad at us. So nobody's going to stop us seeing him out proper." In this case, the wake that followed seeing Dad out proper also upset the staff. One nurse said, "I know a wake is part of their grieving process, but they ought to control themselves until they get out of the building." Most hospitals are not designed to accommodate this sort of clustering and other behavior, but the extended family's attempts to behave in what to them is a natural way might be more readily tolerated if it were better understood.

Beliefs and behaviors that might be thought of as health care counter-cultures also raise barriers the nurse must surmount. The patient, or the patient's family, may belong to a religious cult that forbids specific medical practices, for example, blood transfusions. Postures of this sort in patients and their families are difficult for the scientifically oriented nurse to tolerate. When the patient is a child in critical condition, this difficulty becomes acute.

Sometimes a patient may be convinced that an illness is caused by a spell cast by an ill-wisher. From time to time patients with this syndrome are admitted to hospitals in all parts of the country and, interestingly enough, nurses do not find cases of this sort difficult to handle unless one of them has been given the responsibility of finding someone to remove the spell. The scientifically oriented nurse is not well equipped to tackle this task. The nurse's first response to the hex syndrome is to disbelieve the patient, at least the first time a hexed patient is encountered. As soon as the doctor announces the belief that the patient's condition is caused by belief in a spell, the hexed patient becomes an interesting problem. The patient is too sick to leave the hospital and will not recover until the spell is removed. Removing spells is not a routine hospital procedure. In some cases the patient's family is available and able to hire an appropriate specialist; in other cases a staff member, most frequently a nurse, is assigned the task of arranging to have the spell removed. An anthropologist, if one is available, may be able to remove the spell and, if not, will be able to track down a suitable practitioner. In addition, the anthropologist will be able to explain to the staff how the putting on and taking off of spells is done and why it works.

The health care countercultures suggested above are not new to our society. Ever since the art and science of nursing began to emerge nurses have encountered beliefs and superstitions that made it difficult for them to care for their patients. A new health care counterculture has come out of the women's liberation movement's contention that women rather than physicians should make decisions about what is done to women's bodies. This notion gave impetus to political action legalizing abortion on demand and producing a growing revolt against hospital birth. Both changes have the potential to create cultural barriers with which the nurse must contend. Abortion on demand may violate the nurse's belief system and place a barrier between the nurse and the patient whose medical history reports a self-determined abortion. And it may create barriers between nurses with opposite beliefs about abortion. Barriers rooted in belief systems are most difficult to deal with.

The revolt against hospital birth has the potential to create barriers between nurses and patients. In this particular health care counterculture, expectant parents reject birth in a hospital setting. They do not wish to deprive themselves of medical help, but if the price to be paid for that help is delivery in the traditional hospital setting and the "excessive intervention of the orthodox obstetrician," they will do the best they can without that help. One young woman summed up the situation by saying, "I'd like to have a doctor on call and a qualified midwife delivering me either at home or in a place where birth is not treated like a disease, a place where my husband could be with me and my children would not be excluded. That would be ideal. My choices were to prepare myself as best I could for a home delivery or risk hospital birth."

When asked what she meant by "risk hospital birth," she said, "The ritual cuts: episiotomy for me, and circumcision for the baby if it turned out to be a boy, which it did. Twenty percent chance of having a cesarean." She explained that according to an article she had read, the *national* birth by cesarean section rate had increased to more than 20 percent since the introduction of fetal heart monitoring. Then she said, "They would have tied me down, pumped me full of drugs, and separated me from my baby. I'd rather risk an informed home delivery."

When asked what she meant by an "informed home delivery," she said, "In our case it meant: going to Lamaze classes, getting an English textbook on midwifery, and finding a couple who already had done it themselves. We were lucky our Lamaze teacher gave us advice and helped us white-lie the baby into a clinic for a checkup. We saved ourselves from hospital birth, but we sure could have done with a qualified midwife."

Since that conversation this author has talked with a number of nurses who teach classes designed to prepare parents for childbirth. Apparently from time to time they do have students in their classes who will not enter a hospital to deliver. One of the nurses I talked with summed up the problem all of them had identified by saying, "This sort of thing puts me between a rock and a hard place. I had all mine in a hospital and if I weren't past it I wouldn't have one anywhere else. Maybe the docs tend to go too far, but they're doing their best to protect mother and child. All of them, parents insisting on home delivery, have been nice young people who should have known better. They are well educated and some of them grew up in forty-thousand-dollar homes. All of them could have gone to school with my own children. They are risking so much for so little. We are up against a generation gap."

Death, like birth and women's bodies, also has produced barriers to health care. Advanced technology has created what might be called the death dilemma. When should heroic measures to prevent an inevitable death be abandoned? When should the death of a prospective transplant donor be declared? Physicians have the right to answer questions of this sort. In some cases, patients, their families, and the nurses caring for dying patients are not in complete agreement with the doctor. These disagreements place nurses in a difficult position when they do not agree with the doctor. The following comments by nurses suggest the parameter of this in-house, cultural barrier.

"They say the chief of surgery will go so far as to operate on a corpse."
"Why can't they recognize when enough is enough and let people die in peace?"
"Why waste blood in useless transfusions? We might have a disaster and need that blood."
"If they need a kidney or a heart it's a different story."

Physicians are reluctant to admit defeat, and it may be necessary for the nurse to intervene. The following sequence was a case in point. Robert was a 3-year-old dying of leukemia. Some weeks before he died his mother said to the nurse, "We want to take him home to a few weeks of meaningful life before he dies, but they [the doctors] make us feel like murderers for wishing to do so." The nurse rehearsed Robert's parents before they confronted the doctor and she talked with the doctor before he saw the parents. After that encounter the doctor said to the nurse, "As a doctor I couldn't give up. As parents they were right to demand a more peaceful ending for this child." That peaceful ending included feeding seagulls; swimming in a pool using the frog's feet he put on each day of his hospital stay; a ride in a helicopter; and his favorite foods every last day of his life.

While different subcultures may speak the same language, a single word might have different meanings. The consequence of this state of affairs is miscommunication. For example, in the days when the most frequent failure of the birth control pill was due to a miscount of days, a nurse said to a repeater, "What happened, did you lose count of the days?" This cause for failure was denied, and on further investigation it was found that the patient did not know that when instructed to take a pill one is supposed to put it in the mouth and swallow it. She had assumed that the pill was to be applied to the part of her body being protected from becoming pregnant, and she had conscientiously attempted to do so. The nurse said, "It never occurred to me that there was anyone in the world who could misunderstand when told to take a pill. Now I demonstrate as well as tell." As far as the patient was concerned, it was customary to take a poultice for the chest and ointment for the elbow, so the way she took her birth control pills made sense to her. And an anthropologist who knew anything about the subculture in which she was reared would have been aware of the fact that the instructions about the pill would be misinterpreted.

Another communication hazard is caused by differences in verbal style. For example, misunderstandings sometimes arise when a nurse encounters a person who comes from a subculture in which long pauses punctuated by single words or short phrases are considered good conversation. This verbal style is found among mountain folk and in some rural areas. The nurse comes from and is accustomed to a highly verbal environment, and, when she encounters the naturally nonverbal patient, she tends to leap to the conclusion that the patient is depressed and needs cheering up. In one case, a patient who did not talk was put through a series of diagnostic tests to find out what was wrong. No one asked whether he could talk; it was assumed that if he could, he would. No physical cause was found. Shortly after the tests had been completed, two carloads of relatives and close friends visited the patient; and to the staff's amazement the patient talked to them without apparent difficulty. The staff developed a psychological explanation of the rapid recovery. This theory was abandoned when, in response to the physician's comment that they had been concerned because the patient could not talk after his accident, the patient's brother said, "Wouldn't, not couldn't. Doesn't like strangers." And the patient's father said, "Should have asked the boy."

In this chapter the author has attempted to show how cultural barriers can prevent the care given by nurses from being as effective as it might otherwise have been. The anthropologist is in a position to provide information that will make nurses aware of the cultural barriers they encounter in their patients. These barriers are to be anticipated not only in exotic peoples and ethnic groups, but also when dealing with everyday Americans. The greatest contribution the anthropologist can make to nursing is to make nurses aware that, like all other human beings, nurses leap to culturally conditioned conclusions. It is the author's hope that the nurses who read this chapter will ask a man who doesn't talk whether he can talk rather than start to work on the assumption that if he could he would.

REFERENCES

Brown, E. L. *Newer dimensions of patient care: Patients as people*, Part 3. New York: Russell Sage Foundation, 1964, 56–86.

Taylor, C. *In horizontal orbit: Hospitals and the cult of efficiency*. New York: Holt, Rinehart and Winston, 1970, 151–162.

CHAPTER TEN

BELIEFS OF THE MEXICAN AMERICAN FAMILY

ORA RIOS PRATTES

Because of the numerous religious and ethnic minorities that comprise the population of the United States, it is virtually impossible for a nurse to practice in any part of the country and avoid contact with people in one or more of these groups. The care the nurse renders patients may depend on an understanding of beliefs and a subculture that are foreign. As an example of this type of challenge to health care delivery, the Mexican American family has been selected.

Acculturation and assimilation of a large number of Mexican Americans have been retarded for certain social reasons. One of the most important of these is their segregation in slums or ghettos called *barrios*. In this isolated environment, many folk beliefs of Spanish or Mexican origin persist, and modern medical knowledge and health practices cannot be transmitted. As their economic situation improves, Mexican Americans tend to move out of the barrios into middle-class neighborhoods and are then replaced by newer immigrants from Mexico.

The poor and poorly educated Mexican Americans are isolated in the barrios because they can afford the cheap housing there and do not have to learn English. Since the United States and Mexico share an 1800-mile open border, the Mexican ways remain powerful influences upon these Mexican Americans. A plentiful supply of Mexican literature, movies, material goods, and radio programs further entrenches Mexican culture.

FOLK BELIEFS

Many Mexican Americans in the barrios—especially those who are educated and have had positive experiences with modern health care practices—have accepted the ideas and practices of scientific medicine and allow their children to become immunized, to attend clinics, and to have professional medical care. But many Mexican Americans from the barrios have their own set of folk beliefs about illness and its treatment, which they practice in addition to or before seeking medical care. Many times, when a patient is brought to a clinic or hospital with an illness that seems to have been neglected, he is asked why he did not seek medical care earlier. It is probably because he has attempted to cure his illness with folk remedies.

The folk beliefs of Mexican Americans about diseases and their cures are derived from experience and experimentation and are handed down from generation to generation. Often, two or more cures may be recognized for a single ailment. Clark (1969, p. 164), who investigated folk medicine in California, has identified two categories of folk disorders—those of emotional origin and those of magical origin.

Martinez and Martin (1966), who carried out a study of seventy-five Mexican American housewives living in a public housing project in a Southwestern city, found that relief from ailments recognized in folk medicine is rarely sought from physicians. Healers are relied upon instead. Several women in this study cite instances in which they or others had sought treatment from physicians without disclosing the folk diagnosis. Two-thirds of the women believe that medical doctors do not know how to treat folk disorders because they lack either faith or knowledge and understanding.

Superstition and the Supernatural

Among unenlightened Mexican Americans, there is no distinction between the natural and the supernatural, the scientific and the superstitious. Their folk beliefs are not a separate entity but a part of their daily living. If a folk remedy works, no one is surprised; but, if it does not, the failure is rationalized and some other cure tried. The younger generation of Mexican Americans is becoming more skeptical of the traditional superstitious and supernatural beliefs of their people.

It is common for Mexican Americans to believe that illnesses are caused by external forces. Many think that they are victims of evil forces in the environment or sometimes of the malicious behavior of others. This superstition applies particularly to mental illness. The afflicted (for example, an epileptic) may be the victim of a spell or curse. The belief in *brujas* (witches) is widespread, and even though the majority of the people will admit to knowing someone who is thought to be a witch, they will admit to consulting one only to have a hex or spell cast on a friend or relative removed.

Illness may also be a punishment for sin. If this is believed to be the case, the afflicted will go to confession and carry out penance. Long pilgrimages to certain religious shrines are often undertaken to bring about a cure for a certain illness. The wearing of a habit exactly like that of a certain saint or virgin for a prescribed number of days is also believed to bring about a cure, particularly if the sick person has sinned.

A few years ago, it was believed that by promising not to cut an infant boy's hair until he reached the age of five, the parents could save their baby's life during the first year if he became severely ill. These young boys with long hair were very often mistaken for girls, but if *una promesa* (a promise) had been made to the Virgin, it was kept until the time was up. Any embarrassment or ridicule was accepted as part of the agreement. Today, with the trend toward long hair for boys and men, this practice would not seem so odd.

HEALERS

Espiritistas (spiritualists) practice in the barrios. Not all of them are Mexican Americans; some claim to be from India, Puerto Rico, and other countries. The main reason for consulting an espiritista is to communicate with a dead relative, particularly one who died suddenly. The prestige of the spiritualists is not very high among Mexican Americans, partly because of the high fees they charge, which must be paid before each séance.

The *curandero* (male folk healer) or *curandera* (female) is the healer most often sought. Most of these healers will not deal with the supernatural or with diseases believed to be caused by spells or hexes, but they will treat for simple *susto* (fright) or *susto pasado* (passed fright) and for evil eye. The *curandera* usually sets up practice in her own home. Usually she has installed a small altar in a hall in her house. A statue of a favorite saint and lighted candles adorn the altar. *Curanderas* usually do not charge a set fee but merely ask for donations. Most of them are very religious and prescribe prayers, the wearing of certain religious medals or charms, herbs, baths given with certain herbs, and poultices or teas made with a large selection of herbs.

A respectable *curandera* will not attempt to cure a person that she knows is critically ill. Fearing an investigation by the legal authorities should the patient die in her care, she will usually advise the family to seek professional medical care instead.

The *curandera* consults with all members of the family who are present and attempts to elicit as much information as possible about the patient's daily habits and what the family and the patient think about the illness. She is courteous, attentive, and warm toward her clients, and involves the whole family in her treatments, as the following narrative illustrates:

> A middle-aged woman, accompanied by one son, one daughter, and her daughter-in-law, sought the services of a *curandera*. The woman's chief complaints were loss of sleep and appetite because she had not heard from another son in over 6 weeks. He had been in trouble with the law before this time, and she was afraid that he was in trouble again. The *curandera* asked the woman about her son's habits and listened attentively while the woman explained what a good son he was and that he had just gotten into bad company. She seemed to be deeply depressed about him, even though she had four other sons and three daughters, who were all living either in her home or very near her home. The *curandera* gave her some herbs, telling the daughter-in-law how to fix the tea and when to administer it. She gave the woman a charm and told her to say certain prayers every night. She asked the son if it was possible for the whole family to take their mother to the park or for a walk every day and recommended some warm baths with a certain herb at least two evenings a week. The *curandera* did not guarantee that all this would help the woman to hear from her son; the only thing she promised was that the tea would help her appetite and the exercise and baths would help her sleep. The prayers would be the answer to her main problem. The woman appeared to be more relaxed and serene as the family left, leaving two dollars at the altar.

A few *curanderas* in the barrios combine the usual folk remedies with magical or supernatural rituals:

> A young girl whose engagement had been broken was experiencing severe loss of appetite—she could not eat at all. A *curandera* was recommended to her, and she went to see her. The *curandera* told her to rub herself all over with a raw egg for the next three nights and to repeat a certain prayer three times. She was instructed to then return to the *curandera* and bring the egg. When the girl completed the treatment, she went to see the healer, who took the egg and broke it on top of a newspaper on the floor. Inside the yolk the *curandera* found a dead worm wrapped in some hair. She told the girl that the worm was what was making her sick. Then the healer asked for five dollars and told the girl that she was cured. The girl's appetite improved immediately.

FOLK AILMENTS AND THEIR REMEDIES

Evil Eye

The disease known as *mal de ojo,* or evil eye, is very prevalent. Of magical origin, the effect is most common among infants and children. The belief is that if a person, especially a woman, admires someone else's child and looks at him without touching him, the child may fall ill of the evil eye. Any person who has *vista caliente* (hot vision) is capable of inflicting evil eye, even though unaware of having this power. If possible, the person who inflicted the evil eye should perform the curative treatment.

An object such as a vase or a breakable glass is also capable of having the evil eye cast on it by a person (not the owner) who admires it. Thus, because of the evil eye, a vase or some such object can break even when no one is handling it.

Any nurse who works with Mexican American families should know about their belief in the evil eye. If she admires an infant or a child, she should touch his head, tousle his hair, run the palm of her hand over his face, or touch him in some other manner. This practice will prevent anyone from believing her responsible for giving the child the evil eye.

The evil eye is diagnosed by some or all of the following symptoms: fretful sleep, vomiting, fever, diarrhea, excessive crying. It can be cured by any person who knows how to cure, not necessarily just a *curandera.* The healer is sometimes an older family member, usually a grandmother or an aunt, or someone in the neighborhood.

First the stricken child is rubbed all over with a whole raw egg. He is rubbed in the sign of a cross, two strokes down from head to foot and two strokes across from left to right; prayers are said. The egg is broken and placed in a small saucer under the child's bed. In the morning or after a set period of time (preferably overnight), the egg is examined for signs of an "eye" (a spot, usually white, in the center of the yolk). If the egg appears cooked or a white film has formed over the yolk, the cure is believed to have been doubly effective, the egg supposedly having drawn out all the illness.

The evil eye can also occur in other groups, particularly attractive young females, as the following account illustrates:

A 20-year-old girl working as a nurse's aide had gone to work one day with her hair fixed in two long braids (she normally wore it pulled back in a bun). Everyone admired her braids and commented on how cute she looked. When she got home that evening, she complained to her mother of having had a severe headache all afternoon. Her mother asked her if the girls at work had touched her braids. Her answer was that some had, but she was not sure if everyone had done so. Her mother told her to lie down, and she proceeded to treat her daughter for the evil eye. The young girl took a nap and when she woke up, her headache was gone.

Susto

Susto (fright) is caused by a frightening or traumatic experience. Being scared by a dog or involved in a traffic accident (not necessarily getting physically hurt, just frightened) is enough to cause symptoms of *susto*— excessive nervousness, loss of appetite, and loss of sleep.

Simple *susto* can be cured by a member of the family who is familiar with its diagnosis and cure. The afflicted person is placed on the floor in a reclining position, or on a low cot, covered with a sheet, and then swept in the sign of a cross with palm leaves or a broom while certain prayers are repeated. Afterward the patient is given a drink of water. Usually this procedure suffices to make the person well. In the case of a child, the emotional support, attention, and feeling of importance derived during this ritual is bound to be beneficial psychologically.

If simple *susto* is not taken care of immediately, it can become *susto pasado* (passed susto), which usually needs the services of a professional folk healer.

The following narrative illustrates this malady:

Three little girls, aged 6, 8, and 10, had been riding in the back of a pick-up truck with their father when one of the tires blew out. The father managed to maneuver the truck to the side of the road without an accident. After checking to see if the girls were all right, he proceeded to change the tire. When they got home, the man told his wife what had happened and stated that even though the girls had been frightened, they had not cried. Late that night one of the girls woke up screaming. The other two, who slept in the same bed with her, also woke up and started to cry. Immediately a diagnosis of *susto pasado* was made. The father's older brother and his wife and their five children, who lived next door, were awakened and asked to come over for a family conference about what to do for the girls. It was decided that the uncle should go down the street and ask the *curandera* to come and treat the girls for *susto*. When the healer came, she first asked about everyone's health and was served a cup of coffee. After a brief social visit, she inquired about the girls, chatting with all members of the family and agreeing with their diagnosis. The *curandera* was then taken to the bedroom to see the girls. All the family members followed her into the bedroom, standing quietly along the wall. She covered the girls with the bedsheet and proceeded with her treatment, the girls giggling with delight at the attention they were receiving. As the *curandera* left, the father gave her a couple of dollars from his pocket in payment.

This example of a woman afflicted with *susto pasado* did not end so fortunately:

One cold morning a woman went to visit her neighbor a few houses down the street, leaving her four children in the care of the oldest girl, who was 9. The others were 7 and 5 years and 18 months of age. The infant was strapped in a highchair. While the mother was gone, the fire in the family's wood-burning stove began to die out. When the 9-year-old child put more wood in the stove, the fire appeared to go out completely, so she drenched the fire with kerosene kept in a can beside the stove. As she did so, flames shot out of the stove. The girl dropped the can spilling the rest of the kerosene on the wood floor. The flames started spreading, and the children ran out of the house screaming, leaving the infant strapped in the highchair. The infant died in the burning house. The mother never got over this tragic experience. She was taken to numerous folk healers in the area but continued to be depressed. She could not eat and lost a lot of weight. Folk healers could not bring about a cure for what was believed to be *susto pasado,* and the woman was finally taken to a local hospital. There the diagnosis of pulmonary tuberculosis was made. She had gone without medical help for almost 2 years and died a few months later in a tuberculosis sanatorium.

Sereno

Another common illness is caused by *sereno* (dew or draft). *Sereno* is thought to be produced by some types of evil spirits that live in the night air. Because of *sereno,* a young child is never taken outside in the evening, even in the summer, without first being covered. Exposure to the evening dew may cause a cold or symptoms such as vomiting, diarrhea, and fever. Usually these symptoms go away by themselves, or the services of a *curandera* are sought. She may treat this illness with teas made out of herbs, mainly *ruda* (rue).

Mollera Caida

Mollera caida (fallen fontanel) is a common disorder in very young Mexican American infants. Two main folk causes are recognized. One is a fall suffered by the infant—it is believed that the impact of the fall causes the anterior fontanel to cave in. The other folk cause, which is the more common, is pulling a nipple out of a baby's mouth too vigorously. It is thought that this practice causes the fontanel to be sucked down into the palate of the baby's mouth. The most easily recognized symptom is the infant's inability to suck the nipple. He cannot grasp it, and the sucking reflex is very poor and weak. Other symptoms of *mollera caida* are irritability, crying, diarrhea, sunken eyes, and vomiting.

There are several folk cures for *mollera caida.* One is to insert a finger in the child's mouth (while holding the infant by the feet with its head down) and exert pressure on the palate. Another is to apply to the soft spot a poultice made of soap shavings. Another mixture used for a poultice is egg white mixed with soap shavings.

Most of the babies with a fallen fontanel who are brought to the hospital have a history of diarrhea and show some evidence of the soap poultice having been applied to the soft spot. It is when these remedies have not worked that the parents bring the infant to the hospital. They usually do not mention the treatments they have tried, even though the evidence is very apparent. Once a young intern asked a mother what that "stuff" was on the baby's head. When the mother replied that it was egg white mixed with soap, the intern told her that it would have done the baby more good if she had fed the egg to the baby because the reason for the fallen spot was hunger and malnutrition and not some superstitious belief. Some of the hospital employees, nurses included, thought this remark was very funny. The mother smiled and agreed with the intern even though she was very embarrassed.

Rather than try to "educate" these parents, it is better to institute a program for postpartum mothers to teach them causes and symptoms of diarrhea, inability to suck, and a sunken soft spot, showing actual photographs or films of infants with a fallen fontanel and calling it by its Spanish name, *mollera caida*. Another part of this program could be to show the women how hydration of the infant after intravenous fluids are given "pushes" the fontanel back into place. Their own cures, along with modern medical practice, will assure these parents that everything possible is being done to help their child. The nursing staff should also be cautioned about pulling a nipple out of an infant's mouth with too much force, particularly in the presence of the mother.

Resfriado and Catarro Constipado

Catching a cold or getting chilled *(resfriado)* from exposure to a cold draft or from getting wet and not changing into dry clothing right away is usually treated by applying mentholatum to the patient's body and covering it with warm blankets. For *catarro constipado* (chronic head cold or sinusitis) a mixture of *poleo* (pennyroyal), *mastranzo* (round leaf mint), and *alhucema* (lavender) is made with boiling water. The remedy is sniffed up into the nostrils, where it will supposedly clear the head and open the nose.

Empacho

Empacho is caused by a bolus of poorly digested food sticking to the stomach lining. This condition may occur at any age. The symptoms are loss of appetite, vomiting, diarrhea, stomach ache, fever, excessive crying, and restlessness. The folk treatment is rubbing and pinching the back, or rubbing the stomach. The pinching process involves grasping a fold of skin, pulling it up, and releasing it. This procedure is done with both hands and repeated three times *or* until an audible pop is heard, which means that the food bolus is dislodged. A tea may be given after the rubbing. It is usually made of *estafiate* (larkspur), *hojas de senna* (senna leaves), and *manzanilla* (camomile).

Cleft Palate and Hydrocephalus

There are no acknowledged folk cures for cleft palate and hydrocephalus, but superstition still surrounds these congenital anomalies. A pregnant woman may wear a metal key on a string around her abdomen to prevent cleft palate in her unborn infant, believing the anomaly to be caused by an eclipse of the moon. Plastic surgery is an acceptable cure.

A few Mexican Americans still believe that hydrocephalus is caused by a precious rock inside the child's head. This rock is thought to be very valuable. If the infant dies, most parents refuse to give permission for an autopsy. They believe the doctors remove this rock right after the infant's death and sell it to become rich. The success of surgery, particularly on young infants, in arresting the growth of the head has managed in large part to dispel this misconception. It is still common, though, for Mexican American parents to believe that they are directly responsible for this affliction—that it is a punishment for some indiscretion or sin.

Pain

Pains in various parts of the body are treated by *ventosas* (cupping). A candle, mounted on a coin, is placed over the painful spot and lighted. A small jar is then placed over the lighted candle. When the air is exhausted, the skin is pulled up by the vacuum inside the jar. A prayer is recited during this procedure: *En el nombre de Dios, que salga este dolar* (In the name of God, draw out this pain). The jar is moved around over the entire back. Finally, the patient's back is massaged with *accite de volcanico* (volcanic oil).

Infant Health Problems

The cutting of a baby's fingernails or toenails with a metal instrument such as scissors is believed to cause near-sightedness. So, instead of trimming the baby's nails, a mother may make cotton drawstring mittens and place them over her infant's hands to prevent him from scratching his face. It is also believed that a copper penny hung on a string around the infant's neck will prevent painful teething.

NURSING IMPLICATIONS

The nurse who works with Mexican Americans should always try to involve the entire family when teaching about health care, and should include all the family members close to the patient when giving nursing care. All the relatives in a family usually live close to one another, so this generally is not difficult to do.

Tolerance of the superstition and folk beliefs of some Mexican Americans is very important. It *is* easy to become dismayed and exasperated at their failure to see the benefits of scientific health care practices, such as having children immunized against communicable diseases and consulting a physician in the early stages of illness. But it must be remembered that scientific medical care is often not available to these people in a form that is meaningful to them, and many of them have seen little evidence of the benefits of modern medicine and nursing.

REFERENCES

Clark, M. *Health in the Mexican American culture*. Berkeley and Los Angeles: University of California Press, 1959.

Martinez, C. & Martin, H. Folk diseases among urban Mexican Americans. *Journal of American Medical Association*, 1966, *196*(2), 147–150.

CHAPTER ELEVEN

THE MEXICAN AMERICAN FAMILY AND THE MEXICAN AMERICAN NURSE

MAXINE CADENA

What would the difference be if the term Mexican American were deleted and the title read, "The Family and the Nurse"? Should not the same considerations be taken into account regarding family differences when any nurse is working with any family? It is readily agreeable that the answer would be yes. But it is believed that there are characteristics, though common to many groups of various national origins, that require particular consideration when the nurse is working with the Mexican American family.

The Mexican American people have a rich culture. It is not the purpose of this chapter to discuss the culture of the Mexican American, but to discuss specific cultural factors that are distinct to the Mexican American family and that have an influence on the nursing situation.

There are many generalizations about the Mexican American family. The term "Mexican American" refers to people living in the United States who are of Mexican origin, or whose parents or grandparents were of Mexican origin. They either speak or understand Spanish, and/or the Spanish language was a language of their parents or grandparents. They continue to practice or identify, in some way, with specific customs of their ancestors. Because a large percentage of Mexican Americans are on the lowest of economic, education, and social levels, many times it is believed that Mexican Americans are inferior. They are thought to be illiterate, lazy, and unable to learn. It is assumed that they do not want to work, are very passive, and have a philosophy of *mañana*. These are generalizations believed by a vast majority of the United States population, and they are fallacies.

THE MEXICAN AMERICAN NURSE

The term "Mexican American nurse" refers to persons of Mexican origin, or whose parents or grandparents were of Mexican origin, who have been prepared for either vocational, technical, or professional nursing, as defined by the ANA position paper on nursing education. They either speak or understand Spanish, and/or the Spanish language was a language of their parents or grandparents. In an effort not to be identified with this group and these generalizations, the Mexican American nurse may deny cultural factors that have been a part of the family background. Attempting not to be identified with this group, the nurse may at times work with the Mexican American family in a manner that is most ineffective and runs directly against cultural influences. Or the nurse may be working with a Mexican American family that denies any cultural factors that are Mexican, and the nurse will be just as ineffective by trying to force such factors on the family.

The Mexican American nurse who identifies with the two previous statements may become defensive, and, in so doing, may only deny further that the Mexican culture has many specific factors that can and do influence a role with a Mexican American family. The emphasis here is not that the nurse should not be defensive, but rather that the nurse should examine the working relationships with Mexican American families, and her feelings toward them.

These situations are not without stress and anxiety. This author, too, is a product of two cultures. Where does one end and the other begin? Have they mixed so that one is more dominant than the other? No doubt, there are people who will reject this chapter because the term "Mexican American" is being used. Factually, it is incorrect because we are not speaking of Mexican citizens but rather of American citizens, people who are second- and third-generation Americans. But because this group of people is referred to as a distinct group, the term "Mexican American" will be used. The reasoning for selecting this word has also come from identification—a more positive and comfortable feeling of using the term "Mexican American" and associating with it.

Even though the Mexican American family has taken on American ways and customs, it still is influenced by many beliefs and practices of its ancestors. Mexican Americans have individual differences, just like members of any other group. One will find that they have delinquents and gang leaders as well as college graduates and professional people. There will be some Mexican Americans who will have a firm commitment to their Mexican culture and others who have adopted the Anglo way of life in the United States. But circumstances and situations commonly experienced by Mexican Americans have sometimes placed great stress on the individual. In order to cope with the stress or to be accepted, they may have chosen to play down the part of their culture that has been criticized and labeled as being "Mexican" with all the negative connotations that have gone with it.

Since the role of the nurse demands knowledge of a situation and the factors within the situation, the first step is to know who the Mexican-American family is and what is important to this family. What are their values? What is it that must be considered if the Mexican American nurse or any other nurse is to be effective while working with these families?

CULTURAL FACTORS THAT INFLUENCE NURSING

The specific cultural factors considered to have a direct bearing on the nurse's relationship with the Mexican American are: family life, Spanish language, respect for authority (both inside and outside the family), politeness and graciousness, a sense of modesty, an amount of pride, and the attitudes and beliefs regarding health and health care. The beliefs and practices regarding health and health care will be mentioned only briefly here since Chapter 10 speaks specifically of this topic.

To elaborate with the many references and statements that are available on the role of the nurse and nursing functions would be superfluous. It would also be inappropriate to dwell on the past role of the nurse and to lament over what nursing was not. Time is too short, society is too precious, and the quality of life is too valuable to dwell on the past. Therefore, it is fitting that we look to today and to the future.

For the purpose of this chapter, the nurse is one who has been prepared for vocational, technical, or professional nursing. The nurse, it is assumed, has knowledge of the social sciences and related disciplines, a beginning understanding of the behavior of people, the forces in society that affect the family, and the fact that the family affects society.

When working with the family, the nurse should have the family and their needs as the focal point. In nursing practice and nursing education, we are taught how things should be done; but when we do not follow through in practice, we refer to it as idealistic. Or as can be seen in some settings, our practice is very archaic. If we in nursing and the health services intend to accomplish our purpose for being, then the questions posed in this chapter are important, and an attempt must be made to answer them. Evidence is available that nursing for society is vital and more so with the present discussion of health care systems today (Lysaught, 1971).

Ida Jean Orlando, in her book *The Dynamic Nurse-Patient Relation-*

ship (1961), gives nursing excellent guidelines that can continue to assist us in effectively providing nursing service to people. Her nursing process explains that the nurse must perceive the situation and the patient's behavior, respond to it, and then carry out necessary actions for effective nursing care. An attempt will be made to apply her process to the role of the nurse with the Mexican American family.

Among the Mexican American people, the family is the central focus for social identification. Seldom does the concern for the individual family member become more forceful than concern for the family as a whole (Samora, 1971). This is demonstrated by the gathering of the family members in various situations. Some of these situations are festive occasions, and others are times of illness or hospitalization. When a Mexican American is hospitalized, it is not uncommon for the patient to be visited by his immediate family, aunts, uncles, and good friends. The visitors usually come together. This becomes a difficult situation for the family and the nurse. It is difficult for the family, because they know that not all the visitors will be allowed to visit. It becomes difficult for the nurses, because they are the ones who usually must inform visitors that they may not all enter to see the patient. It will also become difficult for the nurses if they do not understand the closeness of the Mexican American family. The nurse if Mexican American, may be embarrassed by all the visitors, and may exhibit a tendency to be rude in an attempt not to identify with them.

The Mexican American nurse may be embarrassed by cultural traits that differ from those the nurse perceives to be typically American or by behavior of the Mexican American family that is often criticized by the Anglo culture. This embarrassment causes stress, and the nurse's reactions to the embarrassment will have an effect on the family and on the effectiveness of the nursing service provided.

The place of the elderly Mexican American within the family structure is an important family characteristic. The elderly Mexican American family member accepts assistance from children, but this assistance will not be readily asked for. The nurse's perception of situations as they arise when working with the elderly can prove to be very useful when discussing the situation and alternatives with the elderly family members and with the children who are concerned. It is not uncommon to find a great desire for independence among all people who are elderly. They do not want to be dependent on people, especially their children. But with economic costs as they are today, it is found in all cultures in America that often elderly couples or individuals do without the necessary food, medicines, and health care, because they cannot afford it and will not ask for it unless absolutely necessary. But if assistance is suggested or offered in a respectable manner, they will gladly avail themselves of the offer. The nurse, knowing this, can then intervene by suggesting various alternatives and exploring means and methods with the family members. This can be in relation to more adequate or suitable living conditions, necessary medication, and adequate health care.

Authority in the Mexican American family is paternalistic. It belongs to the father or, as is often seen, to the eldest son in the family. This authority deals with permission to do such things as wear lipstick, cut one's hair, date, seek medical assistance, and follow through on health care recommendations.

Nursing contacts with the family are usually made at a time of day when the father and husband is at work. In attempting to meet the health needs, nurses identify situations and needs and then plan for necessary nursing intervention and health care. At the same time, nurses add to the stress of the health situation by demanding that the mother make an immediate decision that, according to their culture, may have to wait until the father is home to discuss the situation and make the decision. What is our goal in nursing? What are the specific goals when working with families? If individual family situations are truly being assessed, and the nursing service provided is being evaluated, then it should be evident that the mother of the family may make a decision; but it may not be carried through. When this happens, nurses usually continue to reemphasize "how important it is to follow through," to make more home visits, to send postcards and reminders. When it is seen that this has not brought results, there is a tendency to conclude that the mother is not interested or that she is "uncooperative." An expression often heard in nursing settings is, "They just don't understand." After proper assessment and validation of the assessment, it is the nurse who usually did not understand or did not realize that other factors were contributing to the situation. Some questions that may prove to be most helpful in such situations are: "What does your husband think of this situation?" "What does your husband think is wrong?" "What do the two of you do when such a situation arises?" "Where does your husband prefer you take the children for medical treatment?" "What does your husband think about your taking the children to the doctor?"

The following is an example that demonstrates the cultural factor of authority within the Mexican American family:

> During a Head Start immunization program, the children were vaccinated against smallpox. Permission had been obtained from the parents by signing an immunization card. In 3 days a father and his 5-year-old son came looking for the nurse who had given his son the vaccination. The father was very upset because there was a reddened and swollen area where the vaccine had been administered. He said that he did not give permission for something like this to happen. To his way of thinking this was an infection, and he felt that his child would become ill.
>
> Realizing that the man was upset for two obvious reasons, the nurse took him and his son aside and explained the normal "take," or reaction, of a

smallpox vaccination. She told him that this was evidence of his child's immunity against smallpox, and that he was correct. This was an infection, but not the type that we usually associate with illness. The nurse, although frightened, did not become defensive. She sincerely told the man that she and other nurses wished that more fathers would get concerned about the type of care and service that their children received. At later meetings regarding health teaching, he and his wife were present and always ready and confident in expressing their doubts regarding certain health care teaching.

Orlando's nursing process can be readily identified in the above illustration.

Mexican Americans know that they are different from the Anglos and that they are not fully accepted. Their language is often different. Does the Mexican American nurse feel the same way? Is this one of the reasons why the nurse sometimes refuses to speak Spanish with a family that has difficulty understanding English, assuming that the nurse knows how to speak Spanish? Frequently the family will be watching for the nurse's response or reaction to the family situation. Two questions Mexican American families ask themselves while waiting for this response are: "Is she like one of us?" Or, "Is she one of those who thinks that she is better than we are?" If the family gets an affirmative answer to the last question, they will not hesitate to ask for a nurse who is not Mexican American.

Working with families would be most effective if, in the nursing situation, the family were approached as a unique group of people with qualities that are important and vital to them. The nurse must work with them to identify needs and then to establish mutual goals. If the family were approached in this manner, then it might not be necessary for the family to set up defenses, attempt to deny some of their own values and beliefs, or accept those that the nurse is trying to force on it.

Recently it was explained by a young person interested in becoming a nurse that her reason for doing this is so she can be helpful, "not like some of the nurses from my own people" who treat poor Mexican American families without any respect. The young person related that she has thought of this ever since she was 5 years old and had to receive medical and health services from a county institution. There her family encountered Mexican American nurses who treated them "very badly," and she felt that this was because the nurses were ashamed of them because they were Mexican American and they were poor. "We didn't speak very good English and we couldn't pay for care."

The Mexican American family is a polite and gracious family. This is especially evident when the family sees that the nurse is also Mexican American, by either name, language, or appearance. One does not have to know or work with a Mexican American family for any great length of time for this to be evidenced. This may be in the form of a hug, a firm handshake, a very flattering statement, or a material gift. If the contact is in the home, this may be shown by offering a cup of coffee, a glass of water, or something to eat. How does the nurse respond to this? Is the nurse embarrassed that this has been offered? Should the nurse accept or refuse? Accept so that the family's feelings are not hurt? Not accept because this is not part of the professional role? Is it what is said and done that communicates more, or is it the way it is said and how it is done that communicates more?

Answers to such situations will depend upon the nurse-family relationship. If the nurse believes that this family is inferior and that accepting this gesture would not be professional, then the response will be very different from that of the nurse who sees this as a sharing with the family and understands professionalism in a different context.

For some reason, when nurses have difficulty in such situations, there is a tendency to act or not act and to refer to this as being professional or not being professional. What is demonstrated and referred to as professional is often dehumanization. The literature has well defined what professionalism is and how this can be attained in nursing. So where do we get our own individual ideas of professionalism that demonstrate a firm, stiff, keep-at-a-distance, and do-not-get-too-involved manner? This too comes from our education and practice in nursing. But now is the time to rectify this, to take a second look, and to change where we see that change is indicated.

There is a great sense of modesty within the Mexican American family. This cultural factor will also be related to beliefs and practices for health care. This sense of modesty is in relation to keeping personal things personal, especially in terms of the body. The nurse has many occasions to work with the family during pregnancy. Oftentimes, individual nurse's values are forced on these families. These are illustrated in the following statements: "You must go to the doctor." "You must go to the clinic." "It is very important that the doctor check you." "You must make plans early for delivering the baby in the hospital." The emphasis in these comments seems to be on the physician, the clinic, and the hospital. It seems that they are the important factors in such statements. Nurses must reexamine the reasons for stressing such issues. Is the family told why these things are so important? How is all of this going to benefit the mother, child, and family?

The institutional way of life and the hospital way of life are American. When we assume that the Mexican American family will avail themselves of this, we are in error. An example of how specific cultural and family clues are missed, and how nurses force their values on families—that all women should be delivered in hospitals by physicians and that this will be best for them—is illustrated in the following:

A Mexican American family was being visited by a Mexican American nurse for prenatal care. This was the tenth pregnancy for this family. All previous babies had been delivered by midwives. No complications or difficulties had been encountered.

When the nurse learned that the midwife delivery was planned, she attempted to talk with the mother so that arrangements could be made for a hospital delivery. The husband and wife chose a hospital that was noted for good care. The nurse felt this was an accomplishment. She had accomplished her purpose, getting the patient to deliver in the hospital.

Time for delivery came, and the patient was taken to the hospital by her husband. She was properly admitted and made comfortable in the labor room. In the hour that she had been there, the nurse had checked her frequently. When the nurse went in to check her again, the mother had her baby lying on her abdomen, but had not yet put it to breast. The woman did not complain, but she did admit that it was more difficult here in the hospital than when she had her babies at home. When she delivered at home, she did not have to do it all by herself. Her husband and the midwife were always there to help her. Here she had to do it all alone. She was very tired.

Do we in nursing credit ourselves with effective nursing intervention in this particular situation? What criteria are used in nursing to determine effectiveness? Is our criterion a count of hospital deliveries versus midwife deliveries? Are our criteria in reference to the family and how the family, mother, and child benefit from nursing intervention and the hospitals available for such care? Some comments from nurses when this situation was discussed were: "She was comfortable." "She had a clean bed." "She didn't have to worry about washing all the bed linen." What rationale do we have for assuming that she was not comfortable at home, that she did not have a clean bed, and that she worried about washing her linens?

If the mother-to-be tells the nurse she is going to have a midwife delivery, does the nurse respond in awe and insist that she go to a hospital? The midwife is an accepted practitioner in the Mexican American culture. She is usually knowledgeable and skillful. Is the nurse aware of this? The nurse, even if not familiar with this aspect of the Mexican American culture, has a responsibility to learn about it. Does the nurse attempt to find out who the midwife is and if she is a safe practitioner? Does the nurse attempt to work with the family and the midwife?

One of the cultural factors of the Mexican American family is pride. One does not expect something for nothing. They want to contribute, to help, and to understand. This desire and willingness to share home, ideas, advice, and food with people whom they trust and respect or who have done them a favor are considered to be a basic Mexican American cultural characteristic. It is a custom among Mexican American families to share different dishes that are prepared for eating. When the food is taken to the next family, the container (plate, bowl, saucer, or pot) is never returned empty. They return it only when they too can send it back with some type of prepared food or gift. To share with one another is basic to the Mexican American culture. The Mexican American family has a need to reciprocate and to show the nurse its gratitude. Perhaps this is the reason why Mexican American families in the lower economic levels do not always participate in various health services that are advertised as *free*.

In connection with immunization programs, it is often heard, "After all, they are free, what more do these people want?" All people feel, or would like to feel, that they too have something to offer. The dignity of persons is destroyed when they are not allowed to share, and to share is to be allowed to give and to receive. Possibly this is part of the problem of lack of participation in immunization programs. Another reason is lack of understanding or information as to what is meant by immunization. In health care practice this is accepted as a part of healthy living. The Mexican American family accepts this concept partially, but in a different manner. They see it as an agent that also causes the disease and feels that the person, usually a child, who received the immunization becomes ill. This too is correct. But nurses must help clarify this a little further so that it can be understood in a manner that is acceptable to the family. The same is true regarding the cost of immunizations. The immunizations are not free. They are usually provided by some level of government if the family is not required to pay cash. This family is living in the United States and also contributes to the taxes that support our health care governmental agencies.

It was mentioned earlier that language is a factor that distinguishes the Mexican American family from the American and Anglo culture. What is the role of the nurse in this regard? The nurse's foremost role is to determine whether the family identifies with the Mexican American culture in this respect. As there are Mexican American nurses who tend to deny any cultural traits with the Mexican American culture, so are there families who do this. How can this be determined? This will depend upon the nurse, the family, and the situation. Is the nurse working in a community where it is the belief of many people that English should be spoken at all cost? If this is so, then the nurse must reexamine personal thinking and practice. If the nurse too believes this, there will be difficulty in delivering nursing service to a population that speaks and understands Spanish better than English. A nurse who comes from a background that is more Anglo, and where Spanish was not spoken in the home, may not know how to speak it, or at least not well enough to assist in service. In order to improve communications and nursing service, the nurse should then do whatever is necessary to learn how to communicate with the Mexican American family. It has been reported by Mexican American families that they prefer an Anglo nurse who knows a few words in Spanish or makes an effort at it to a Mexican American nurse who denies knowing Spanish and makes no attempt to speak it or understand it.

There is a large population of Mexican American families throughout the Southwest. Depending on the specific states and regions, some people have continued to speak Spanish, and others do not use it at all. It is the nurse's responsibility to determine the practice of other individuals at work. One part of the Mexican American culture deals with health beliefs and practices. Although the health practices of these families have already been covered, they will be mentioned briefly because of their impact on and importance to the effectiveness of nursing service. Even today there are practices with evidence of results that imply better health or at least a relief from the symptoms of illness. One will find these health practices believed and practiced by economically poor, middle-class, and professional Mexican American families who identify with this cultural trait. The family will not admit to these practices if the nurse working with the family is going to ridicule and downgrade them. In an effort to keep the nurse from knowing of these practices, they will hold back information important in the assessment of the family health situation.

There is one isolated characteristic that has been observed while working with the elderly Mexican American. This is in relation to the regularity with which medications are taken. They do not take medications for hypertension and cardiac conditions that must be taken daily as prescribed by the physician because, if the pills are taken this often, the patient will then "get used to them and will have to take them the rest of my life." This is a most difficult barrier; even after explanations regarding addiction and the taking of these medications are discussed, experience has not shown any great change in relation to this particular problem. One other reason for not taking the medications regularly is that they are very expensive and will be used up too soon.

SUMMARY

This chapter has concerned itself with the Mexican American nurse's role in working with the Mexican American family and has considered cultural characteristics that influence the nursing care provided. We in nursing can achieve our purpose for being if we continue to assess individual situations *with* the family concerned, and then mutually plan for the necessary health care desired and needed.

REFERENCES

Aranda, J. The Mexican American syndrome. *American Journal of Public Health,* 1971, *61*, 104–109.

Burma, J. H. (Ed.). *Mexican Americans in the United States.* Cambridge, Mass.: Schenkman, 1970.

Lewis, O. *The children of Sanchez.* New York: Random House, 1961.

Lysaught, J. P. *An abstract for action.* New York: McGraw-Hill, 1971.

Madsen, W. *The Mexican Americans of South Texas.* New York: Holt, Rinehart and Winston, 1964.

McWilliams, C. *North from Mexico.* New York: Greenwood Press, 1968 (first Greenwood reprinting: copyright 1948).

Orlando, I. J. *The dynamic nurse-patient relationship.* New York: G. P. Putnam's Sons, 1961.

Samora, J. *Los mojados: The wetback story.* Notre Dame, Ind.: University of Notre Dame Press, 1971.

Sanchez, G. I. History, culture, and education. In J. Samora (Ed.), *La Raza: Forgotten Americans.* Notre Dame, Ind.: University of Notre Dame Press, 1966.

CHAPTER TWELVE

LOW-INCOME FAMILIES AND THE PROFESSIONAL

JEAN L. SPARBER

What a pity this chapter should have to be written at all! If health care were, indeed, the right of everyone, then we should not have to separate our thinking about assistance to low-income families from help to those more economically endowed.

Indeed, there is a tragic gap between what should be and what is. This requires straight talk, not pretty talk.

PUTTING IT BLUNTLY

Working with low-income families is a professional field for people capable of growth, personal warmth, and maturity. It is hoped that those who cannot measure up to these standards will have the common decency to get out. The poor have troubles enough without having to cope with square professionals working in a round hole.

Generally, the person who works in the world of the poor goes home at night to a vermin-free bed. Close contact with poverty and deprivation is often shocking to new students—especially those brought up in protected wealthy and middle-class homes. At first, the deluge of negative impressions tends to disturb the student to the point of taking the situation personally. A first impulse might be to organize a neighborhood brigade to mop, replace smashed window panes, or plan an overkill assault on the rat and roach population.

Unfortunately, the new health worker's enthusiasms are often chilled early. A cool response from both community and professional people may come. Righteous indignation can sputter out into a sheepish feeling of foolishness. After all, indicates the community, how can this arrogant stranger eradicate problems that have defied so many experts before? Unless the new health worker can retain some of the felt initial indignation, an adjustment or truce with the job environment will soon be made. The new health worker will gradually learn to forget the day's problems upon going home at night. Submerged frustrations might take the form of occasional nightmares about injustice and wasted human lives. Unfortunately, the "poor" health consumer wakes each morning to find that the bad dreams are *true*.

Warm, sensitive supervision and understanding are essential to the young worker. In the beginning, it is easy to become cynical and bitter about inequalities that appear to defy correction. A student from a protected background with limited life experience can be emotionally traumatized by exposure to writhing misery. These devastating feelings must be worked through if this person is to become an effective health care helper.

Nastiness exists. Those who study to ameliorate health conditions of the poor must be trained to "take it" while retaining their warm humane concern. This is no small order!

GIVE ME YOUR TIRED AND POOR

The United States may have got itself into some of this trouble through generosity. Historically, the country advertised itself as a haven for the world's underdogs. Millions of destitute immigrant families rose out of poverty by climbing Horatio Alger's ladder.

But the fabled land of opportunity did best for strong, clever, lucky, and racially acceptable families. Some people never got to the first rung of the ladder. And those who failed to meet the tests of success and status were somehow considered unfit for first-class citizenship. What a paradox that we have permitted generations of elementary school children to pledge their allegiance daily to a flag promising liberty and justice for *all* (Hurley, 1971, p. 6)!

Eventually, middle-income people began to wake up to some frightful truths. Social infections originating in neglected, rejected areas were spreading to "nice people's" children. Then, *horrors,* the costs of inhibiting the disease began to hit middle-income wallets!

Emotionally and socially crippled families not only tended to perpetuate themselves, they also resisted suggestions about cutting down their birth rate! Welfare costs, prisons, and police protection cut into funds that might have been used to promote preventive measures. To be sure, there were always humanitarian programs that sought to maintain dignity and snatch families from the jaws of pathology. Slowly, social reforms were legislated. Private and government agencies and church organizations launched pilot projects. Some steered straight courses. Others hit the rocks.

At this moment, remedial action remains fragmented. Misery exists on a massive scale. And some of that misery is that of sincere, thoughtful, intelligent professionals who are frustrated by their inability to deliver quality health services to low-income families.

Today, one cannot work with low-income families without becoming aware of gigantic forces for change. The Constitution and Bill of Rights are taking on new meaning to the disadvantaged. Reactions range from nonviolent legal efforts to revolutionary resistance using desperate tactics. Families are changing, too, along with divorce and abortion laws, communal living experiments, and women's liberation (Wheeler, 1971, p. 19).

The nurse working in a hospital, making a home visit, or working in a storefront clinic must become involved with these larger socioeconomic problems in order to understand those who are to be served. At this time in history there can be nothing routine and sterotyped about working with low-income families. In fact, it comprises a new interdisciplinary frontier—as wild and challenging as steering a covered wagon across a rampaging stream.

WHO ARE THE POOR?

One chilly evening after Thanksgiving, a dozen sorority sisters on an urban college campus called a traditional meeting. The agenda was simple and seasonal: What good work shall we perform this Christmas?

Being a sociable, sentimental group, easily touched by the plight of needy children, the decision was an easy one.

"We'll have a Christmas party for poor children!"

"Great! I can't wait to get started."

Plans thrust ahead rapidly. Animated committee heads urged their followers into enthusiasm. Soon, a storage room bulged with new and reconditioned toys, games, and dolls. A gigantic Christmas tree dominated the sorority house living room. Cheery notices went up all around town, proudly announcing the free event—the untold treats and surprises and the treasures available for needy children. What a welcome! What warmth and goodwill!

At 2:30 P.M. on that sunny pre-Christmas Saturday, the sorority sisters had every cookie and goodie in place. A costumed and very perspiring Santa fanned herself, especially around the pillowed stomach.

By 3 P.M., the truth had dawned. No one was coming. What red-blooded American child wanted to be considered "needy"?

DEMOLISHING THE STEREOTYPES

We have plenty of low-income families, and the public has created an overabundance of stereotypes to describe them.

The Deserving Poor

The most acceptable of all, epitomized by the characters in Charles Dickens' *A Christmas Carol,* are the deserving, uncomplaining, and grateful poor. They reward their benefactors with blessings and cause us pangs of the deepest guilt that the "Little Match Girl" should have frozen to death unnoticed in the midst of plenty.

The Lazy, Shiftless Poor

These are a supposedly clever lot. They are unmotivated people who have made a career of leaning against shovels and avoiding work. The *Congressional Record* speaks of them on many occasions, especially when liberal health and welfare bills are ready for the vote.

The Loud, Complaining Poor

These people are never satisfied with the taxpayers' contributions. They grumble at low-quality goods and services as though they had a right to consumer protection.

The Unexplainably Wealthy Poor

Some of the shiftless poor acquire color television sets, drive luxury cars, and own products that most certainly could not be purchased on a welfare budget. Poverty seems to agree with them. They have a lot of fun, make noise, dance with joyous abandon, and let others take care of their rainy days.

The Lying Poor

These are the professional poor. They have every angle figured and know whom to approach when grant money is being handed around.

The Scary Poor

This is a new kind. Oh dear, the anxiety they are causing! This is the "political-legal" poor. They can quote the Bill of Rights and the Constitution with no effort. Some can spout ordinance numbers and have been in personal contact with elected officials and the Civil Liberties Union. There are some members of the public who fear what would happen if these people really got the equality to which they are entitled.

The Nouveau Poor

You've heard of the "nouveau riche," now learn about the "nouveau poor." Here is a brand-new stereotype we are creating with every rise in inflation. The elderly, with what they considered to be secure pensions, are joining this group. Educated men with obsolete jobs are edging in. These people simply will not permit you to put them in their "low-income" place! They will resist even the most temporary labels and make a big fuss about how they always had private doctors and never had to stand in line for food stamps. This is a growing group. Watch out, *you* might even qualify for it yourself someday!

The Hereditary Poor

This is a lot of hogwash. Exciting new research is being done on the deteriorating effect of poverty on health, IQ, culture, family structure, emotional illness, and character formation. The temptation used to be to lump the families who tended to stay poor from one generation to another as a sort of Juke-Kallikak syndrome. This granddaddy of stereotypes is one of the hardest to break. Evidence is emerging that indicates our gross undervaluation of these families for too long. Unfortunately, the families with visible racial charactertistics appeared to have got the worst of the deal (Hurley, 1971, p. 8).

The Criminal Poor

Facts are beginning to come out, especially through the Fortune Society, that we have been manufacturing criminals in our so-called reformatory system. We took fathers out of their homes and finally returned them to their families without a shred of dignity and no way of making a decent living or changing the factors that got them into prison in the first place.

There are also the unfortunates who never made it at all as criminals. Not only were they unsuccessful thieves, but they could not even learn criminal techniques from the skilled conmen they met while serving their prison terms.

The Voluntary Poor

An emerging low-income group, now coming up strong on the poverty scene, and just as stereotyped as the rest, are the people who are simply antimoney. They do not value materialistic goods. Motivations differ, and very little is known about how the voluntary poor will develop. They might figure out some solutions we can use.

IMPLICATIONS FOR PRACTICE

The above-mentioned categories of poor are stereotypes because they do not take into account the individual circumstances of the family being described. It is not our purpose to size up families and attach to them tags reading "poor risk," "fun to work with," "uncooperative," etc. It is our function to assemble as objective and fair a social history as possible. We should try to understand how the family feels about itself, what problems it thinks it has, and how it perceives the health care worker.

If the health care worker is to be of any positive assistance whatsoever in working with low-income families, the crucial test will be one of attitude. It is for this reason that this chapter concentrates on challenging the feelings and preconceived notions of those of us who are currently working or planning to work with low-income families. You may be assigned to a family with a "bad" reputation. It is your job to observe, record, evaluate, and to try to see them as human beings deserving dignity and the chance for rehabilitation.

In other words, we professionals are not entitled to preconceived, judgmental opinions. This does not mean we approve, but it does separate us into a clinical group capable of maintaining fairness as one of our major tools.

MAJOR PITFALLS AMONG HEALTH CARE WORKERS

We hereby list five of the most obvious and commonly found "characters" who, perhaps without realizing it, fall into habits not in the best interest of our clients.

The Defrocking of Lady Bountiful

In the long-gone years of garden parties, demure lawn frocks, and flowery picture hats, there was once a lovely Lady Bountiful whose serene reputation rested on her good deeds to the deserving and grateful poor. We hereby rip off her many-buttoned, floor-length dress and strip her down to a Godiva nude.

You see, Lady Bountiful gave her gifts in a capricious yet charming manner. She might donate a basket of luscious pears to a child with a desperate need for eyeglasses, or distribute flower seeds to the villagers in need of basic tools for the cultivation of vegetables.

Do not think for a moment that Lady Bountiful has not been reincarnated among us. She exists among both experienced and uninitiated health care workers. She lives on, providing sturdy, unglamorous, prep-school-type sweaters and skirts to young girls desperately yearning for bellbottoms, hot pants, or whatever the current styles demand. All of us have the capacity to give unwanted services to families while enjoying the illusion of having done a good deed.

The Lady Bountifuls who occasionally remain backbones of our institutions and agencies carry the infection into higher-echelon decision making. This can be exceedingly dangerous.

The victims of her gifts, on the other hand, can be caught in a treacherously embarrassing bind. Should they be grateful or speak out for their real needs?

Take the case of a Lady Bountiful who pounces on a federally subsidized plan to retrain low-income mothers on welfare for semiskilled jobs. All the lucky applicant must do is pass a small battery of tests and be evaluated for a variety of jobs. The proposed new careers hold the promise of a fast elevator ride from lower-to-middle-income living. This is an ingenious scheme for free education, and a subsidy to the student's family will be covered at its previous level of poverty while mother studies.

"How could anyone in her right mind refuse?" thinks Lady Bountiful. But the old girl is astounded to discover that Mrs. J., a most intelligent woman with a cooperative record, vetoes the plan at first hearing. She will not listen. Lady Bountiful becomes annoyed, surly, almost rude. Her negative attitude is not lost on Mrs. J., who now has a big conflict on her hands. She really does want to advance, but the J. family is so constituted that Mr. J. prides himself on supporting his family whenever possible. Now, if Mrs. J. is trained and advances to a higher-paying job, Mr. J. will lose confidence in himself. Mrs. J. is ashamed to admit this. Lady Bountiful is not sensitive to this, nor does she bother to explore it further with Mrs. J. If Lady Bountiful were a bit more concerned about the family, she might be able to dig up a similar training opportunity for Mr. J. Then, perhaps they both could be advanced, and the story might have a happy ending.

Lone Rangers

These are a breed unto themselves but also pop up occasionally in the best of us. We try, singlehandedly, and preferably without consulting with others, to solve a problem by ourselves. The results are occasionally gratifying but ordinarily stir up more trouble than they are worth.

The Eager Beaver: A Close Relative of the Lone Ranger

Eager beavers go around slapping their tails vigorously over minor issues. These give them a fine sense of importance and give everyone else a gnawing sensation that they are out for their own glory rather than that of the client. They can never see the forest for the trees.

The Establishment Preservers

These dear people are dedicated to the preservation of triplicates and interminable meetings to discuss grammatical trivialities. They also enjoy propounding policy statements destined for rehashing at annual delegate assemblies. They look very important.

The Sob Sister (or Brother)

Each of us has a soft spot. Some low-income families become experts at discovering these areas and learn to play one agency against another. Flattery can get them somewhere. Beware.

Undoubtedly one will find even more of these prototypes as one piles up years of service. Just be careful that *you* do not turn out to be one.

HONEST SERVICES POSSIBLE

Real, bona fide service can be and is being performed every day. You must be open to the opportunity to get in and do your bit. This is only possible if you become increasingly sensitive to what people really want you to help them do.

FIRST STEPS IN OPENING ONE'S EYES TO REALITY

Millie and Mollie, experienced, long-term welfare recipients, leaned their gritty elbows out of the peeling lead-paint window sill and smirked at the student social worker retreating from their house four flights below. The interview had been a short one. Miss Watchamacallit had been nervous. She asked the same tired old questions, and Millie answered them mechanically. Miss Watchamacallit tried to smile with sympathy, but the general effect was self-consciousness.

Mollie thought the interview had been rather entertaining. Mollie did a hilarious and fairly accurate imitation of Miss Watchamacallit's unsuccessful attempt to ignore a cockroach crawling out of the sugarbowl.

"She'll be an easy one to twist around our little finger," observed Millie.

Meanwhile, several blocks away, Miss Watchamacallit, professionally known as Miss H. R. Watchung, collapsed onto a coffee shop counter stool. While waiting for the murky beverage to cool, she envisioned grand and glorious social changes in store for Millie and Mollie. She would personally lead these crumpled, unmotivated women toward better lives.

"By George," thought Miss Watchung, "I'm the one to do it!"

The preceding paragraphs are typical fantasy fragments in our current health care collection of illusions. Millie and Mollie have become cynical and "wise" to the young, idealistic, and inexperienced workers. The clients are tired of the solutions promised by fervent predecessors. They reject both excuses and panaceas. In some areas, because of high agency turnover, some families are lucky to get the same health care worker two times in a row.

On the other hand, the young, inexperienced worker may be in danger of promising too much and of indulging overoptimistic fantasies. The worker can be "used" by the experienced low-income client. The result can be a mighty disillusioned young professional. It can drive good people out of the field, challenge them to become really good workers—or turn them into cynical, red-tape-loving health care robots.

ALL IS NOT LOST

The low-income family was not born yesterday. It has become adept at pulling heartstrings. There are both passive and active resistant methods of foiling the best worker's attempts to be of assistance.

While the low-income family is sizing up the professional, however, it might be in for a few surprises. For one thing, even a green health care worker may be a talented and trustworthy listener. He might not know the answers or make promises, but the consumer might find him to be exactly the right person to hear problems. If the health care listener is nonjudgmental and supportive, the relationship could easily take a positive turn.

What we are trying to achieve, then, is a nonstereotyped, sensitive give-and-take relationship between two or more human beings. This is true in working with families in all income brackets and also when working with individuals. However, the poor tend to have low self-images. This complicates the formation of the simple dignified relationship. The health care worker must, therefore, be especially scrupulous in respecting the family and avoiding every trace of condescension.

Words alone cannot communicate these qualities. The nonverbal undertones and overtones take courage to control. For instance, the aforementioned Miss Watchamacallit might have broken through to Mollie and Millie if she could have openly admitted her discomfort about the cockroach. By simulating an "I don't see the roach" approach, the trio never grappled with what was really happening around that table.

Most people appreciate honesty, even if they are sometimes suspicious about it. Part of honesty may be the frank admission by a health care worker that the environmental conditions are uncomfortable. This gives the client or consumer the opportunity of verbalizing the problem. By allowing the "underdog" health consumer to be the expert in explaining hardships, there is a subtle switch of roles. The professional is no longer the "giver," but can receive advice and counsel. The disadvantaged consumer can teach the professional how to work in disagreeable neighborhoods. The low-income family can give tips to the inexperienced worker on how to walk a street or climb dark tenement stairs with greater safety. Why can't the professional relinquish authority to the point of establishing a true working partnership with the family?

REALLY LOOKING AT A FAMILY

Each family is different. We see families changing in structure and wonder whether the institution will survive in the future. There are migrant families, rural families, and woman-dominated families. Then there are ethnic and racial differences. These factors are important if we do not permit these labels to become stereotypes.

Working with a family is different from caring for one individual. One must size up that family's power structure. Who proposes decisions? Who appears to make the problems? Who blocks their solutions? Is some family member being protected at the expense of all the others? Is one member unconsciously terrorizing the family by using illness, martyrdom, or control of money?

Why have these people been classified as low-income? Were their parents poor? Do they have areas of untapped strengths? Perhaps there are longings and hopes just waiting for some skillful, kind, and sensitive worker to explore. Are there undiagnosed emotional or physical problems?

Most important, and this cannot be emphasized too strongly, what are the family aims? Some homes show interests in several directions simultaneously. The mother wants material goods. The father wants simplicity and solitude. Be careful. Siding with one member of the family might upset the balance among the other relatives.

Then, one must think very hard about how the family fits into the social structure. It is possible that a family is an antisocial one. Think hard. Are they harmful to others? Should the family be evaluated by experts to determine if they are unfit to exist freely within our society? A dangerous family can harm other families trying to live decent lives. These are extreme examples, but nonetheless real. They will require help from wise and experienced supervisors and many social agencies.

On the other hand, what if a health care worker discovers a treasure—a family member of such positive potential or talent that it would feel like a crime to waste it? Again, one must return to the true aims and motivations of the family. The parents might not wish the child's gifts to be developed. It is their right to refuse.

Getting to know a family's real interests and motivations may not be impossible. There are ethnic, racial, class, language, and intelligence barriers, to name a few. We are not always able to achieve communication. It is a bitter pill to swallow, but we can fail.

Nevertheless, a loving health care worker can often get across complex ideas by exercising the simple human force of caring. Trust can grow in the most unlikely places. Did you ever see a fragile, beautiful flower growing from a rock crevice hardly wide enough to contain a fragment of soil?

AVAILABLE RESOURCES

Health care workers meet the recipients of our services in many settings: hospitals, streets, migrant labor camps, furnished rooms, social agencies . . . anywhere.

There is a continuing controversy. Should we reach out to families or wait to be asked in to help? There is some virtue in crisis intervention. On the other hand, many families are much more apt to accept service when they state their wish for it. Let this controversy be resolved for the present in a simple, basic way. It would not hurt to at least start to establish a friendly, nonthreatening relationship with a family. It could be the basis for a genuinely needed relationship at some future date.

Referrals to existing social agencies is a usual way of handling problems. There are many available community resources. In this day and age, it is difficult to keep up with the new ones springing up in low-income areas. Older agencies are reevaluating their purposes and sometimes abandoning long-term policies. Referrals can be valuable. But again, they cannot be done in a stereotyped or thoughtless way. For example, one might suggest that the Jones family solve an after-school problem by enrolling 10-year-old Benny in an afternoon play group in a local schoolyard. Mrs. Jones goes there and finds there is a waiting list. Or maybe Benny is too young. The fee may be more than they can afford. Maybe the play group has a reputation for starting kids off on drug experimentation. Look harder. A mechanical referral may make the worker feel good, but it may be no solution. Also consider that Mrs. Jones might only be trying to please the worker, and might actually prefer Benny to stay home, where she can keep an eye on him.

A referral looks good on paper. It can enhance an agency record. If there is enough volume, perhaps the agency will have its funds renewed. But be honest—nothing replaces the family's complete participation in the plan and the health care worker's sensitive follow-through. If the plan turns out to be a poor one, get rid of it with the family's consent and look for something better.

This boils down to something simple and basic. Be friends with your families. This should not be confused with unprofessionalism. Just be real friends. The families and you will know the difference and everyone can benefit.

WHERE MATURITY AND COMMON SENSE COUNT

Standing on One's Own Principles

Principle 1: You are the tool for serving others. Be as clean, sharp, and true as possible.

Principle 2: Be tremendously concerned. Listen very hard to what the family is trying to tell you. Try to understand it from their point of view whether you agree with them or not.

The health care worker will grow in the job if good sense and sensitivity permit it. Agencies, hospitals, and institutions at this point in history appear to be in a state of flux. One can no longer rely on the mimeographed policy book for the answers. Some agencies are in decay and do not know it. You might find yourself working in an organization, doing a job, and suddenly be hit by a thunderbolt of insight! The agency may be perpetuating more wrongs than righting injustices!

What is the next step for you? Do you quit in a huff? Is it more courageous to stay and try to work out positive change from within? This can sometimes be the wisest course.

Now here is another touchy one. Can you trust your supervisors? Are they unalterably aligned with the old established policy? Have they forgotten the needs of the people? Can you discreetly work with an authority figure and reawaken some of his former sensitivities?

Every day one is bound to hit a problem that is not in the rule book. You will bump into unspeakable, embarrassing situations that are not supposed to happen, or that workers in the past have chosen to ignore because there was no ready answer for handling them.

Here are some examples and a sprinkling of comments to stimulate your thinking about how to find some sort of solution of your own.

1. "Your family" on welfare seems to have plenty of cash for toys. The kids have the latest gadgets advertised on television. You do not want to be suspicious, but it is strange. You see evidence of numbers slips. You think the oldest brother is involved in illegal gambling. *Comment: First of all, do you know anything about the numbers rackets, how they are set up, why low-income people seem to enjoy playing the numbers? Shouldn't you learn more about the legal side of the situation? What is considered proof? If you decided to bring this to the attention of the legal authorities, would you have to appear in court? How does your suspicion about this illegal process affect your feelings about the family? Do you think all of them sanction dishonesty? Might not the parents be concerned about having the numbers in their home? Would you rather forget the whole thing than "rat" on the family? Would you go off and say, "I'm only here to be a health care worker, the numbers aren't my business."*

2. The mother listens carefully to your detailed explanation of how she should administer medication to a child recuperating from surgery. You check her records. Everything seems in order on paper. Something tells you to look at the medication bottles. There seem to be many more pills than there should be. Is she lying? *Comment: The medication is very important, and it would be an excellent idea to straighten this out for the patient's sake. What are the facts? If the mother is not giving the medication properly, why not? Is she afraid it is habit forming? Is she suspicious of side effects? Is she using this as a way of showing unconscious hostility to you? Does the medication taste bad and is the child have trouble swallowing it?*

3. You accompany your "family" on a visit to the out-patient clinic of a hospital. You have waited for almost 2 hours on the hard benches. Little Jackie needs a change of dressing and a treatment. The mother spots the physician who customarily treats little Jackie. As he passes, she gently reminds him that her son is becoming exhausted from the long wait. Dr. X is furious. He snaps back that he is overworked. Besides, he says loudly, clinic patients cannot expect the same service as private patients. *Comment: It is usually not good policy to sock a physician on the nose in front of a lot of witnesses. Can the entire problem of long waits, discourtesies, etc., be opened for discussion with medical students? Can a coalition of students and sensitive workers challenge this outrageous, undignified kind of treatment? Can any of us afford to let it stand as a tradition?*

4. You are sending a report to a social agency asking them for additional services for a member of your "family." The forms are complex. One of the questions, if you answered it honestly, would indicate that the child is ineligible for service. In confidence, the mother has indicated that

while she was married she had an extramarital affair, and the boy is not legitimate, in the strictest sense. Meanwhile, you hear rumors that the social agency in question has a reputation for carelessness with handling confidential material. Do you manipulate your report to disguise the facts? *Comment: This is an "elegant" compounding of establishment errors. One must consider why legitimacy has any bearing on the child's current needs. More urgently, how can our society permit erosion in the area of confidentiality? The health care worker is thus put into the position of stretching the truth or perpetuating outmoded values. As for confidentiality, is there no longer a reliable check and balance system within our institutions? Or is this only reserved for middle- and upper-income families?*

5. An unmarried woman, supported by the state, has produced six children out of wedlock and has become pregnant again. You broach the subject of family planning. The woman becomes furious, claims you are suggesting genocide. She feels strongly that you and your kind are trying to eradicate her group from the world. *Comment: If you find a way of answering this one, let us know.*

6. Your "family" makes grammatical errors to the point of murdering the King's English. They also use a colorful lingo, liberally sprinkled with terms related to waste elimination and sexual activity. Do you attempt to make them feel more at ease by falling in with their method of speaking? Or do you maintain your ordinary high school English syntax and refrain from adding "in-trend" phases? *Comment: It depends upon how comfortable you are in the dramatic arts. Ordinarily, one makes fewer errors if one stays in one's own character.*

7. Would you sincerely congratulate a 14-year-old girl on the birth of her second illegitimate baby? *Comment: How does the girl feel about the blessed event? If you think a new baby entering the world is cause for joy, then why not say so? If you are adversely affected, then no one says you have to be a hypocrite.*

8. If a teen-aged boy in your "family" confided to you that he was "splitting" and moving out of the state as soon as he got his high school diploma, would you feel it important enough to tip off his family? What if the family was depending on his presence in order to survive? *Comment: This is a much more complex problem than meets the eye. For instance, it indicates an awesome lack of communication within the family. There are depth-charged feelings behind his decision to leave without giving his folks a chance to prepare for an alternative solution. One could try to find out why the young man felt the way he did, but offhand, this is a matter to be handled by an experienced and very sensitive professional. Try to find one to help you out.*

9. A 10-year-old has an odd look in his eyes, and you wonder whether he has been experimenting with drugs. In numerous casual discussions

with the family, the parents openly pride themselves on their kids being strong enough to resist temptations of the neighborhood. *Comment: You will need more than a hunch to go on. There are other knowledgeable people who may have contact with the boy. Maybe you can piece the facts together. Who knows, you might be wrong.*

10. Your "family" is sheltering a son who has broken parole. Do you feel obligated to report him to the police? *Comment: Try to contact a member of the Fortune Society, a fast-growing group of former convicts with a firm grasp of the heres and nows of parolee situations. You need not reveal the name of the parolee to them, but the society might be able to track down the man's parole officer and give you a line on whether the man is going to get a fair shake. It might be that by careful handling, the young man could get into some worthwhile rehabilitation situation. Also consider what you discuss with your "family." After all, it's their son, and there is a trust relationship involved.*

11. Do you accept a cup of coffee from the lady of the house when you visit a low-income home? What if you preferred tea? Would you ask for it instead? Would you offer her one of your cigarettes if she were out of them? *Comment: Some of this has to do with agency policy, but it is pleasant when one can do what comes naturally.*

12. Should you accept or buy underground newspapers, handouts, and giveaways on the streets near where your "families" live? Might not people think you are some sort of radical or maybe even belong to a bunch of bombmakers? *Comment: How can you ever know what is going on if you never try to find out? Perhaps you and your close friends will want to go a few steps further and speak with the people distributing the ideas? You might be surprised to learn that your families may have either positive or negative feelings about these ideas. Your interest may also lay the groundwork for further talks.*

YOU ARE THE EXPERT; YOU ARE THE TOOL

Skim through professional journals, résumés of seminars, or conference critiques. Can you sense the fear about our crumbling institutions and agencies?

There is no longer a confident clear-cut way to "solve problems." Consumers do not always trust agencies enough to use their services.

You will find plenty of speakers and writers with exciting new theories on how to eliminate poverty and the misery it causes. Some of the ideas undoubtedly have merit. Each of these solutions is subject to interminable debate. The discussions appear to be as savage among the friends as the enemies of the ideas. There is so much vested interest. There is so much status to protect. It is very easy to become confused.

And if everyone agreed, then there would still be laws to be passed and funds to be appropriated. Who would get the cash, and how much of it would get into greedy hands instead of into the pockets of hungry people?

Things Are Changing

Well, maybe something new is happening and changes will be forced upon us. Poverty exists on a worldwide basis. Our mammoth agencies and traditional institutions may not exist in a few decades.

This may sound hopelessly overwhelming. Perhaps it is a new opportunity if we use the situation in the best interests of all people of all races and nationalities.

How Can We Salvage the Situation?

Perhaps we must simply return to ourselves. To be sure, there are many frightening aspects of change going on. Yet that is the most important time to become even more sensitive than before. We must find small groups of people willing to open themselves up to trust.

Who Are You?

We all have a lot to learn about ourselves. Working with low-income families, especially those with troubles, can be personally difficult to tolerate. Partially submerged fears and anxieties begin to surface. This is another good reason to become allied with sensitive and mature people with aims similar to your own. You will need emotional support.

Look at Your Motives

Are you in the "helping game" because you want power over others? Are you essentially a gullible kind of person who wants exposure to "real life"? Will encountering harsh realities tend to change you into a cynic? Will it make you hard? Or, with the help of others, can you grow in sensitivity and compassion?

How will you handle frustration or discouragement? Would working in difficult areas give you a ready-made excuse for tantrums and other regressive behavior?

After a day of meeting people living in squalor, would you go home feeling guilty, almost wishing you could ease your conscience by desecrating your own comfortable home? And then, there are the daydreams of glory—how you personally will salvage an entire neighborhood and earn the praise of all!

What Is Professionalism?

Whether you are being trained for nursing, medicine, social work, physical therapy, rehabilitation, etc., you will get certain basic skills and knowledge. Let us hope it is useful. Being professional, to some extent, encompasses much more than having the right training and the right degree of license. Professionalism is not too different from good manners.

For instance, a professional would approach a $1,000-a-year family with the same attitude as one with a $20,000-a-year income. You would hesitate to invade the privacy of either. One would certainly not betray confidences. It is only right to give equal respect to rich and poor alike.

This may seem simple. It is not. How many times have you been softened up by a high-status, well-to-do person? So watch it.

What to Watch For in Yourself

Try for a "here and now" realistic view of the family. Your sight will often be clouded by past experiences. You will not immediately recognize submerged prejudices. Don't be alarmed. All of us have these. We must have the patience and courage to root them out. Our sensitive friends can often point them up. You need not change your prejudice or point of view if you are aware of it and take it into account when making a decision.

For instance, if you come from a home where the bathtub is usually clean and the garbage pail routinely emptied, will it make your skin crawl on entering a smelly, infested house? If so, face it. How will your personal disgust affect the way you relate to the family? Will gamey socks and a stained undershirt on a man admitted to the emergency room alter your attitude toward him as the patient? Will you find it more difficult to give him his due as a first-class, full-quality patient?

Watch yourself and ask trusted coworkers to help you spot these personal reactions. Many observations will become obvious to you as you continue watching for them. For example, will you accept a reply to your questions from a neatly aproned housewife in the same way as from a slipshod one with a hint of beer on her breath?

How about judgmentalism? Are you turned off by a loud shrill voice?

Does a person who uses a four-letter, sex-oriented vocabulary seem less credible to you? Do you learn how to cut through the language and hear what may be attempted desperately to be communicated to you?

As if this were not enough, are you aware of your own stake in the situation? Do you expect some sort of thanks or reward in a spiritual, if not a concrete, form? If a family deteriorates while under your care, do you tend to repudiate it—to look for ways of blaming them or yourself? Are you working to help the family, or to get praise and a good rating from your supervisor?

This is why only a person capable of growth, warmth, and maturity should attempt to work with low-income families. It is not that you could not hold down the job, pass the tests, fill out the forms, etc. We owe these people superquality service until we can get them up to par with the rest of our citizens.

Rewards

We should speak of humility. It is not taught and some people never learn it. Warm human contact with those who survive and occasionally thrive under awful conditions can start you on a path to humility. Observe those with so much less than you, who make so much more of what they have. You can learn from a family and let them know about it. How wonderful for all of you to share an experience of coping with life.

Maybe you will be a creative health worker and find a better way to give assistance. There is a psychiatric hospital somewhere in New York State that offers vacations to the families of chronically emotionally ill patients. They simply take the patients back as short-term guests. This gives the ill person's relatives a chance to stretch, enjoy, and prepare for the continued battle against mental illness.

So many new ideas are needed: more free clinics, new kinds of half-way houses, day care, night care, etc. Could you be the one to develop something original, simple, and inexpensive?

Never Forget You Are Only a Tool

A capable carpenter keeps work tools in good shape and stores them in a proper place. Should not the health care worker take the same care to keep skills, knowledge, and attitude in fine working order? We can all get stale or fall in with the easy routine established ways of working. This is very easy to do while working with low-income families because a "who cares" attitude so often prevails among the professionals.

Find others like yourself among all the health care disciplines. Groups of mixed peoples can check on each other in a spirit of maturing relationships.

THE ULTIMATE AIM

Would it not be best if each family could decide its own aims and work out its own problems, financial or otherwise? Is not our job to help and then get out?

There are ideas under discussion about ombudsmen—neighbors of families who are friendly, trained visitors. These should be thoroughly acceptable to the family and used as resources as needed. Could not such a trained neighbor refer a sick child to a specialized agency as well as prepare the family for what it can expect? We are not sure that people prefer to receive assistance from racially or ethnically similar professionals, but we could learn to be more sensitive to what they do feel and do more about establishing a more realistic basis of trust.

Working with families in low-income areas is so huge a subject that it cannot be covered in a chapter of this size. But it can be explored as one human being to another and as one increasingly aware person learning to live with himself.

REFERENCES

Fromm, E. *The art of loving.* New York: Bantam Books, 1967.

Hurley R. *Poverty and mental retardation.* New York: Random House, 1971.

Jonas, G. *On doing good, the Quaker experiment.* New York: Charles Scribner's Sons, 1971.

O'Gorman, N. *The storefront.* New York: Harper & Row, 1970.

———. Storefront, *Columbia Forum,* 1970, *13,* 3.

Wheeler, G. R. America's new street people: Implications for the human services, *Social Work,* 1971, *16,* 19–24.

CHAPTER THIRTEEN

URBAN FAMILY HEALTH CARE

JEAN HUFF GALA AND HELEN REISCH MOORE

INTRODUCTION

The urban environment and its relationship to the health of its families is a puzzle that, to date, appears to have been studied in a piecemeal fashion. In addition, there is very little evidence that the findings of studies done on the various segments of the population (such as the poor, ethnic minority groups, the culturally deprived, stress factors, etc.) have influenced to any great extent program planning and provision of health services. The challenge to find new methods and approaches for improving the level of health not only of the various segments of the urban population but of the urban population as a whole must not be shelved. The reality is that an increasingly larger proportion of the world's population will be living in urban areas rather than in the countryside.

NUMBER OF FAMILIES LIVING IN URBAN AREAS IS ON THE INCREASE

The exact percentage of the population that is considered urban is dependent upon the way in which "urban" is defined. In recent years, the problem of how to classify people who live in suburban or rural-urban fringe areas has caused the Census Bureau to develop the concept of "urbanized" areas, and to define some 212 standard metropolitan statistical areas (SMSA). An urbanized area may lie outside the legal boundaries of the city, but it is characterized by urban residential density and is concerned primarily with the business, commerce, or communication activity of the central city. When the census was taken in 1790, about 5 percent of the population lived in urban places. By the year 1900, about 40 percent of the population lived in urban areas, and by 1960 the percentage had risen to 70 percent (Kommeyer, 1971).

Examining cities from an historical perspective, Toynbee (1970) predicts the emergence of a world city that he calls *ecumenopolis*. In contrast to ancient cities, our present-day mechanized cities are not stationary; they are dynamically on the move and changing into new types of cities, which he calls megalopolises. He defines the megalopolis as a "conurbation" of several very large cities such as Boston, New York, Philadelphia, Baltimore, and Washington along the northeastern seaboard of the United States. Toynbee views this development in North America as part of a trend that is worldwide. Toynbee believes that eventually the various megalopolises will stretch out their tentacles toward each other, forming a world city. In addition to these observations, Toynbee notes two currents, both of which are flowing in the same direction, which for him makes the coming of the world city a certainty. One current is the rapid growth of the world's population. The second is the simultaneous migration from the countryside into the cities that is taking place in "developing" and "developed" countries alike. If, in fact, this world city becomes a reality, we would then need to think about family health care on an international or global scale. Mind-boggling? Indeed! We have not yet come to grips with planning and meeting the health needs of families on a much smaller scale, i.e., for an urban area.

THE URBAN FAMILY—HEALTH PROBLEMS OBSERVED

In looking specifically at the health of an urban population, the authors must speak to the overwhelming and complex maze of problems compounded by poverty in the ghetto or transitional areas. However, "ghetto" is a misleading generalization for the mosaic of unique neighborhoods that form a city—each demonstrating unique variables in health and illness beliefs, risk factors, genetic traits, and social-structural conditions that influence levels of health. Indeed, one of the strongest biases of these authors is that, in viewing a population and planning to meet its health care needs, a model of "multiple causation of illness" as proposed by Cassel (1964) is urgently needed.

Historically, the patterns of disease affecting the urban dweller have changed over time.

> In 1900, the leading causes of death in the United States were communicable diseases, such as influenza, pneumonia, and tuberculosis, and these deaths occurred with disproportionate frequency in cities. The reduction of mortality

from such diseases has eliminated this historical relationship. The present leading causes of death, however, are again most frequently found in urban areas; this is particularly true of coronary heart disease and cancer. Generally, higher death rates from degenerative diseases are now associated with urban regions and those from communicable diseases with rural regions (Griffin, 1975, p. 15).

There are a number of health-threatening factors that emanate from an urban environment and impinge indiscriminately upon rich and poor alike. For example, various chemicals pollute the air that is breathed by all the residents of a city. Smog, smoke, elevated ozone levels, and exhausts from motor vehicles put healthy respiratory systems at risk and seriously impair the functioning of persons with chronic lung and heart disease. Chemically contaminated water and foodstuffs are increasingly linked to various types of cancers and genetic malformations. Occupational health hazards are being identified at an increasing rate and more and more public pressure is being placed on industry to protect their workers from identified hazards. Unfortunately, a backlog of court cases frequently enables industries to drag their feet on instituting the protective and preventive measures mandated by such governmental regulatory agencies as the Occupational Safety and Health Administration and the Environmental Protection Agency. Lead, especially in older homes near automotive dumps and expressways, presents a significant source of poisoning, particularly for young children.

Concern for physical safety and fear of bodily injury on the part of city dwellers is undoubtedly understandable. The evening news reinforces this fear on a daily basis. Fatalities and disabilities in significant numbers result from accidents on city streets, expressways, and mass transit systems. Conflicts within some ethnically mixed neighborhoods frequently escalate into open violence. Open warfare between rival neighborhood gangs is not uncommon. Drug-related crimes are on the increase. People of both lower- and higher-income neighborhoods are gradually becoming equally vulnerable to bodily harm. When the vast majority of the urban population perceives the city and the people in it as potentially dangerous, it is not surprising that many city health agencies are experiencing great difficulty in the recruitment of public health nurses for work in these neighborhoods.

The authors, in their work with families in a variety of urban neighborhoods, have observed the impact of the high crime rate on family life. For example, many families find it necessary to hire a sitter for their flat so that their furniture will not be stolen while they go grocery shopping or keep a clinic appointment. Children in many of the families are forced to pay "protection" money to local gangs—the price for refusing to join a gang. Signs are posted on apartment buildings warning the occupants that they must vacate the building by a specific time because the building is going to be set on fire. Well-kept neighborhood parks are not used by mothers of young children because of threats of violence from neighborhood gangs. Thus, the mothers and their children are prisoners in their own apartments. Under these circumstances, a kind of situational paranoia can be observed. People are fearful of, and alienated from, each other. How can parents simultaneously facilitate the development of trust in their children and at the same time teach them to protect themselves from all of the potential dangers in the environment? If the effort to promote mental health is to be successful, we cannot continue to ignore those factors in the environment that are working against positive mental health.

Lack of desired private space appears to provide additional sociological and biological stress to the urban dweller. Although these stresses have been well documented in animal experiments, we have as yet no definite answers for the effects on man. Basic information sufficient to establish human levels of tolerance for crowding is being sought by the Institute of Mental Health and by other agencies of the Department of Health, Education, and Welfare. It is known that the highest incidence of aberrant behavior—including crime and delinquency, drug abuse, and illegitimacy—and of other social and mental health problems occur when human beings are most densely packed. Obviously, people with higher incomes have the advantage of escaping from their crowded surroundings from time to time through travel. Poor families must live with what the core city holds for them (NIMH, April 1969).

Rodents and insects frequently come furnished with older apartment buildings and houses, and are difficult, if not impossible, to eradicate. In addition to the illnesses directly transmitted through bites by the infestors or their mites, another stressor often accompanies their presence. The authors are familiar with family members who shared chronic loss of sleep as they traded watches to protect sleeping infants from rat bites.

The necessity to accommodate to the rapid changes in the urban environment is another stress. Renewal programs, construction of expressways, problems of arson in the community, and racially changing neighborhoods convince the urban dweller that this place of residence cannot be considered permanent. These forced relocations often produce prolonged grieving from a profound sense of loss. The result of this grief poses a considerable threat to emotional health and social functioning (NIMH, April 1969).

PROBLEMS SPECIFIC TO THE NEW IMMIGRANT IN THE URBAN SETTING

A weighty challenge to the health care provider in any city is the presence of the family newly immigrated from either a totally different setting in this country or a foreign country. In addition to the general stresses and problems mentioned earlier in this chapter, the family's survival is placed at risk by separation from and loss of familiar structures, support systems, and important relationships. Language is not the only barrier to understanding vastly different customs and protocols. The type of housing initially chosen may be structurally unsound, crowded, and rodent- or insect-ridden. These accommodations are frequently viewed as temporary, while the family saves to become upwardly mobile. The fact remains, however, that all families do not have equal opportunity to become upwardly mobile.

It has long been true that the newest migrants to the cities of the United States come directly to the central core of the city. (This pattern does not seem to hold true universally, since, for example, in Latin America, the new migrants tend to settle first on the fringes of the city.) It is interesting to note that as the various migrant groups made economic gains they tended to move out of the central city and into the suburban areas. If the predominantly black and Puerto Rican populations presently occupying the central cities move out as they make economic gains, they will be following a well-established pattern in American migration. This is essentially what the migrants from Ireland, Germany, Italy, and the Eastern European countries did in earlier years. Blacks, however, face the problem of discrimination in the sale and rental of housing and in employment, so that it is more difficult for them to escape the central city, even when it is economically possible for them to do so (Kommeyer, 1971).

It is not uncommon to see a mutual avoidance pattern established between health workers and people they view as "different." Very different illness beliefs and behaviors often cause the health professional to label immigrant families as resistant or noncompliant to medical care. Conversely, the impersonal, rushed atmosphere of the health department or hospital clinics often does not meet the expectations or needs of families for personal caring, and produces an equally angry labeling of health services as cold, impolite, and money grasping. Differences in parenting practices, family composition, and routines also exist, and must be studied on an individual basis if the health professional would intervene constructively into the family life-style.

Another fairly common problem encountered by health service agencies and institutions is that of providing interpreters, advocates, and representatives for the specific immigrant groups. Optimally, these personnel should be chosen on the basis of skill and acceptability of the community they will be representing.

A large percentage of the newly immigrated find that the only jobs readily available to them are within factories, and involve manual skills and body mechanics that they do not have. Out of urgency to achieve financial support, they may claim competency, and suffer either mutilating injuries to the hands or back injuries due to strains. It is important for the health professional working with the newly immigrated to become knowledgeable about symptoms of significant illnesses within the geographic area of origin, so that signs of hookworm, leprosy, malaria, etc., are not overlooked or misinterpreted.

THE URBAN FAMILY AS IT RELATES TO THE COMMUNITY

An attempt has been made thus far to present a case for the importance of recognizing that the urban setting, in fact, has no "typical" family with a characteristic quality or brand of relationship to a "typical" community. It is fairly evident, however, that within the myriad communities comprising an urban area, some families survive, whereas others become victims of a discouraged or disruptive life-style.

It would seem highly appropriate at this point to hypothesize salient skills that enable families to survive, functioning cooperatively and contributively within a given community. One very important skill would be ascertaining how and whereby daily needs could be met—including such basic needs as food, employment, shelter, health care, and assistance in problem solving. A second skill that assists survival is the ability to identify and utilize a support system; be it kin, friends, neighbors, or agency-network. A rather complex challenge to family survival occurs when the sole support system exists in a far distant location, such as Puerto Rico, Mexico, or Tennessee. Another important skill that facilitates survival in the urban setting is utilizing available resources to the family's best advantage. A highly operant level of functioning of this skill might even include the creation of new resources. An example would be the organization of a neighborhood baby-sitting pool. A second example might be the use of block clubs, which constitute the banding together of neighbors to solve certain neighborhood problems. Finally, the family with a sense of some power to make desirable changes in its own world, and the ability to adjust to external changes that affect its environment, is more likely to survive within a given community in the urban setting, where neighborhoods are constantly being pressured for entrance by groups with different color, race, religion, customs, and values.

THE COMMUNITY AS IT RELATES TO THE URBAN FAMILY

Obviously, if health and health-related resources are to be effective in promoting a high level of wellness in the population served, they must be utilized. To be utilized, they must be easily accessible to families, render a high quality service, and communicate a sense of genuine caring.

How do health and health-related resources bridge distances between themselves and individual families? There is no simple answer to this question; however, the first step would be willingness and readiness on the part of health care professionals to see a problem of consumer disenchantment when it does exist. The second step would be to determine consumer's perceptions of the problem(s). Finally, a mutually agreeable solution would be actively sought. Advisory boards composed of health care providers and consumers are mechanisms frequently used by neighborhood health centers to bridge any distance that may exist. To determine if the advisory board is effective, one need only be sensitive to families' attitudes about the health center. If the residents feel the neighborhood health center is theirs, one can be fairly sure the goal of bridging distances has been attained. One example is the Mom and Tots Center, which was the only building in a block spared from destruction in the Detroit riots of 1967 (Milio, 1971).

Characteristically, urban areas have an abundance of health and welfare resources. Lack of coordination of efforts between agency representatives when more than one resource is being utilized by a family is a very common problem. Duplication of services, working at cross-purposes, confusion in the family, and weakening of the family as a unit may be the end result. Although it takes time and effort to establish collaborative relationships in these situations, it is time well spent, and a positive outcome for the family usually is the end product. Some urban neighborhoods have organized health and welfare councils composed of representatives from all the health and welfare agencies serving a defined geographic area of the city. The council members meet on a regular basis to share with each other. They keep each other informed about their programs, policies, and problems encountered in the community. Meetings are kept as informal as possible, so that workers from the various agencies have the opportunity to get to know each other by name and face. This facilitates the development of collaborative relationships when the need arises with individual families in the community.

FLAWS IN THE FAMILY HEALTH CARE SYSTEM

In looking specifically at urban family health care, fundamental debits appear to be most glaring in the areas of: lack of identification and attention to actual need, a limited definition of health that fails to take into account social factors that directly or indirectly affect health, feeble attempts to gear service to the differences in life-style and health and illness behaviors encountered, and the need for revival of the element of caring.

The first debit, lack of identification and attention to actual need, seems to relate directly to the second debit, a limited definition of health.

Public health programs in general are aimed at populations who have been identified as being at risk to a certain disease or condition. However, the process of instituting new programs by responsible boards and agencies often seems geared largely to discovering in what categories funds are available, and then jumping on that bandwagon. One need only look at the proliferation of proprietary home health agencies in the metropolis, and note the high instance of Medicare fraud, to realize that health care can make money at the expense of the consumer. The categorical grant has gotten in the way of planning programs based on actual need in a broad spectrum of the population. With these grants, monies are often withdrawn prematurely; e.g., in the mid-1950s, monies for programs to combat venereal disease were drastically cut at a point when the prevalence had dropped to an all-time low. Today, we see the folly of that decision, as these diseases are once again on the increase.

The germ theory, with its fairly clear-cut cause-effect relationship, provided the basis for highly effective programs for populations at risk to communicable diseases. However, in noncommunicable diseases and health conditions, the cause-effect relationship is not so clear-cut and the problem of identifying populations at risk is, therefore, more difficult.

Griffin (1975) makes a very strong case for the need to develop a model of multiple causation rather than continuing to rely on the germ theory. A working hypothesis based on a century of documented evidence states that stress contributes to increased susceptibility to disease. A number of the stressors alluded to earlier in the chapter arise from the social environment. Examples of these are problems of adaptation to urbanization, social disintegration (i.e., people living as neighbors, but having no patterned relationships with each other), cultural conflicts, and loss of familiar life situations and support systems via the uprooting process. Studies by Holmes and Masuda (1972) have shown that stress, resulting from significant life changes, not only increases susceptibility to illness, but actually results in illness and/or death if enough of these changes occur within one year and the cumulative stress value reaches a high level. They found that as the number of life change units increased, the connection between life crisis and illness became more certain.

The third debit, failure to gear health care services to cultural differences, is expressed in a variety of negative behaviors on the part of consumers. Health departments, outpatient clinics, and family practice groups ponder agonizingly over missed appointments. Lack of compliance with prescribed treatment regimens is common. Health teaching efforts frequently fail to bring about desired changes in health behavior. Interest in disease prevention holds little appeal to the family burdened with the magnitude of "here and now" problems. Frequently, health workers who hold to a limited definition of health, fail to concern themselves with those "other problems," which they believe have no relationship to health. Once again, a mutual avoidance pattern sets in: The health worker is angry because the family does not change its health behavior, and the family is angry at the health worker's insensitivity and lack of concern about problems that are so important to the family. Whose priorities are more important? Success or failure on the part of health care providers may depend to a very great extent on how that question is answered. It is ironic that provider agencies frequently maintain hours of operation, regulations, structures, and regimens that, at best, display little understanding of cultural mores, value systems, and usual illness behavior. At worst, these methods of providing urban family health care frequently mystify, alienate, or disgust those persons supposedly being "helped."

Finally, the element of personal caring on the part of the helping or health care agency would seem to be a treasure no longer available to the consumer of urban health care (Fuchs, 1974). The lack of a readily available familial support system would seem to accentuate an even greater need for caring on the part of the professional agency. In the hospital emergency room, or outpatient clinic, which has become their access to a physician, consumers meet with irritating waits, minuscule allotments of time, cursory attention to underlying problems, and, at times, an atmosphere of hostile impatience or enmity. If admitted to inpatient units, they suffer care that probes and pokes at an interesting specimen rather than a person. It is the authors' bias that the "rent-a-nurse" agencies, that provide nurses who work a night here and there, abet this impersonality.

RADICAL CHANGE VERSUS BAND-AIDS

The percentage of the population living in urban areas is expected to continue to increase not only in the United States, but throughout the world (Toynbee, 1970). Cities offer families a mixed diet. Nowhere else is life so stimulating, transportation so convenient, jobs so plentiful, and advancement so possible . . . at least for some urban families. For other urban families, life in the city does not offer such a positive experience. Stresses that arise from the social setting present hazards to family health. There is considerable evidence that stress is significant as a causative factor in diseases of many types, including chronic and disabling diseases (Griffin, 1975; Holmes, 1972). Thus far, health professionals who work within the health care system have not yet decided to share the responsibility for eradicating those causes of illness. Is this the fault of the health care system?

There is a general agreement among providers and consumers that our current health care system has many shortcomings. Some critics are so dissatisfied that they are convinced an overhaul of the system would not make it better and that it should be traded in for a whole new system. The authors, on the other hand, have implied that there are problems more basic than the system itself that need to be addressed. Health care planners and providers must take a more comprehensive view of health and the multiple factors that influence health. Germs are no longer the leading cause of illness. At the present time, the causative factors of illness are part and parcel not only of the physical environment but of the social environment. Therefore, health promotion activities, if they are to be genuinely effective, need to reflect an understanding of the influence of many different social, emotional, and cultural factors on health and health behavior. Finally, if family health status is really to be improved, health professionals must learn to function as social change agents by providing leadership to harness the various political, economic, and social forces necessary to bring about change in the social environment. Conditions that are known to have an adverse effect on the health of urban families must be attacked with the kind of zeal that was so well demonstrated in, for example, the fight against poliomyelitis. Band-aid approaches have lost their credibility for consumers. The authors believe that providers of health care have their work cut out for them regardless of whether the health care system is revamped or remains the same.

REFERENCES

Cassel, J. Social science theory as a source of hypotheses in epidemiological research. *American Journal of Public Health,* 1964, *54,* 1482–1488.

Fuchs, V. R. *Who shall live?* New York: Basic Books, 1974.

Griffin, R. N. Jr. Social structure and urban diseases: Need for a broader base for health planning and research. *The Urban & Social Change Review,* 1975, *8*(1), 15–20.

Holmes, T. H., & Masuda, M. Psychosomatic syndrome: When mothers-in-law or other disasters visit, a person can develop a bad, bad cold, or worse. *Psychology Today,* April 1972, *6,* pp. 71–106.

Kommeyer, K. C. *An introduction to population.* San Francisco: Chandler, 1971.

Milio, N. *9226 Kercheval—The storefront that did not burn.* Ann Arbor: University of Michigan Press, 1971.

National Institute of Mental Health. *The mental health of urban America.* U.S. Department of Health, Education, and Welfare, Publication No. 1906, April, 1969.

Toynbee, A. *Cities on the move.* New York and London: Oxford University Press, 1970.

CHAPTER FOURTEEN

CHANGING NUTRITIONAL STYLES WITHIN THE CONTEXT OF THE MODERN FAMILY

NORGE W. JEROME

Nutrition, particularly that aspect largely concerned with food selection, provides an excellent vehicle for understanding how the family or domestic unit facilitates or hinders an individual's health. Family influences on nutritional health begin at birth and continue throughout life, although the level of influence will vary with the psychosocial and cultural situation and the individual's stage of development.

For example, the young child up to the age of 6 years is greatly influenced by the dietary styles of the immediate family, including full- and part-time nonkin caretakers. However, as the child expands his or her horizons beyond the home and the family to include peer and other social groups, the influence of the family on dietary styles diminishes appreciably. However, these influences will continue to be felt and expressed periodically in connection with religious and family rites and ceremonies.

The psychosocial situation surrounding eating during the early formative years may also have immediate and long-term nutritional consequences. The young child, and indeed all members of the family, is likely to enjoy and derive nutritional benefits from meals that are served in a peaceful, pleasant, and nurturing environment. By contrast, a disruptive, distracting environment often leads to various eating syndromes and their attendant nutritional problems. Force feeding, and constant eating in a tension-filled environment, for example, could lead to a persistent "fear of eating" syndrome and nutritional disorders.

Family influences are especially evident in the young child's food selection and consumption patterns. In early life, individuals are initiated to materials labeled food by the family and culture; over a period of time, through repetitive behavior they learn to combine food items, colors, textures, and flavors into patterns deemed appropriate by the family and culture. At the same time, where the family setting is noncoercive, each person is encouraged to develop and cultivate his or her personal dietary tastes along lines that promote the individual's nutritional health.

The family setting is particularly influential in teaching social rules governing food etiquette and eating schedules, meal-eating and snacking, food preparation, distribution and exchange, and helping and serving sizes. The family also provides guidance in differentiating home-based from away-from-home eating, nutritious from "junk" foods, prestige from taboo foods, male foods from female foods, children's foods from adult foods, and foods for the sick from those for the healthy. The family therefore functions as a microculture by filtering from the larger culture those values and patterns it deems appropriate for nutritional health and gustatory satisfaction of its members.

The transmission of foodways and diet patterns is far from unidirectional, however. It follows multiple pathways from the larger external macroculture to the family as a microculture, from the older to the younger generation, and from young members of the family to adults. Developments in the macroculture are first filtered through the various individuals comprising the corporate structure of the family before they become established as a family diet pattern. For example, family food styles and diet patterns respond to changes in group ideology, social interaction, and communication patterns, and to changes in national policies and programs particularly as they relate to agriculture and commerce. Food styles of families also change in response to changes in the production, trade, processing, marketing, and distribution of foods. Family members respond to these social and technological developments individually and usually act on them in the family setting. Thus, each learns from the other by observing, sampling, and experimenting with new ideas and novel foods and food combinations. In time, new nutritional patterns emerge that are simultaneously unique to the individual and to the family as a microculture. Family dietary styles and nutritional patterns are therefore dynamic, since they are constantly undergoing change.

The rapid pace of social, technological, and other changes in contemporary U.S. society forces the health practitioner to pay special attention to variations in family nutritional patterns. Important clues on health status may be missed if the practitioner assumes that nutritional uniformity obtains when variation is often the rule.

This chapter describes how changing ideologies and life-styles in the

1960s and 1970s, a period of rapid social change in the United States, influence food use and nutrition of American families. This chapter is therefore concerned with dietary responses to social change.

The 1960s and 1970s will be recorded as an era marked by rapid social change, and distinguished by two major social movements: (1) *self-assertion* and its accompanying activism, individualism, and expansion of consciousness, and (2) *revitalization* with its attendant theme on self-reliance, the search for practical purpose, and the validation of the person as a member of small, close groups. The revitalization movement is best recognized by "return-to-roots" themes and activities.

Both movements have had an effect on family structure and relationships, which in turn have influenced patterns of food production, marketing, and exchange, and the selection, distribution, and consumption of foods. Any change in traditional food-use patterns has important nutritional health consequences for the individual.

The self-assertion movement had its beginning with the Civil Rights movement for blacks in the 1960s, but by the early 1970s had expanded to include other "minorities." By 1977 the rights of other ethnic minorities, the elderly, women, children, youth, homosexuals, individuals with visible physical and mental impairment, and those who had been confined to institutions had been addressed. The assertion of individual rights for highly visible subgroups within the society has had its impact on family organization and structure, the redefinition of roles, relationships, and responsibilities, and a reconceptualization of self. Trends away from institutionalized health care toward self-care in health and nutrition are prime examples of the self-assertion movement. By actively asserting the self, personal goals change, as do living styles and arrangements. These changes are reflected in patterns of food use and in nutrition.

A study on the American family sponsored by the Consumer Center of General Mills, Inc. and conducted by Yankelovich, Skelly and White in 1976 provided some insight on the topic of changing family styles and nutrition. The results are based on a national probability sample of 1230 families; interviewees included children between the ages of 6 and 12 years and parents. According to this study, American families fall into two distinct groups—the "new breed" parents, representing 43 percent of all fathers and mothers of children under 13 years of age; and the "traditionalists," who represent the majority (57 percent) of all parents.

New breed parents tend to be better educated and more affluent, and have adopted a new set of attitudes toward the relationships of parents to children. They epitomize the goal of self-assertion. Compared to previous generations, new breed parents are less child-oriented and more self-oriented. They regard having children as one available option that they have chosen freely and not as a social obligation. New breed parents question the idea of sacrificing in order to give their children the best of everything and are firm believers in the equal rights of children and parents. They believe that boys and girls should be raised alike and that children should be free to make their own decisions, including food selection.

The beliefs of new breed parents have important nutritional consequences, since their doctrine places the responsibility of diet selection on young family members who are often ill-equipped to make appropriate decisions on diet and nutrition. Furthermore, the decisions made by children are often influenced by many external forces, including print and television food advertisements, peer groups, and other nonfamily members. Also, like adults, children's food selection and consumption patterns are further influenced by the available food supply. Thus, the unsupervised child in American society is placed in a very difficult position of trying to select dietary items away from home from among a wide array of attractive, ready-to-eat foods and beverages of varying nutritional quality. New breed parents have therefore abrogated their roles as filterers of the macroculture in an important aspect of health.

Self-assertion through diet selection has many dimensions. This phenomenon has been described by Jerome (1972), Fine (1971), and Kahn (1976). Jerome labeled the phenomenon "dietary individualism" and went on to describe that this dietary style was a peculiar response to food abundance, complexity, and diversity in a modern Western society (Jerome 1975, 1976).

In a study on dietary patterns and food habits conducted by the author in 1971, a sample of 150 households (575 individuals) included 1466 items in the customary diet. The respondent households represented a 5 percent random sample of households in a low-to-middle-income community in a midwestern city. The 1466 items were fairly evenly distributed within four consumption cycles (very high through very low frequencies), thus indicating either the selection of a wide range of foods by the group as a whole, or intrahousehold variation in food selection. Both theories were upheld in further in-depth study of a subsample of 26 of the original 150 households. The subsample of 54 individuals (17 percent of the households and 9 percent of the individuals in the original study sample) provided detailed records on individual activities, eating sites and schedules, and on food and beverage items consumed during 3 to 7 consecutive days. Records were analyzed to determine what items were included in each person's diet at the time of eating, and whether eating was communal or individualized.

As a group, the respondents consumed 87 different items at breakfast, 186 at lunch, and 199 at dinner. Individuals in each household either sat together at mealtime or ate separately either at home or away from home.

When eating together, each person consistently selected fewer than the total number of items available to the group; individuals rarely chose identical items. Eating separately was a frequent occurrence; each individual maintained his or her own primary schedule for work, school, avocation, and recreation and then adjusted eating into that schedule; the result of such individuated schedules was an individualized diet selection and consumption pattern.

Obviously, food abundance and diversity, easy access to foods and beverages, and the varied schedules of family members have direct links with the individualized eating patterns. Some authors have commented on the rapid disappearance of the traditional three-meals-a-day eating pattern. Breakfast is particularly vulnerable to that trend (LaChance, 1973). Eating today, according to Fine (1971), should be viewed as a nonstop activity of the many, minimeal pattern.

A recent article by Kahn (1976) reported additional trends toward *dietary individualism* for younger small households, i.e., young single men, young single women, and young couples. Members of these younger small households espoused individualistic food and eating goals: fewer meals, less emphasis on a particular time to eat, and eating in response to hunger. Statements made by the respondents indicated that while eating is viewed as a necessary activity, it is secondary to self-realization.

For these younger small households, eating is a daily choice with no ritualistic three meals a day at appointed times; the items consumed at a given time depend on whatever the individual feels like eating at the time and whatever suits the needs of the moment. Jerome (1972, 1975) had found similar attitudes and practices among the 150 respondent households. When volunteering information on dietary practices, few were willing to commit themselves to a firm dietary practice; responses were conditioned by "it depends on how we feel at the time," or, "sometimes we do and sometimes we don't . . . it depends on what else is going on." Questions concerning traditional practices yielded responses such as "most times . . . depending on the . . . children . . . mother . . . husband . . . friend," etc. In fact, the individual food records of the subsample of 26 respondent households are a direct result of these conditioned responses from the larger sample.

Some consumers see a direct relationship between the difficulties they encounter in providing a nutritious diet for their families and assertiveness of family members. A consumer study on nutrition conducted by the A. C. Nielson Company in 1976 revealed that while 88 percent of the 1000 households surveyed indicated that they did not have problems in providing a proper nutritional diet, the 12 percent with problems linked a significant number of their problems to dietary individualism. For example, 12 percent of those with problems cited "the family doesn't like what is good for them"; 7 percent stated "work—hard to prepare a meal in a hurry"; and 4 percent gave as a deterrent "everyone likes different things." Although the latter response was reported as a problem, in light of other observations referred to previously, this expression might have been viewed positively by the 88 percent of the households who reported that they had no problems in providing a nutritious diet for their families.

Dietary individualism is apparently reinforced by the self-selection style practiced in restaurants, cafeterias, and fast-food establishments. Away-from-home eating has shown a sharp increase during the last two decades. The share of food dollars going for away-from-home eating rose from 20 to 21 percent in 1950 and 1960 to 23 percent in 1970 and 25 percent in 1975 and 1976 (NFS, 1977, p. 25). Away-from-home eating is popular among younger households. A 1976 Department of Agriculture Survey of 1400 United States households revealed that in the previous year, 90 percent of those surveyed had eaten out. The majority (96 percent) of those eating out in 1975, were under 50 years old; only 74 percent of those 65 years old had eaten out that year. Fast-food restaurants were favored by the younger (under 50) respondents. Over 60 percent of the households who ate away from home did so in restaurants where the main course was under $5.00. These moderately priced restaurants were favored by all age groups and were the most popular kind of restaurant with the elderly (NFS, 1977, p. 25).

Fast-food establishments have grown appreciably between 1965 and 1975. During that time, their share of the away-from-home food market grew from 10.5 to 26 percent. At the same time, the share of conventional restaurants, lunch rooms, cafeterias, and caterers declined from 45 to 39 percent. This development represents an interesting social and economic phenomenon, and it has been attributed to "rising consumer incomes and continued increases in the number of working wives" (NFR, 1978, p. 33).

Undoubtedly, families utilize fast-food establishments as family kitchens and dining rooms—a new and important trend in U.S. foodways and dietary patterns. The health practitioner must take into account this new trend in eating style by the modern American family in order to act realistically and appropriately in nutritional care programs.

The assertion of self as a factor in diet selection is rooted in ideology but facilitated by food abundance and diversity, and by social and technological developments. The bounteous food supply permits individuals to pursue their goals for self-enchancement without being burdened by the quest for food. It is of interest to note that dietary individualism parallels the dietary style of the ancient fruit, nut, and insect gatherer whose individualized mode of food procurement and consumption was dictated by periodic scarcity and primitive technology rather than by the bounteous harvest of a highly industrialized, modern society. Obviously, we have turned to some of the dietary methods of our ancestors as a result of supertechnology.

Revitalization[1] as a movement in social change symbolizes an attempt to recapture a fading culture or a glorious past in order to explain an unsatisfying present and point the way to a more fulfilling future. Cultural revivals often accompanied threats to group identity. This "return to roots" movement is manifest in dress, art, music, coiffure, life-style, and diet. The movement assumes variant forms in both life-style and diet. With regard to food use and diet patterns, the two extremes are recognized in the search for *pure foods,* preferably home grown and prepared, and in the preparation and enjoyment of *exotic dishes* in gourmet fashion. Health, pleasure, and conscious, sophisticated dining are the key interests in the two forms discussed here.

In its extreme form, the revitalization movement peaked in the late 1960s and early 1970s with public protests by the "flower children" and the strident voices of young adults who "dropped out" of society for a different life-style in rural and urban communes. This "back to nature and people" movement represented an attempt to neutralize the threats of "big government," "big business," and "big technology."

The environment and humanity were at stake. More importantly, the quality of the food supply was questioned, and food became a focal issue. "The forces at work," states Hall (1974, p. 38) " were public awareness, and an uneasiness that the new food technologies were somehow getting out of hand; scientists' lack of interest in studying and assessing the secondary effects of new technologies; and the government's inability to monitor the rapidly changing technology in food and agriculture."

The economic recession of the early 1970s coupled with heralded world scarcities in basic resources—energy and food—literally added fuel to the ferment by providing a well-defined rationale for conserving the food supply and improving health at relatively little cost. The "vegetarian way" addressed all the issues and solved as many problems. It was an attempt by American youth to redress the "greed and wantonness" of previous generations. Parents reacted with concern because the new dietary style did not conform to their ideas of "the basic four" or "three squares."

New labels and terminologies were specially developed to describe the value systems and diet practices of those subscribing to alternative dietary styles. Unquestionably, the goal was to achieve or maintain health. Thus, foods were classified as being "natural," "organic," "health," or "junk," and systems of food production, processing, marketing, preparation, and consumption were similarly classified.

During the past 10 years hundreds of new industries have been created to cater to the needs of the millions of individuals and families

[1]The term was used by Anthony F. C. Wallace, "Revitalization Movements," in Barry McLaughlin, ed., *Studies in Social Movements: A Social Psychological Perspective* (New York: The Free Press, 1969), pp. 30–52.

who eschew the fabricated items of chemical food technology. These industries provide services in the production and processing of food and beverages at home, and centers for securing nutritional supplements and commercially prepared health foods. Growth of these establishments has been phenomenal.

A 1977 U.S. Department of Agriculture report indicated that sales of health foods are growing not only in the United States, but in Europe as well. It is estimated that by 1980 sales should reach 1 percent of the nation's grocery bills, double the sales of such items at the beginning of the 1970s (LeBovit, 1977). A 1972 report showing that year's sales by health food outlets at $500 million, projected an increase in sales by these outlets to $3 billion in 1980 (Wolmak, 1972). Recently, *Newsweek* projected 1977 sales of the 3500 health food stores in the United States at $900 million. Differences in the figures and projections reflect the difficulties inherent in making determinations in new developments that are not clearly defined. It is clear, however, that the health food industry has grown by leaps and bounds and will continue to grow. To developers and users of the industry, such interest and awareness are revitalizing.

These recent developments have added an important dimension to food use and nutrition in contemporary America. In addition, social interactions surrounding food and eating are being redefined and strengthened as individuals take time out to develop relationships with others and with the natural environment; this strengthening of relationships occurs as people produce foods, exchange sources, ideas, and recipes, and create food products and dishes.

The current popularity of gourmet foods and exotic dishes is closely linked to the health food movement. The two developments have much in common—both provide creative outlets for their adherents and underscore a movement away from the mass production of foods and ingredients and toward the creation of special dishes that are "better" and "healthier" because they are produced or prepared by one's own hands, in intimate surroundings, or under known conditions.

How do those apparently opposing developments in food use and nutrition—the self-assertion and revitalization movements—influence the nutritional health of individual family members? How do family members accommodate to an increase in the use of fast-food *and* health-food establishments? Are family relationships affected by these developments?

It must first be pointed out that social change and the resultant dietary change do not proceed in linear fashion. Individuals vary, and the opportunities and preconditions for change vary within the population at large, among subgroups, and within families. Inter- and intragroup variations and inter- and intrafamily variations are the norm. It is to be expected that the self-assertion and revitalization movements as they influence food use will have a different impact on each family.

Variations among subgroups and families and within subgroups and families will reflect the propensity of each family to filter selectively from the macroculture only those elements that "fit" into the family's microculture. Factors influencing selective filtering include religion and ideology, location, age structure, family composition, and patterns of interaction among family members. Interfamily and intergroup variations will also reflect the quality and nature of contacts with other members of the society; the personal goals and life-styles of each member of a family will also influence variability within the family. These variations add to the complexities of modern family life and present serious challenges to the individual in his or her quest for health in general and nutritional health in particular.

Dietary patterns do not develop or change in isolation. They are integrated into society's fabric and follow recognizable societal changes. By understanding the moods, themes, and changes in society one gains insight on behaviors that impinge upon the diet, nutrition, and health of individuals in the society.

The health practitioner must develop skills that would assist each client in the assessment of the biological, psychosocial, and cultural dimensions of nutritional health on a continuous basis. The individual should be made aware of how certain social developments, actions, and decisions may have positive or negative consequences on nutritional health. Each person should learn how to complement and supplement dietary items in accordance with existing sociocultural conditions in order to maintain or achieve nutritional health. The family setting is ideal for implementing these nutritional and health goals.

REFERENCES

Fine, P. A. Modern eating patterns—the structure of reality. Presented at the *American Medical Association* symposium on "Eating patterns and their influence on purchasing behavior and nutrition," November 1971.

Hall, R. H. *Food for nought: The decline of nutrition.* New York: Harper & Row, 1974.

Jerome, N. W. Individualized home diets: Response to food diversity in an "economically depressed" U.S. urban community. *Federation Proceedings* (Abstracts), 1972, *31*(2), 718.

———. On determining food patterns of urban dwellers in contemporary U.S. society. *In Gastronomy: The anthropology of food and food habits,* M. Arnott (Ed.), Mouton Publishers, 1975, 91–111.

———. Individuals, not families, are the key to nutrition. *Community Nutrition Institute Newsletter,* 1976, *6*(36), 4–5.

Kahn, P. One and two-member household feeding patterns. *Food Product Development,* October 1976, *10*(8), 22.

LaChance, P. A. The vanishing American meal. *Food Product Development,* 1973, *7*(9), 36.

LeBovit, C. The Health Foods Market. *National Food Situation*–161, 17–18 September 1977.

National Food Situation–161, September 1977. p. 25

National Food Review–1 January 1978. p. 33.

Newsweek, December 19, 1977.

Nutrition . . . food for thought: Is the consumer getting the message? A. C. Nielsen, 1976.

Wallace, F. C.: Revitalization movements. In B. McLaughlin (Ed.), *Studies in social movements: A social psychological perspective.* New York: Free Press, 1969.

Wolmak, B. Food industry and FDA face fad food threat. *Food Product Development, August*–September 1972, 6, 28.

CHAPTER FIFTEEN

DENTAL HEALTH AND THE FAMILY

CHARLES L. DUNLAP

Dental diseases are among the most prevalent of diseases. They are also the most preventable. Caries and periodontitis and their sequelae account for the bulk of oral disorders. Though they seldom represent a serious threat to the individual patient, the sheer number of people they affect makes them a major nuisance to public health. Toothaches, abscesses, and cellulitis arising from dental infections cause much suffering and account for thousands of lost school and work hours each year. Americans spent $8.6 billion for dental care in 1976.

Because caries (decay) and periodontitis (pyorrhea) are the major diseases, they will be discussed first. A section will be devoted to oral cancer. Two "nuisance" diseases, herpetic lesions and canker sores, will be covered because they are so common and frequently confused with each other.

CARIES

Though there are several inheritable and environmental factors that may cause diseases of the teeth, dental caries is virtually the only disease that attacks teeth after they have erupted into the mouth. Caries may start any time in life, but commonly occur soon after the teeth erupt. Both deciduous and permanent teeth are affected. In one survey (*Decayed*, 1971) 14 percent of children age 6 had at least one decayed tooth; by age 17, 90 percent had caries (*Decayed*, 1974).

Untreated caries leads to progressive destruction of teeth followed by painful infections requiring extraction of the infected tooth. Decay, thus, is one of the major causes of tooth loss, especially up to middle age, when periodontitis (pyorrhea) becomes the leading cause of tooth loss. One survey conducted by the Department of Health, Education, and Welfare showed 20 million people, 18 percent of the nation's adult population, had lost all of their teeth as a result of caries and periodontitis (*Total Loss,* 1967).

Cause of Dental Caries

Many factors influence the development of dental caries. The most important factor is a sticky film of material that accumulates on teeth. The material is called dental plaque. It consists of tenacious polysaccharide secreted chiefly by streptococci. Literally millions of bacteria live in dental plaque. These bacteria convert sugar in the person's diet into acid, which demineralizes the tooth. The defect in the tooth surface permits proteolytic bacteria to destroy the organic matrix of the tooth.

Plaque tends to accumulate in the sheltered areas of the teeth such as grooves on the biting surface of molar teeth and the "in-between" surfaces where teeth touch each other.

Other than plaque, major factors that influence caries formation include diet, fluoride content of teeth, and salivary flow. Common sense tells us not to consume excessive sugar, which is a substrate for acid production. Fluoride makes the tooth less susceptible to decay, probably by decreasing solubility. It is most effective when given during the years the teeth are forming, because the fluoride is incorporated into the entire tooth. More than a 50 percent reduction in decay can be expected when the teeth have optimum fluoride content.

An especially severe type of decay is seen in individuals who have received radiation to the head and neck, usually for oral cancer. Within a few months to a few years, the salivary glands slowly cease to function and the person develops dry mouth. Brown et al. (1976) reported a 93 percent reduction in salivary secretion. This leads to caries on virtually every tooth, especially around the neck of the tooth at the gum line. Wescott et al. (1975) have shown that postradiation dental caries can be prevented by daily topical application of 0.4% stannous fluoride gel.

Sequelae of Caries

Decay will eventually destroy the tooth substance and expose the dental pulp in the center of the tooth. This leads to infection of the pulp, which usually causes severe pain. The infection will spread down the inside of the tooth and exit into surrounding bone. Severe infection will lead to abscess formation and osteomyelitis. Mild infections accompanied by good host resistance may keep the infection localized around the root end, where a cyst may form.

Prevention of Caries

Nothing beats good dental hygiene. Daily removal of bacterial plaque with toothbrush and dental floss is the first line of defense. The next best thing is daily consumption of approximately 1 mg. of fluoride. This is best achieved by drinking water whose fluoride content is approximately 1 part per million. Since total intake depends on the amount of water consumed, the fluoride content of community drinking water should be adjusted to take into account the average temperature of the community. People who live in hot climates drink more water and the fluoride content should be reduced. A discussion of adjusting fluoride levels in public water supplies can be found in the References (Richards et al., 1967).

Topical application of fluoride is also beneficial. This may be in the form of fluoride toothpaste or periodic application by a dentist. Recently a fluoride mouthwash has become available. There is no set rule as to how often topical application should be done. Those with extremely high caries susceptibility should have daily application, whereas once a year may be adequate for others.

A SPECIAL DENTAL PROBLEM IN INFANTS

An unusually severe type of decay occurs in some infants who fall asleep with a nursing bottle in their mouth. It is called the "nursing-bottle syndrome" and is characterized by rapid and widespread decay of the deciduous teeth. Although all teeth may decay, the upper front teeth are most severely effected while the lower front teeth are usually spared. Apparently, liquid pools around the upper front teeth in a sleeping child.

This condition affects slightly less than 1 percent of infants and is usually seen in those from 18 months to 5 years of age. Fruit juice, milk, soft drinks, and sugared water have been implicated (Powell, 1976).

Treatment consists of prevention. Children over 10 to 12 months of age should not be permitted to sleep with the bottle in their mouth.

SPECIAL PROBLEMS IN THOSE WITH DENTURES

Those who are edentulous and wear dentures may have problems with chewing, speaking, and appearance. Dentures also may produce lesions of the oral mucous membrane. Friction from constant pressure may produce a painful traumatic ulcer. Reducing the thickness of the denture will eliminate the "pressure" and allow the ulcer to heal.

A lesion of the mucosa of the hard palate, called papillary hyperplasia, occurs in those who wear dentures. The mucosa is red, thick, and papillary. It is a painless condition and may require no treatment. The surface epithelium may become quite hyperplastic. In the past, this exuberant but benign hyperplasia has occasionally been mistaken for malignancy or premalignancy.

PERIODONTITIS (PYORRHEA)

In health, the teeth are firmly anchored in bone, which in turn is covered by gingiva. The gingiva attaches to the necks of the teeth to form a seal. The space between root and bone is filled with fibrous connective tissue similar to periosteum. It is called the periodontal ligament. It holds the tooth in the socket and also acts as a cushion.

Inflammation of the periodontal ligament, bone and gingiva is called periodontitis. The term pyorrhea (flowing pus) is no longer in use because in most patients with this disease there is no pus production.

Cause of Periodontitis

Bacterial plaque on the tooth surface acts as an irritant, which induces inflammation in the adjacent tissues. In the early stages, the inflammation is confined to the gingivae (gingivitis). The gingivae are swollen, red, and bleed with slight trauma such as toothbrushing. The gingival inflammation silently spreads to adjacent bone and periodontal ligament, causing slow, progressive destruction of these tissues. As ligament and bone are destroyed, the teeth lose their anchor, become loose, and may drift. The gingivae may recede. Periodontitis is a painless disease and may be advanced when discovered.

Sequelae of Periodontitis

Other than the cosmetic defect produced by tooth migration and gingival recession, these are only two problems caused by the disease: (1) the infection may become intense and localized, producing a painful abscess requiring immediate treatment and (2) if allowed to pursue its natural course, periodontitis will destroy all of the supporting tissues of the teeth, leading to loss of all teeth. It is largely because of this disease that approximately 20 million Americans have no teeth.

Treatment of Periodontitis

This disease may be arrested, but cure in the usual sense is not possible. Once supporting bone has been destroyed, it will not regenerate. When the disease is discovered, the teeth should be cleaned and be kept clean, not an easy task. If the gingival crevice has become abnormally deep because of destruction of underlying bone and periodontal ligament, surgery may reduce this crevice depth. This eliminates the deep, hard-to-reach surface of the tooth where excessive bacterial plaque tends to build up.

Prevention of Periodontitis

Periodontitis ordinarily starts in the teens or twenties and progresses sluggishly over the next 20 to 40 years. The daily elimination of bacterial plaque by using toothbrush and dental floss is effective in preventing this disease. Thus, prevention of the two major oral diseases, caries and periodontitis, is achieved in essentially the same way.

PUBERTY, PREGNANCY, AND THE PILL

It has long been held that there is an increased risk of gingivitis during those times when there is an increase in the level of circulating sex hormones. Clinicians have used the terms "puberty gingivitis" and "pregnancy gingivitis" to describe this condition. The gingivae are red, swollen, and bleed easily.

There is epidemiological evidence that puberty gingivitis does exist. Sutcliffe (1972) studied 127 children between the ages of 11 and 17. He found the incidence of gingivitis to peak at age 12 when 25 percent of the boys and 38 percent of the girls were affected. The incidence decreased as the age increased after 12 years.

Sex hormones probably will not provoke gingival inflammation but will worsen gingivitis that already exists. The metabolism of sex hormones, especially estrogens, provokes the release of chemical mediators of inflammation, including histamine, bradykinin, and prostaglandin. An increased incidence of gingivitis during pregnancy and in those taking birth control pills has also been reported (El-Ashiry, 1970; Loe and Silness, 1963). The reported frequency ranges from 30 to 100 percent. Gingivitis starts around the second month and reaches a peak during the eighth month, declining after parturition.

Pregnant women are also more prone to develop localized enlargements of gingivae called "pregnancy tumors." These are red, easily bleeding nodules of granulation tissue. Because they also occur in children and men, the term "pregnancy tumor" is not entirely appropriate. Pyogenic granuloma is a more acceptable term.

Because of the increased risk of gingivitis associated with puberty, pregnancy, and the use of oral contraceptives, these are times when especially good oral hygiene should be maintained to minimize the problem.

ORAL CANCER

About 3 percent of all human cancers arise in the mouth. Males are more commonly affected and most patients are over the age of 40. There is an increased risk of oral cancer associated with tobacco use and excessive alcohol consumption.

Squamous cell carcinoma accounts for 90 percent of all oral cancers. Carcinoma starts on the mucous membrane as a chronic red patch, white patch, or persistent ulceration. Any lesion matching this description lasting more than 3 or 4 weeks, especially in an adult, should be biopsied to rule out cancer.

Some areas of the oral mucous membrane are more prone to develop cancer than are others. The mucosa under the tongue and on the side of the tongue are especially susceptible. Tonsillar pillars and soft palate are also likely targets. While the upper lip is virtually never the site of cancer, the lower lip has more than its share. Direct rays of the sun striking the lower lip presumably account for this.

Treatment of oral cancer consists of irradiation or surgery or a combination of both. Chemotherapy is palliative. The prognosis depends on the stage at time of diagnosis. Stage 1 tumors (those under 2 cm with no clinical evidence of cervical node metastasis) have a relatively good prognosis, probably 75 to 80 percent 5-year survival. Advanced carcinoma (greater than 4 cm primary lesion with palpable cervical nodes) have a poor outlook, as low as 20 percent survival.

Little is known about prevention. Avoidance of tobacco and alcohol helps but is no guarantee. It has long been held that dentures that do not fit well, chronic infection, and jagged teeth are irritants that may play a role in the etiology of cancer. There is no evidence to support this belief.

HERPETIC LESIONS AND CANKER SORES

These are different diseases, but even experienced clinicians often do not distinguish between them. The herpes virus usually will produce two types of disease: (1) crops of small fluid-filled blisters, incorrectly called fever blisters, that occur on the lip or adjacent skin and (2) a generalized eruption of the gingiva and entire oral mucosa called herpetic gingivostomatitis. Whereas the lip infection tends to be a recurring disease in teen-agers and adults, herpetic stomatitis is chiefly a disease of young children in the preschool or early school years. Also, the generalized mouth infection is accompanied by fever, lethargy, and pain so exquisite that eating and drinking are difficult. This type of herpes infection apparently confers some degree of immunity, because second attacks are rare. Such patients are not immune from recurrent lip lesions, however.

There is no good treatment for either of these two types of herpetic infections. The efficacy of topical application of idoxuridine is yet to be proven. Photodynamic inactivation of lip lesions is claimed to be effective, but there are counterclaims that the treatment is carcinogenic. Fortunately, herpetic infections are self-limiting in persons with an intact immune system.

Health care personnel should be aware that the virus is transmissible. Painful infections of the skin of the finger (herpetic whitlow) are seen in physicians, nurses, and dentists who work with patients with active disease.

Not as much is known about aphthous stomatitis (canker sores). Though clearly not caused by the herpes virus, canker sores are frequently misdiagnosed as being of herpetic origin. Most evidence points toward an infectious agent, possibly the L form of *streptococcus sanguis*.

Though the lesions may bear a resemblance clinically to herpes lesions, there are major differences. Whereas herpes forms a blister that bursts to produce mucosal ulcers, aphthous lesions do not blister. Aphthous lesions start as a white-yellow ulcer surrounded by a red halo of inflammation. The number of lesions is extremely variable, ranging from 1 to over 100. The typical patient has a solitary lesion. More than three lesions per episode is uncommon. They are painful, but the patient lacks the extreme pain, fever, and lethargy seen in herpetic gingivostomatitis.

Recurrence is a hallmark of aphthous stomatitis, but intervals between recurrence are extremely variable. Some unfortunate patients have them almost constantly, whereas others go months to years between episodes. Patients with continuous lesions are frequently and incorrectly diagnosed as having chronic herpes infection.

The age of the individual is of little help in distinguishing between herpetic and aphthous lesions, since all ages are affected in both diseases.

Treatment for aphthous stomatitis consists of the combination of topical steroid and tetracycline mouthwash. For patients with few lesions, palliation may be achieved by frequent topical application of triamcinolone acetonide or hydrocortisone acetate. Topical anesthetics such as a benzocaine provide short-term relief. Patients who have multiple lesions with frequent recurrences are treated with tetracycline and topical steroid as outlined by Stanley (1973). This treatment is no cure, but provides long-term relief in many patients.

Because of the difficulty in differentiating between aphthous and herpetic lesions, Table 15-1 summarizes and compares them.

CONCLUSIONS

For those who practice health care, it should be remembered that many oral diseases are preventable. The simple practice of good oral hygiene

Table 15-1 A comparison of aphthous stomatitis and herpetic stomatitis

	Aphthous	Herpes
Etiology	Unknown. Mycoplasma? Hypersensitivity to L-form of *Strep. sanguis?* Auto-immune? Neurophysiologic?	DNA virus called herpes virus hominis or herpes simplex (herpes type I)
Type of lesion	Single or multiple ulcers exclusively on oral mucosa, mostly on "loose" mucosa such as labial and buccal mucosa. Typically a disease characterized by multiple recurrences.	"Primary" form causes acute febrile illness characterized by diffuse stomatitis, chiefly in children but sometimes in adults. "Secondary" form characterized by recurrent lesions on vermilion of lip and adjacent skin. "Primary" form is a "one-shot" disease (i.e., you don't get it again except in very rare instances).
Constitutional signs (fever, malaise, leukocytosis)	Absent	Present in "primary" type. Absent in "secondary" type.
Histology	Ulceration of oral mucosa with nonspecific acute exudative inflammation in mucosa around the ulcer.	Intraepithelial vesicle with intra-nuclear viral inclusion bodies (Lipschutz bodies or Cowdray type A bodies) and polykaryo-cytes. Vesicles break eventually and an ulcer forms. Lesion may resemble an aphthous lesion.
Treatment	For patient with just a few lesions, frequent topical application of triamcinolone acetonide in orabase to the lesion or lesions. Tetracycline mouthwash (held in mouth at least 3 or 4 minutes and then swallowed) 4 times each day for 7 days then once a day for 2 to 3 weeks. After each mouthwash, a heavy coat of triamcinolone acetonide in orabase is applied to each lesion until they disappear. When tetracyclines are used, be alert to the possibility of superimposed candidiasis. Do not use tetracycline in children under 8 years because of tooth discoloration.	*Primary herpes*—topical anesthetics to kill pain and antibiotics to prevent superimposed bacterial infection. Application of 0.1% idoxuridine solution painted on the lesions with a small brush every 2 hours for 3 days has been recommended. *Secondary herpes*—idoxuridine, ether application, or photo-inactivation.

will eliminate most of the pain, cosmetic problems, and expense associated with caries and periodontitis.

Oral cancer is not yet preventable, but early diagnosis is lifesaving and can be achieved with currently available methods. The mucosa that lines the mouth avails itself to thorough clinical inspection. Oral examination should be a part of every physical examination.

REFERENCES

Brown, L. R., Dreizen, S., Rider, L. J., & Johnston, D. A. The effect of radiation induced xerostomia on saliva and serum lysozyme and immunoglobulin levels. *Oral Surgery*, 1976, *41*, 83.

Decayed, missing and filled teeth among children. Washington, D.C.: U.S. Department of Health, Education, and Welfare, Vital and Health Statistics—Series 11 No. 106, August 1971.

Decayed, missing and filled teeth among youths 12–17 Years. Washington, D.C.: U.S. Department of Health, Education and Welfare, Vital and Health Statistics—Series 11, No. 144, October 1974.

El-Ashiry, G. M., El-Kafrawy, A. H., Nasr, M. F., & Younis, N. Comparative study of the influence of pregnancy and oral contraceptives on the gingivae. *Oral Surgery*, 1970, *30*, 472.

Loe, H., & Silness, J. Periodontal disease in pregnancy. *Acta Odontologia Scandinavia*, 1963, *21*, 533.

Powell, D. Milk, is it related to rampant caries of the early primary dentition? *Journal of the California Dental Association*, 1976, *4*, 58.

Richards, L. F., Westmoreland, W. W., Tashiro, M., McKay, C. H., & Morrison, J. T. Determining optimum fluoride levels for community water supplies in relation to temperature. *Journal of the American Dental Association*, 1967, *74*, 389.

Stanley, H. R. Management of patients with persistent recurrent aphthous stomatitis and Sutton's disease. *Oral Surgery*, 1973, *35*, 14.

Sutcliffe, P. A longitudinal study of gingivitis and puberty. *Journal of Periodontal Research*, 1972, *7*, 52.

Total loss of teeth in adults. Washington, D.C.: U.S. Department of Health, Education, and Welfare, Vital and Health Statistics—Series 11, No. 27, October 1967.

Wescott, W. B., Starcke, E. N., & Shannon, I. L. Chemical protection against postirradiation dental caries. *Oral Surgery*, 1975, *40*, 709.

CHAPTER SIXTEEN

THE FAMILY WITH A CAREER MOTHER

GEORGIA S. DUDDING

INTRODUCTION

Family systems are undergoing change in our society, and the viability of
the institution known as the family has been questioned by many (Elliott,
1970). Changes in our society have influenced the evolution of the family.
Change is a response to needs as well as opportunities, available in any
area, and one change facilitates or instigates others. One of the more significant changes over the past several years is the increased number of
adult female family members who pursue projects, paid or unpaid, outside
the family constellation. This is a reflection of other social changes, one of
which is increased freedom for all individuals. The "pursuit of happiness"
is more likely to be an active process if individuals are not threatened with
loss of "life or liberty." Our society as a whole demonstrates less immediate concern with mass death or loss of freedom and promotes more
self-actualization of all individuals. Since survival no longer depends upon
each family member carrying out a specific function, as in pioneer or early
farm life, people are more free to develop their own interests and pursue
their own goals. Children now exist not for what they can do to help the
family, but rather for themselves as growing persons with rights,
privileges, and values recognized as uniquely theirs (Duvall, 1971). As
individuals who have experienced this kind of freedom become adults, the
life-style they pursue will be different from that of their parents or grandparents. This difference creates new benefits to all family members, but

213

also creates new problems to be faced and dealt with. The approach to the problem will be compounded if people attempt to compare their family life and experiences with that of their neighbors, their own as children, or other more traditional views. The problems cannot be solved by one family member, but instead must be assessed and managed by all those members experiencing conflict. Some families do that as a unit better than others, but all families will find a solution despite their success or failure to attain harmony or maintain their unit status.

Just as individuals go through predictable phases in the course of their lives, so do families as a whole. Families have responsibilities, goals, and developmental tasks that relate directly to the life cycles of their members. If a family can successfully meet the challenges of its growth responsibilities, there will be not only unit satisfaction, but also motivation and good morale among its individual members. If the family fails to successfully complete a task during the course of development, the unit will experience disharmony, more difficulty with subsequent tasks, lack of support for individual growth, and possibly disintegration.

The success or failure of the family to grow as a unit is greatly influenced by the ability of individual members to interrelate their own development in a mutually supportive way. If individual goals and needs are not assessed and planned for by the family, the development of family members may be so diverse that it will produce constant conflict, which will be destructive to the unit.

Changes that take place in society as a whole greatly influence individual development, and consequently family development. The case of worldwide mass communication alone instigates or facilitates changes that would otherwise be much slower to evolve. This puts much more stress on families to keep pace, as a unit, with societal changes and its individual members' vulnerability to those changes.

One very significant change society is experiencing is that of adult women pursuing commitments outside their home and family constellation. According to the U.S. Department of Labor Statistics in 1976, 49 percent of all mothers were working outside the home. Approximately three-fifths of these were mothers of school-age children and two-fifths had preschoolers. This 49 percent compares with 35 percent in 1965, 27 percent in 1955, and only 9 percent in 1945. This change is a response to many needs and opportunities—some individual, some family, and some societal.

Because of changes in the traditional life-styles of families, progress has been made in redefinition of male as well as female roles. It is the opinion of one author (Salk, 1974) that the challenge brought about by this change has been positive, because more people are experiencing greater fulfillment, which eventually improves family life in general.

FACTORS INFLUENCING DECISION FOR MOTHER
TO PURSUE OUTSIDE COMMITMENT

Outside commitment is not always in terms of a career, but may include involvement with school, hobbies, volunteer programs, or anything else one may enjoy. If it is salaried, the money may be a motivating factor or it may be a secondary benefit. Many families, whether single- or two-parent, depend upon the woman's paycheck to obtain the necessities of living. Other family units could buy necessities without the additional income but enjoy the extras or luxuries they could not experience if the woman were not employed.

If financial gain is not a motivating factor, the "pursuit of happiness" or "self actualization" very often is. If a woman has acquired a formal education, she very likely will be eager to use it in some way outside her home, where she can derive satisfaction and pride from success in her job. If her job is satisfying and a positive experience for her, she will most likely want to continue it or return to it once it has been interrupted by other stages of development in her family. Women frequently respond to questions about their reasons for employment with statements about the need for adult contact (Curtis, 1976). This is a very real need for a woman who is used to spending most of her time with children.

Several years ago, magazines were liberally sprinkled with articles promoting motherhood as the ultimate fulfillment of women. It was promoted as an end in itself instead of as a stage in individual development. The importance of mothering or the satisfaction it brings should not be in conflict with other needs of a woman. Many women have difficulty defining their own attitudes and philosophy about this subject even when assimilating only their own data. This is further complicated for individual women as well as family units when two or more people begin to contribute input from their own knowledge and experiences. Since the trend in our society has been to promote self-actualization and parents have often encouraged children to do those things they themselves were never able to do or to improve upon what they did do, individual women grow up with strong and often conflicting messages. Many young girls were encouraged by families to pursue an education, but grew up in a society where women did not work outside the home, unless they had to, at which time it became acceptable. The message perceived by many was that education was pursued in order for a woman to have "something she could fall back on" in case she needed it. Society continually changes the prevailing attitude, however, and with the promotion of a new self-awareness, our culture is making it more and more acceptable for women to be people with a capacity for response to needs and opportunities for commitment outside the home.

Individual vulnerability to societal factors or other external attitudes varies greatly, and any family unit may experience conflict during a period of growth for any one individual. All individuals within that unit have attitudes shaped and molded by their own experiences within a family and society during childhood, and much of it may not yet be at a conscious level. As a family anticipates the wife/mother committing her time to involvement outside the home, everyone may undergo extensive stress. Many times the stress is greater if she is initiating or implementing an outside commitment to meet an individual stage of development as opposed to a direct family unit need. The psychological demands are also compounded if her family or close friends oppose her decision to work. If other women and mothers in her life question her ability to be a "good wife and mother" and work or go to school at the same time, she will need help in assessing her own sensitivity to external attitudes promoting maternal guilt and a great deal of support in planning how to defuse guilt. Many family members, especially adults, need help with this assessment, because so much of the data, functioning strongly within them to influence feelings, attitudes, and expectations, elude awareness, and may not be a conscious but nevertheless vital part of their decision-making process.

It is vital, when counseling parents, to remember that their concerns and feelings are valid and the tapes[1] they bring into adulthood include perceptions, feelings, and distortions of their childhood experiences. Therefore, if either parent has strong attitudes regarding maternal activities outside the home, it was shaped and molded by childhood experiences of which they may or may not be consciously aware. For instance, if a parent values a memory of coming home from school to encounter the aroma of freshly baked cookies, it may affect expectations of mothering often without realizing it or being able to define "good mothering." We can help parents to broaden their expectations and more closely define mothering by directive questioning and guidance about problem solving.

When discussing the problems surrounding maternal self-actualization, it is important for the woman to involve her spouse as much as possible. One author has attempted to group husbands into categories that may be helpful in understanding and assessing families, but one should keep in mind the rule that in any attempt at typing human personalities, there are no absolutes. The following are the types described by Jean Curtis (1976, p. 169).

[1]In TA terms, parent tapes include "everything a person experienced in childhood, all that he incorporated from his parent figures, his perceptions of events, his feelings associated with these events, and the distortions that he brings to his memories. These records are stored as though on videotape. They can be replayed, and the event recalled and even re-experienced" (James and Jongward, 1971, p. 17).

Type A: "Professionals"

1. Informed on feminist issues.
2. Do what needs to be done at home.
3. Take the demands of husband and father as seriously as the demands made on them at the office.
4. Work hard at becoming as much a psychological parent as the wife and are protective of the children.
5. Can manage the housecleaning, laundry, and cooking.
6. Would not hire a maid to avoid exploitation of a female.
7. May be strivers because they have to work hard at affirming equality.
8. Planning must be done by both to preserve spontaneity, humor, and sexual fun.

Type B: "Amateurs"

1. Know little about feminist jargon, literature, and issues—are more traditional.
2. Believe women "ought to be treated well."
3. Married for "love," open doors for their wives, are satisfied with their marriage, and treat their wives as "special."
4. Do a share of the household management but division of chores is more traditional—i.e., woman does light work, man the heavy work.
5. Would rather hire a maid or housekeeper if affordable than share household responsibilities.
6. Value their wife's salary for running the household.
7. Take pride in wife's accomplishments
8. Expect children to carry their own responsibilities and experience stress when it occurs.
9. Wife needs sense of humor, healthy ego, and responsiveness to passion.
10. An identity crisis or new needs for wife may threaten marriage.

Type C: "Supportive" (not totally hostile)

1. Say it's O.K. for wife to work as long as she can keep up with kids, house, and their social life. Do not usually hassle regarding working.
2. Wives usually accept this type as "the way men are."
3. Grateful for extra income wife brings in.
4. Usually offer to "help" in some special way—such as preparing one meal/week, but not cleaning up.
5. Feel pride in contribution to working and often boast about it.
6. Praise wife for "doing something" with her life.
7. Women with this arrangement should be aware of the burdens on her and the possible implications and stress if she accepts that role.

Type D: "The boys"

1. Anxious and embarrassed that wife works.
2. Feel like a failure because of wife's working.
3. Threatened about what she does when she is away from home.
4. Never help out at home unless the job is "manful," i.e., painting outside or fixing a large appliance.
5. Can't stand to help with laundry, cooking, or house, but can't stand seeing wife work so hard.
6. Usually take up an active hobby or sport so they don't have to watch her work so hard or be alone while she is.
7. May undermine wife's abilities at work.
8. Women may develop problems with own self-worth.
9. If marriage fails, husband never takes any blame. Children are often caught in the middle of the bitterness.

These stereotypes are included as information meant to be helpful in assessing and planning for the possible problems that come with maternal employment as a stage of development. Even if the type of marriage is assessed and danger signals are brought to awareness, couples may be too threatened about trying to change their roles and routines in order to prevent problems. The health care provider then must continue to care, support, and confront constructively as danger signals increase. Many women, because of their own background, are willing psychologically to accept the responsibility for the house and children, because they feel guilty about doing anything else.

Usually, the event of the maternal commitment to school or career is not an isolated factor that induces conflict. As each individual or family unit develops, mutually supportive growth depends upon previously successful completion of developmental tasks. If those tasks have not been successfully completed, they do not build a firm foundation for growth, and families find themselves trying to conquer a new task with many unfinished matters still producing conflict and unhappiness. Health care providers need to be aware of the possibility that this may be why a woman is choosing to return to school or work. She may be encountering so much dissatisfaction, sometimes unaware of it at a conscious level, that she sees this as a necessary step in her own growth.[2] At this point she must be helped to assess her reasons.

[2]Within my own practice and those of my colleagues, this has become more and more apparent. Many, certainly not all, women do become divorced within two or three years after making the decision to return to a career or school. More research is needed in this area, but the possibility of viewing self-induced change in a woman's career growth as symptomatic of her own need for independence and fulfillment should be considered.

Care should be taken not to prejudge the situation, but instead to maintain openness and support in helping meet her needs. It is important not to make her more vulnerable with confrontation, unless one can offer her the necessary support to develop through that vulnerability. Society does offer the possibility to women today to be divorced working mothers—perhaps happy for the first time in their adult life. Although that is a group to be considered and not overlooked, there are many others who work for many other reasons.

According to Rich (1976, p. 19), as she reflects upon the work of Margaret Sanger, women have asserted their courage for generations on behalf of their own children and men, then on behalf of strangers, and finally for themselves. With the onset of the women's liberation movement, more and more women are beginning to have the courage to grow for their own fulfillment—fulfillment that does not preclude but expands beyond motherhood. Even as recently as 1971 many women were still in agreement with psychoanalyst Clara Thompson, who was quoted (McBride, 1973) as describing fulfillment for "women as receiving economic security and a full emotional life centering around her husband and children in return for being a man's property." Thompson was also quoted by McBride (1973) as saying woman has little cause for discontent and would be happily fulfilled if she had the opportunity to express her capacities in the management of her home; further, she could not be troubled by feelings of inferiority even though she lived in relative slavery.

Most people do not subscribe to that philosophy today, and many women do want more out of life than that. Some women, however, are very happy being at home with their children, and they in no way should be made to feel anything but valued and self-confident. If, however, a woman plans to return to work at some point after the children have begun school, etc., appropriate counseling for both parents should include equal parenting from the beginning, despite the manner in which other responsibilities are divided at that time.

BENEFITS DERIVED FROM MATERNAL EMPLOYMENT

Commitment outside the home offers a greater exposure to peers and opportunities for interpersonal growth and relationships. This can awaken or arouse dormant interests as well as provide achievement in previously identified areas of interest. Success in any area helps increase a person's sense of self-worth. Often, mothers will find that once they are having some of their needs met at work—needs that are different from those that can be met at home—they are better able to meet the needs of those around them. Once this begins to happen, self-satisfaction is increased and experienced not only at work, but at home as well. This side effect certainly is supported by a review by Stolz (1960) of more than fifty studies, all of which pointed to the same conclusion—that a mother's working is, in itself, not a significant factor in mothering, family adjustment, or development of her children. Whether a mother's working is a problem or not seems to depend much more on many personal or family factors than on her being gone from the home for a period of time every day.

When a woman begins spending more time out of the home, everyone in the family unit must adjust. This can be fostered and encouraged as a growth process for all individual members. Children can become more independent and responsible for themselves and household chores at a very young age. If the decision has been made for a woman to go to work or school, and both parents are comfortable with that decision, the children can adjust comfortably. When a mother/wife is spending less time in her home, her children may very well become progressively more responsible for at first simple, then more complex tasks. If, however, a mother feels guilty about working and views it as a negative stage in her development, she is likely *not* to expect even the most simple tasks to be carried out by her children. When this happens, parents may overcompensate for their own negative feelings by being more permissive with their children. For the health care provider, this may be an initial clue to unsatisfactory adjustment to maternal employment. Instead of reinforcing the fears that the employment is causative, it will be more helpful to the family unit and certainly to the parents and children individually to deal with control of the unacceptable behavior than to suggest that mother stay at home with the children.

Authors who have written on the subject of maternal employment frequently point to the problems it causes with the children and have discouraged employment. Fortunately, today's parents are beginning to reassess the validity of that advice, partially because of the support they receive from other "successful parents," health care providers who either are, or are married to, working mothers, and literature that is more supportive of working women. Dr. Benjamin Spock (1974a) suggests that a child is more secure when its mother is in the home and caring for it full time. Simultaneously, however, he offers that when mothers *have* to work, their children usually "turn out" all right. According to one author (Curtis, 1976), Dr. Lee Salk is also widely quoted regarding adjustment of children when both parents work. He suggests that disturbed children sometimes result from that situation without comparing the number of those children with those who come from homes where mothers have no outside involvement. Jean Curtis (1976) questions the statements made by these and other authors and suggests the answers to the problem are gravely oversimplified. She states, "Among the families I interviewed, only a handful had children who were not adjusting to school as well as other children. Statistically speaking, their experience could indicate that Salk's thesis is not valid."

Husbands have been mentioned previously in this chapter, but only in respect to the way they view their working wife. Being a father in addition to a husband and having an outside commitment is also not an easy task. Traditionally, the father in the home has not been the "psychological parent."[3] Rich (1976) suggests that under the institution of motherhood, the mother is the first to blame if theory proves unworkable in practice or if anything goes wrong. Historically, those statements are true, but within changing families, those traditional roles are taking on new appearances. Children are reaping the benefits, even if the changes are slow, of less stereotyped images and experiencing lives with parents who are more willing to share responsibilities beyond the very rigidly defined roles of the past. Fathers are also experiencing fuller lives as a result of increased sharing. Spock (1974a) begins the easement of increasing awareness of "fathering" with the message that fathers have been brought up to think caring for babies and children is entirely the mother's job, but that a man can be a warm father and still remain a *real man*. He validates the fact that a father's closeness and friendliness to his children will have a vital effect on their characters for a lifetime. He goes on to say that it is easiest for fathers to begin at the start of the child's life and that both parents learn together. If Spock's awareness promotion had stopped there instead of going on to suggest that the father's involvement might be making formula on Sunday, many parents might approach the problem more realistically. He suggests that many fathers get "gooseflesh" at approaching a new baby and should not be forced. He apparently never asked mothers if *they* got gooseflesh. Mothering is not a natural phenomenon for women either.

Spock offers a different slant to the problem in a more recent book (Spock, 1974b) in which he offers the idea that it is better that a child strives to be an adult with adult interests than that an adult strives to succeed in the world of a child! If both parents help the child in this maturation process with everyone taking part in all aspects of jobs around the house, the child will have a much broader definition of marriage and family unity. It is important, however, for parents to continue meeting the emotional and developmental needs of their children and not expect them to function totally as adults.

The financial flexibility that a salaried woman offers to her family can take several forms. There is certainly a greater ease in meeting the financial "needs" in the family, and if the mother is a single parent, the income certainly is a necessity. If the family is able to live and meet financial

---

[3]The person who is always mindful of—who always feels a direct responsibility for the whereabouts and feelings of each child . . . who knows what emotional supports they need, etc. (Curtis, 1976).

obligations without a second income, the second salary may be a bonus for recreation, vacations, or other expenditures benefiting the family as a unit. Thirdly, she may simply have the satisfaction of an independent source of income that offers flexibility in her own purchasing power and satisfaction regarding her fiscal contribution, whether it is necessary or not.

RISKS AND CONFLICTS ENHANCED OR INDUCED BY MATERNAL EMPLOYMENT

As discussed earlier, change by its very nature affords benefits to those experiencing it, but also causes risk and conflict that must be assessed and planned for.

People find themselves tied to many traditional roles that may or may not be valid for them. Often men and women behave within a family structure with attitudes they do not enjoy or even find desirable, but seem to be locked into as a result of experience, perceptions, and feelings accumulated during their own growth process. Many men have come to adulthood with expectations of themselves providing financially for their families and avoiding showing a soft, emotional side to their children. Ginott (1965) warns fathers not to get too involved with feeding and diapering children because a child might end up with two mothers. Likewise, women often carry with them the idea that if they can only do their job well as mothers, read the right articles, and solicit the right professional opinions, their children will be "right." Mothers seem to have this expectation of themselves, especially if they are intelligent, read what the "experts" have had to say during the fifties and sixties, and are achievers in general. During the past 20 years, multiple books and magazine articles have freely offered advice that women should find total fulfillment in motherhood, especially if mothering is done properly. Many child care books suggest that only mothers can do that job and that if a mother shares her child's care with someone else, both mother and child will suffer. Whether this is true or not possibly depends on how dedicated the family members are to believing and accepting it. Because men and women have heard that philosophy for so long, they are apt to accept it without ever examining it for themselves. It is that acceptance, many times, that causes so much conflict over a decision for a woman to be more than a wife and mother. It is the opinion of Biller and Meredith (1975) that working wives can better balance work and mothering than husbands can balance work and fathering.

When women do pursue outside commitments, the redefinition of traditional roles must occur to some extent. Depending on the development of that family to that point, the redefinition will take place in varying degrees. Curtis (1976) found, by interviewing working mothers and their husbands, that even if the traditionally maternal tasks were divided among family members, or if external help was sought, the responsibility for those tasks remained with the mother. It is important to recognize this prevalent attitude, because it does seem to occur frequently and causes a great psychological demand on mothers. Women are often reluctant to give up those psychological responsibilities and to expect others to complete them successfully without their guidance. This, too, is a result of years of societal conditioning, for which no one is to blame, but which must be recognized.

DECISIONS TO BE MADE

Substitute Child Care

Choosing a child care substitute can be a major problem area for parents. It is important to encourage fathers to share in the decision-making responsibility and the active selection. There are limited, but increasing alternatives for solutions to the problem. The Department of Labor shows that approximately one-half of preschool children of working mothers are cared for in their own homes, less than one-third are cared for in other homes, and about 5 percent are in group day care centers. The remaining 10 to 15 percent are cared for in some other manner. Day care is often limited in what it offers and therefore many people seem to use it as a last resort. Day care centers are often open for a limited number of hours, leaving parents who commute or work irregular (not 8:00 A.M. to 5:00 P.M.) hours unable to use them. They often are staffed in such a manner that parents find them unacceptable as parental substitutes. The difficulty may include a ratio of caretakers to children that is too low, or caretakers who have different values regarding discipline, etc. When centers are acceptable in all these areas, they are often very expensive, and that offers additional conflict. Parents should be encouraged to visit day care centers they are interested in, taking with them a list of criteria they have previously decided on, and compare not only price, but the staffing ratio and the comfort they and their child feel there, and observe the interaction between the children and staff.

Parents with infants or young toddlers may have more difficulty than others in finding a suitable solution to child care. Many centers are not staffed for the extra care infants require and most will not take a child unless the child is toilet trained. Parents who find a center that will take an infant are often tempted or feel forced to accept it regardless of whether or not it meets their other criteria.

There are a number of women who care for children of all ages in their own homes, and this alternative can be either very positive or a disaster. When parents are considering this alternative, they are often dependent solely on the personality of the caretaker involved. They should be encouraged to visit the home and be suspicious if they have to schedule their visit in advance. They should be aware of licensing requirements and whether or not the home meets those standards.

If parents are considering employment of a caretaker in their own home, they should be encouraged to advertise and interview applicants thoroughly. It is important to be aware that people often need someone to care for their child so badly that they are insecure about insisting on the kind of person they really desire. Consequently, they often settle for someone they do not have complete confidence in and then feel very guilty about it. Parents have difficulty enjoying their jobs if they are worried about the care the child receives at home in their absence.

People who come into the home may do so only during the hours the parents are away; or they may live with the family. Either way, the family should all have some time with the prospective employee and feel comfortable with the choice.

Children who are of school age pose a special problem. Sometimes parents of classmates can be an alternative, or a housekeeper who is present when the child comes home. Often, children are responsible enough to carry their own key, call a parent when they arrive at home, and do specific tasks in the time they have before a parent arrives home. Children can learn a great deal of independence and responsibility with this arrangement if they are comfortable doing it. Parents should be encouraged to talk with the child openly to assess the child's attitude about this. Children can be very active contributors in the decision making. Many children would rather have this arrangement as they get older than have a babysitter. Parents need to be aware of the child's activities after school and be able to assess the degree of responsibility the child can comfortably handle.

It might be suggested that an older preschooler or school-age child visit both parents' offices and be allowed to hang a picture they've created, see the telephone, and otherwise get a feeling for where their parents spend their time. In that way the child feels more a part of the *other world* of its parents.

As a health care provider, one should become aware of the resources in the community, encourage parents to consider seriously what kind of care they desire, make that a priority, and be very discriminating as a unit until they are satisfied. They might be encouraged to interview, using the criteria they would use if choosing for a close friend. That approach facilitates objectivity and helps eliminate compromise arising from anxiety or urgent need.

If a preliminary choice is made to have someone live in, a week-end trial with the family might be considered. This would allow interaction among the children and caretaker and give both some time to assess the viability of the arrangement. As a result, the confidence they feel will free them to enjoy the time they, as a family, have together much more than if their energies were being used processing and rationalizing the guilt over inadequate child care. Their awareness of the various alternatives can be increased and suggestions can be made. For instance, if a family is considering a college student to help part time or to live in, might they consider a male as well as a female student? A retired man might enjoy being a grandfather substitute after school and an older couple who enjoy children might offer a very satisfactory solution. It is important that the entire family be involved and comfortable with the decisions made, however, or frustration and conflict manifested in other areas may be the result.

Housekeeping

Housekeeping seems to be much less a problem than responsibility for child care. It does, in general, however, remain the psychological responsibility of the woman. Again, this may be because she is unconsciously unwilling to let go of it, or because people simply fall back into living the way they observed their parents live. Both statements probably overlap, and change will most of the time have to be a conscious process. The solution as to who does the laundry, marketing, cooking, or cleaning the house will probably relate directly to how successfully the family handles this stage of development. If the family members value the mother going to work or her own growth in that area, they will be more likely to share in cleaning, marketing, doing the laundry, or cooking. The family should be counseled to avoid making these decisions or changes based on political issues, e.g., women's rights, but instead to assess what the needs are and plan for who can best execute them. Depending upon each individual's stage of development, the solutions will differ from family to family.

Just as decisions regarding child care and housekeeping must be managed, it is also important for parents to discuss who will provide transportation to and from activities outside school and see that music lessons are practiced and homework done. Unless these are also discussed, mothers may find themselves assuming the psychological responsibility without an actual decision ever being made.

Finances

Another potential source of conflict may be a financial one. The benefit of an extra salary has been discussed, but often the hidden or unrecognized costs of employment cause confusion when the budget doesn't balance the way both spouses expected. Parents may have to be reminded that it also costs something for either of them to work outside their home. The most obvious expense, of course, is child care and good child care is expensive. When parents work outside their home, they also have to have an expanded wardrobe. There is also the increased cost of transportation, whether for a second car, payment to a car pool, or fare on a mass transit system. And, even if people take their lunches every day, it still may add costs to the budget. These things should be brought to awareness, not to deter or discourage families, but so they can be planned for in order to avoid unexpected conflict at a later time.

If a husband has a "need" to provide for his family financially and sees his wife's working as a threat to his own ego, both may be in need of counseling. It could perhaps be suggested that she either begin a hobby or volunteer work that she enjoys if her need is for some time away from home. On the other hand, if her needs include fiscal contribution, perhaps a compromise could be suggested that allows for her salary to be put into a savings account for a few months. Whatever the solution, their talking about the attitudes involved needs to be facilitated, and in some cases if one or the other is very rigid, caring and support of each by different people may be indicated. No health care provider should promote guilt in parents who find themselves in a situation where individual growth is so conflicting that positive unit growth is no longer feasible and potential destruction of the unit seems inevitable.

Family, Work, and Community Responsibilities

Attitudes of family and society can either be a benefit or a source of conflict. Society is in a stage of transition where women are concerned, and some sectors will be more supportive than others. It would be helpful, of course, for all women to be employed by people who believe in working mothers and understanding of necessary family responsibilities. However, that is not usually the case. Women, however, need to be encouraged and to some extent educated by the health care provider to at least make her needs known. The working mother should not prejudge her employer any more than she would want to be prejudged. If a woman can be helped to organize her approach in a realistic, mature manner and not an already defeated apologetic, or aggressive manner, she is more likely to communicate with the adult side of her employer when she has a sick child or other needs. According to men who have written in this area (Biller and Meredith, 1975), neither parent should be reticent about presenting special needs to their employer. It should be explained that special time off may occasionally be needed, or even that there will be a need to bring the child to work occasionally. They believe the most essential factor is that men realize fatherhood is as important as the father's career and that he take an active part in parenting. This same approach is important when dealing with neighbors, families, teachers, etc. Because of their own data regarding working mothers, many women feel guilty before they ever begin to interact with others about it. They find themselves so vulnerable to outside criticism that even if it doesn't materialize, they will imagine it or impose internal guilt.

Mothers will often suggest that because of their working hours, they cannot attend school-related functions for their children. They do value the school activities, and sometimes the suggestion that a father attend when possible is a new idea to a family. Often, working mothers are more keenly aware of and more involved in school activities than nonemployed mothers. They often try harder to carve time out of their schedules to participate, because they want their children to know they care. Working mothers should be made aware, however, that very few parents, working or nonworking, attend *all* school-related functions.

Another area of conflict applies to husbands of women who return to work after several years at home in a nonworking role. Marital partners who have enjoyed a great deal of flexibility in their lives may find the increased demands on the wife's time very stressful. Women may handle this much better than their husbands because of their increased fulfillment in their work. Even when a husband is supportive of the changes being made, he will have adjustments to make that either partner may not understand. Marital partners need to be reassured that the negative feelings they have are normal and must be verbalized and dealt with together. Recognition and acceptance of feelings is a first step toward planning for the changes in order to maintain an intact relationship. A woman may need to be alerted to the need for her to be patient and understanding of the growth her husband is experiencing at a time when she is excited and highly motivated regarding her own activity.

A personal risk caused by women returning to work after becoming used to an at-home life-style is the alteration of the already fulfilling factors in her life as well as those factors she would like to change. Established friendships will be altered and sometimes may disintegrate. If a woman is not free to participate in the activities of her friends during her working hours, she will feel some loss regarding that contact. The attitudes of her friends may not be accepting of her employment, and she may need support and counseling in order to cope with changes in close friendships at a time when she feels she needs her friends the most.

Some authors (Biller and Meredith, 1975) have pointed to the fact that children of working mothers compare favorably as a group to the children of nonworking mothers in terms of emotional, intellectual, and physical development. They suggest this is probably because mothers who work *are* conscious of the need to spend time with their children, whereas nonworking mothers do not feel the need as keenly. Therefore, many working mothers find themselves spending time on weekends with their children and friends for an occasional outing or sponsoring scout troops when nonworking mothers cannot find the time.

RESOURCES FOR COUNSELING

McBride (1973) points out that the expectations mothers carry of themselves, when successfully accomplished, can be motivation for attaining their goals, or a form of torture when they cannot feasibly meet those expectations. Often, the main source of support for working mothers is other working mothers. Much of the psychological stress with which mothers have to deal comes from their perpetual effort to bolster their own convictions. Just as other working women can provide support, very often women who do not work can perpetuate the conflict that working mothers experience. The health care provider, especially if a working mother herself, can be a source of support and facilitate much personal growth by sharing personal problems and solutions, as well as teaching families some problem-solving techniques of their own.

Any individual who faces a change in life must recognize that regardless of whether the change is seen as positive or negative, it is potentially painful. Change is continuous and cannot be avoided; therefore, the recognition and planning of it is to an individual's or family's advantage (see Table 16-1). If a woman decides to work, she should, with her family, identify as clearly as possible what changes will have to be made in order for that to happen or as a result of its happening. They must next accept the responsibility for the change and make a conscious commitment to that change. Many women do this and do it alone, but seem to stop here. That may be the reason so many women accept the psychological responsibility for parenting and running the house at the same time they are working full time.

The next step may be a vital one, and that includes identification of

Table 16-1 Steps for creating change in family unit

1. Accept fact that change is continuous and potentially painful.
2. Identify specific goal that is bringing about change.
3. Accept responsibility for wanting change.
4. Make a conscious commitment to that change.
5. Identify support system and other resources.
6. List as a family unit, all problems or problem areas regardless of currently recognized significance.
7. Seek solutions to problem, as a family unit.
8. Reallocate tasks, using appropriate resources.
9. Maintain changed system, using the support system and established resources.

her support system and other necessary resources for herself and others. Next the specific problems should be listed by everyone involved, no matter how large or small they may seem at the time. Based on that problem list, solutions must begin to be sought and tasks reallocated with the help and use of appropriate resources. This may include finding appropriate child care, reassignment of household duties, or transporting children to music lessons. It may all be accomplished within the family or it may include use of outside resources.

The remaining step may be the most important of all. Too often, people forget that any working system needs maintenance. The family must continue using the support system and the resources identified.

If the family is satisfactorily developing and undertaking this developmental task of maternal employment, there are interrelated functions occurring. Each will be perceiving new possibilities for their own behavior, some of which will be positive, some producing conflict. These possibilities will be based on expectations others have of that individual. During this time new self-concepts will be forming, and individuals will begin to cope effectively with the conflict they are feeling. If the family is successful and supportive, each member will become motivated to achieve this task by assuming the new responsibilities and will be rewarded for their success by other members of the family unit.

COUNSELING

Some authors (Gillis and Mitchell, 1975) suggest that health professionals do not know enough about effects of maternal employment on children to offer advice. Some suggest a "conservative" approach and recommend part-time employment if it is necessary at all. Furthermore, Howell (1973) points out that most articles on maternal employment are written with marked negativism and that hypotheses and questionnaires have often been phrased so that only ill effects can be demonstrated. If a mother perceives the need to work, whether it is an emotional, financial, or some other type of need, she is facing a decision and a stage of development. The information health care providers do have available may make the transition an easier one for all concerned. Families should receive support for whatever stage of development they are facing. Currently, only limited resources are available to health care providers trying to support and guide these families. When there is a lack of supportive literature available, working mothers can at least share the experiences they and other employed mothers have had. Until more long-term data are available, experience and sharing may be our best resources, along with newer and very readable literature available to both mothers and health care providers. These are designated in the bibliography by an asterisk (*).

CONCLUSION

There are no conclusive data to suggest maternal employment is good for a child or a family, nor are there data to suggest that it is not. The literature is full of opinions and speculations by people who are not working mothers. More and more writing is being done by working mothers sharing information from other working mothers and their families.

If one does accept the fact that each successfully completed developmental task is a strong foundation for the next one (Duvall, 1971) and views maternal employment as a developmental task, then the success of the family developing as a unit seems to be more important.

To say that health care professionals cannot advise parents because of a deficiency in knowledge about long-term effects seems to be a lack of response to development. If health care providers can advise parents about bottle weaning or toilet training without knowing what long-term effects any one method may have on the child, can health care providers not at least offer help with decision making, resource identification, and continuing support as families take on new tasks in our ever-changing world?

As a working mother, as well as a nurse, this author believes that not only is it vital for professionals to recognize increased maternal employment as a changing and very realistic factor in our society, but that it is also extremely important to respond to the needs it invokes. Only when professionals can help parents deal with the reality of their own lives, instead of imposing biases or prejudices on them, will they be really facilitating optimal growth and development of that family. Our profession must also demonstrate viability by growing and expanding our perspectives as society changes and grows. When outdated attitudes no longer provide answers to questions raised by today's life-styles, new information must be sought through expansion of attitudes accomplished by research and sensitivity to the needs of the very people we profess to help. Mothers with careers are a part of society's changing life-styles. Can we afford to ignore the needs of those families (sometimes our own and those of our colleagues), when caring is a part of our philosophy?

REFERENCES

*Biller, H., & Meredith, D. *Father power*. New York: McKay, 1975.
*Curtis, J. *Working mothers*. Garden City, N.Y.: Doubleday, 1976.
Duvall, E. M. *Family development*. Philadelphia: J. B. Lippincott, 1971.
Elliott, K. (Ed.) *The family and its future*. Ciba Foundation Symposium. London: Churchill, 1970.

 *Recommended as resources for career mothers and their families.

Families and the rise of working wives—An overview. Special Labor Force Report 189, Washington, D.C.: U.S. Department of Labor, Bureau of Statistics.

Gillis, S., & Mitchell, A. *Pediatric alert.* 1975, *1* (1), 3.

Ginott, H. *Between parent and child: New solutions to old problems.* New York: Macmillan, 1965.

Howell, M. C. Employed mothers and their families I. *Pediatrics,* 1973, *52* (2), 252–263.

———, Employed mothers and their families II. *Pediatrics,* 1973, *52* (3), 327–343.

*James, M., & Jongward, D. *Born to win.* Reading, Mass.: Addison-Wesley, 1971.

Labor force patterns of divorced and separated women, Special Labor Force Report 198, Washington, D.C.: U.S. Department of Labor, Bureau of Labor Statistics.

*McBride, A. B. *The growth and development of mothers.* New York: Harper & Row, 1973.

Marital and family characteristics of the labor force, March 1975. Special Labor Force Report 183, Washington, D.C.: U.S. Department of Labor, Bureau of Statistics.

*Rich, A. *Of woman born.* New York: W. W. Norton, 1976.

Salk, L. *Preparing for parenthood.* New York: McKay, 1974.

Spock, B. *Baby and child care.* New York: Pocket Books, 1974a.

———. *Raising children in a difficult time.* New York: Norton, 1974b.

Stolz, L. M. Effects of maternal employment on children. *Child Development,* 1960, *31* (4), 749–782.

Working mothers and their children, Washington, D.C.: U.S. Department of Labor, Employment Standards Administration, Women's Bureau,1977.

*Recommended as resources for career mothers and their families.

PART THREE

APPROACHES TO ASSESSMENT AND INTERVENTION

This section introduces the readers to some of the general approaches to assessment and intervention useful with families for whom they are providing health care. Specific approaches that can be applied to families undergoing developmental (maturational) and situational crises are explored in Volume II of *Family Health Care*.

Chapter 17, *Humanizing Health Care,* challenges us to provide a more human approach in delivering care, regardless of, or perhaps in spite of, our complex health delivery system. In Chapter 18, *Community Health Family Nursing,* the author presents a structural model for providing primary health care nursing. She uses a systems theory approach in an attempt to untangle part of the maze of our very complicated health care system. The next two chapters suggest guidelines for assessing families. The *Family Assessment Guidelines,* presented in Chapter 19, provide a comprehensive tool that could be used with any family. The instrument suggested in Chapter 20, *Assessment of the Chronically Ill Child and Family,* uses the developmental task framework as a basis for assessing the needs of chronically ill children and their families.

Chapter 21, *Principles of Family Counseling,* presents the reader with general guidelines for counseling. A specific application of counseling principles is described in Chapter 22, *Genetic Counseling and the Family.* With the increasing awareness of the need for human sexuality education at all stages of development, we have chosen to include Chapter 23, *Sexuality, Education, and the Family.* This chapter provides the reader with

233

information regarding areas of childhood and adult sexuality. In Chapter 24, *Behavioral Pediatrics,* the author suggests a practical, problem-oriented approach to the prevention and early detection of behavior problems. The final chapter, *Legal Aspects of Nursing and Medicine,* discusses the legal aspects of primary nursing care as it pertains to the nurse's relationship with patients and physicians.

CHAPTER SEVENTEEN

HUMANIZING HEALTH CARE

JOY PRINCETON CLAUSEN

Humanizing health care is a current social issue in the United States. Some anthropologists theorize that the human mind operates in terms of binary oppositions, continually dividing phenomena into two dichotomous categories. This is a helpful theory when we consider humanization of health care, for almost automatically the opposite of humanization—dehumanization—comes to mind. In other words, each concept is simply one side of the same coin, and it is difficult if not meaningless to discuss one to the exclusion of the other.

Definitions have been set forth for humanized, hence dehumanized, health care (Howard and Strauss, 1975), and although they differ to some degree, there is a universal thread that runs through the fabric of the definitions: Whereas humanized health care recognizes the personalized inherent worth of each consumer and his or her individualized needs and wants, dehumanized health care does not. Only through further research can the definitions be sharpened and operationalized, illuminating the rather uncomfortable fact that humanized health care for one person may very well be dehumanized care for another because of distinct individual differences in their biological, psychological, and sociocultural makeup. It may be most disturbing for some health professionals to realize that there can never be a finite checklist of variables that determines if care rendered is humanized or not; that at best the concepts must be operationalized in accordance with specific individuals comprising specific groups that are target populations for health care. Clifford R. Barnett (Howard and

Strauss, 1975, p. 269) spoke to the importance of operational definitions when he wrote "Humanization and dehumanization are labels that may be useful in rallying popular support for changes in certain medical care practices, but are hardly useful for designing research." He goes on to say that each scholar who has discussed humanization research has had to redefine it in order to operationalize the term meaningfully for distinct individuals and populations.

Dissatisfaction and frustration with what has come to be known as a dehumanizing health care process is expressed in different ways by consumer groups. For example, some couples in the prime of their childbearing years from all socioeconomic groups are opting to deliver their children at home rather than in the sterile atmosphere of hospitals. They are voicing their protests against rigid hospital policies regarding anesthesia and analgesia, visiting hours and visitors allowed, and access to and care of their newborn infant. They are demanding that they be included in assessment of their physical and psychosociocultural state, and that they be allowed to codirect their health care in conjunction with health professionals. Alternative systems of health care are being developed in some cities in which women's centers are constructed that enable a family to experience the birth process in a homelike atmosphere focused on health, in contrast to the pathological orientation of a hospital setting. In some locations where the building of such a new center is not possible, hospitals are remodeling a labor room into a "birthing room" that closely resembles a home environment, and in which family members may be present to assist and aid with the birth.

More and more consumers are entering into litigation for what they believe is inadequate, incompetent health care received, and they are no longer content to allow health care personnel and the agencies under which the latter practice to control their health care totally. The premise upon which health service has been delivered in the past, i.e., the health professionals "know best," is readily meeting its demise.

Rather than define humanized health care in concise terms, some scholars have attempted to describe the process through which health care is humanized and dehumanized. Jan Howard (Howard and Strauss, 1975, pp. 60–65), for example, cites a series of definitions used to describe the dehumanization process in which some recipients of health care find themselves; these are summarized in Table 17-1. Howard then utilizes these definitions to form a basis from which to derive three components of humanized health care (pp. 66–67).

The first component is based on the proposition that men and women have biological needs and humanized health care behaviors are oriented toward fulfilling these needs. Conversely, dehumanized behavior works against fulfilling these biological needs. Insofar as the fulfillment of needs is on a continuum, there are degrees to which behaviors are humanizing and/or dehumanizing. For example, when working with expectant

Table 17-1 The dehumanization of consumers of health care

Process	Definition and characteristics
Clients as things ("thinging")	A human being is reduced to a nonhuman entity, and may be referred to as "the 2 o'clock appointment," "the partial previa," and like terms.
Clients as extensions of machines	The health caretaker may be absent while the client interacts with a machine; hence the former is replaced to a large degree by the machine. When labor patients are electrically monitored, and when newborns are attached to various equipment in the high-risk nursery, it may become questionable where the person leaves off and the machines begin, particularly when the patient is inactive and passive.
Clients as guinea pigs	This concept is frequently used to describe medical research on human beings, and/or when techniques like amniocentesis and intrauterine transfusions are being developed and perfected.
Clients as problems	Health professionals over time tend to become problem- rather than people-oriented. This process is intensified when professionals focus on specifics of client care without attempting to incorporate a holistic approach. The medical model of health care with focus on pathology and disease conditions reinforces this process.
Clients as lesser people	Health professionals develop the attitude that clients are inferior due to social and cultural differences such as level of education, economic factors, ethnic group affiliation, age, and sex. These attitudes in turn directly affect the quality of health care delivered.
Clients as isolates	This process is similar to the one immediately above in that clients and patients are seen as totally unique from the health workers, so different that too little time and effort is expended talking or intermingling with them. This is primarily manifest in the waiting room of doctors' offices and clinics in which the clients are literally abandoned for long periods of time.
Clients as recipients of substandardized care	Care becomes haphazard and spotty, of a generally inferior quality given the knowledge and technology available. Often this substandard care is rationalized as the outcome of health workers being overworked; more than not, however, there are other more truthful reasons, such as noninitiative and complacency on the part of the health workers that better account for the phenomenon.
Clients without options	This is manifest by the *powerlessness syndrome* among clients and patients, and signifies loss of control over one's own destiny. This occurs when health consumers are not included or only menially included in their plans for health care, and implementation and evaluation of the care.

Table 17-1 The dehumanization of consumers of health care *(continued)*

Process	Definition and characteristics
Clients interact with icebergs	Often health care personnel are seen as cold and aloof, with an air of omniscience and omnipotence. Personnel rationalize that this results from their attempts to remain objective and emotionally distant from the consumer of health care, an unfounded premise.
Clients in static, sterile environments	Clients often view the health care environmental setting as one of sterility, one in which there is a general feeling of coldness, depersonalization, as well as physical austerity. This is primarily one reason why some consumers opt to deliver babies at home.
Clients and the preservation of life	The central question here is concerned with death and the responsibility for preserving life. This reflects the ethical question of the quality of the life that health professionals attempt to maintain. Theologically, some clients argue that health professionals deny them the right to continue a life hereafter by maintaining the life on earth.

Source: Adapted from Jan Howard and Anselm Strauss, *Humanizing Health Care,* New York, John Wiley and Sons, 1975, pp. 60–66.

couples, nurses may overlook the importance of thorough anticipatory guidance related to nutrition, even though other biological needs during pregnancy are being met via the health team. Thus, the pregnant woman is not able to reach her full human potential because she may not understand or perhaps does not have sufficient knowledge of nutritional requirements expected of her during pregnancy that would ensure a healthy self and baby. The end product of this is dehumanization of the client.

The second component of humanized health care is the psychological, equally as important as the biological, and might include such needs as self-expression, self-image, self-actualization, affection, and empathy. When a client's psychological needs are not met, the degree of dehumanization that occurs is more difficult to measure than with biological deprivation. This is in part because of difficulty in accurately measuring psychological processes and the relativistic nature of this type of need. Often such needs are based on ethnic group values and are culture-bound, which in turn prevents generalization from one subgroup of clients to another.

The third and final component closely integrated with the psychological is the sociocultural, which defines needs in terms of relationships with fellow human beings. This component is no less important than the other two, and as with the psychological, measurement of the degree of humanization or dehumanization is difficult because of the relativism of the model. That is, one's viewpoint of relationships with others fluctuates over time and space, between individuals and cultural groups. This difficulty does not negate the fact, however, that health professionals must recognize and acknowledge social and cultural variations among ethnic groups, and they must not assume there are universal viewpoints concerning health and illness. To erroneously make this assumption nurtures the delivery of dehumanized health care to clients.

As can be gleaned from the above, of the three components of humanized health care, the one that at present can best be measured to determine the degree of humanization of health care is the biological. Related to this notion, Andreoli and Thompson (1977, p. 34) point out that while there is much overlap between the emphasis of medicine and that of nursing, "the differentiation appears to rest in . . . nursing exhibiting a greater emphasis on the psychosocial nature of man." If this is, indeed, true, it is more than ever the responsibility of nurses to develop research methods by which the psychological and sociocultural components of health care can be accurately measured to determine where this care falls on the humanized/dehumanized continuum.

Goals germane to humanized health care that must be operationalized, according to Howard (Howard and Strauss, 1975, pp. 73–86), include appreciation of the client's inherent worth as a human being and recognition that the client is irreplaceable. Then too, health care must utilize a holistic perspective of the client situation, one in which clients have the freedom of choice and action, and status equality with health professionals. Clients must share in decision-making and health care responsibilities, empathy is unconditionally present, and health personnel reflect a positive affect. The focus of each of these goals is ultimately upon the client, as they should be.

It is not difficult for health professionals to be misled into thinking that in some instances there are simple solutions to complex problems. For example, in order to promote parent/infant bonding, rooming-in for all mother/infant dyads should be established in hospitals and all fathers should be present at delivery. What such thinking does in essence is to replace one rigid system with another, when indeed the focus of health care should be on individual choice. Barnett and others (William and Oliver, 1969; Barnett et al., 1970) have clearly illustrated the validity of individualized health care through research conducted in the late 1960s and early 1970s.

Beginning in 1965, intensive-care nurseries throughout the United States began the unprecedented practice of allowing parents into the nursery to touch and interact with their sick baby. This was a humanistic movement based on the theory that such parent/infant interaction is psychologically necessary for both parents and infant to promote and nurture a healthy relationship. Barnett and his colleagues conducted research about this practice, which, although it focused on increased infection rates, eventually illustrated the humanized qualities inherent therein. An experimental group (mothers allowed into the nursery) and a control group (mothers kept out of the nursery) were utilized in the research design, and it was found that there was clearly a negative impact on the primiparous mothers separated from their infants immediately postpartum, but little effect on multiparous mothers. A finding equally important was that regardless of the mother's parity, if she had low self-confidence as a mother and in that related role, the separation resulted in her maintaining a low degree of self-confidence and in some cases it dropped even lower. Conversely, those with low self-confidence initially gained assurance after contact with their infant in the intensive-care nursery. Thus, the research defined a specific population that was at risk and who could definitely benefit from interaction with their infant. Mothers in the experimental group were given a choice of when to enter the nursery, depending upon when they themselves felt they were ready, thereby eliminating the possibility that one rigid system (all mothers enter at X time) would be substituted for another (no mothers allowed in nursery). The results of the research indicated that individual choice for mothers in the experimental group was one of the most important variables considered. Barnett (Howard and Strauss, 1975, p. 271) summarizes these findings in his comment that "If humanization is to mean anything, institutions designed to serve human needs must allow maximum choice and maximum alternatives to match the great variety of human desires."

Taking a devil's advocate role, Eliot Freidson (Howard and Strauss, 1975, pp. 223–228) argues that some types of dehumanization in health care are not detrimental, as is the case when people want "convenience and simplicity much more than solicitous human contact." This includes the group of people who primarily manage their own health care and who buy nonprescription medicines for their discomforts and disorders. He argues that self-care for this group should be nurtured in every way possible, thereby releasing health professionals for care of those who desire and seek humanized, individualized health care. Ethnic group membership and subscription to cultural norms do indeed dictate to some individuals the degree of humanized health care sought and that is able to be accepted comfortably, illustrating once again that what for one person is humanized care may for another be dehumanized care. The theory of proxemics, developed by social scientists, which describes how social distances are culturally prescribed, lends further light on how people perceive health care as humanized or dehumanized.

This author recently conducted research that further illustrates how what appears to be humanized health care for one group is for another group dehumanized (Clausen, 1977). The research population was comprised of a group of people, members of a religious sect located in a Rocky Mountain state, who do not seek private or public health care and who actively refute much of what modern medicine has established as scientific fact. Two children under the age of 5 years died from diphtheria within 16 months, and sect members entered into a conflict situation with local and state health department officials as well as local and surrounding townspeople.

These sect members' health/illness beliefs are based upon their religious orientation, which in turn is founded upon scriptural passages. Quoting from Isaiah 55:8–9 and Proverbs 14:12, sect members, or brethren as they call themselves, state that they believe God's ways are not man's ways, and that there is a way that seems right to man, but the end thereof are the ways of death. Medicine and health care as subscribed to by members of the dominant population are seen as the "arm of the flesh," and according to members' interpretation of the Scriptures, the arm of flesh destroys man.

The problem under study in this research was not to determine the validity of either the sect members' scriptural interpretations or the tenets espoused by health professionals in relation to health/illness behaviors. Rather, it was to determine the effects of interactions between the two groups insofar as change of health/illness behaviors of the brethren was concerned. The findings revealed that although brethren had become more knowledgeable about communicable diseases as a result of interactions with health professionals, they did not anticipate changing their behaviors relative to communicable diseases as the result of this increased knowledge.

An interesting finding arises, therefore, regarding humanized/dehumanized health care pertinent to this research population: It becomes clear that what health professionals believe is humanized health care in the form of immunizations and other preventive measures, as well as treatment for active communicable diseases, is seen as dehumanized care by religious sect members. The latter in no sense of the term have a death wish, nor do they accept death complacently when it strikes a member, no matter what the cause may be; in that respect brethren are no different from most members of the dominant population. Life is maintained, however, through good nutrition, exercise and work, rest and recreation, and living as dictated by the Bible. Interference into this life-style by health professionals and scientific medicine is viewed by brethren as decreasing their quality of life and inflicting a dehumanizing process upon them. This supports other research indicating that health/illness attitudes, beliefs, and behaviors that seem so valid and humanized to one sector of the population may have a completely opposite connotation for another.

Health professionals' concern with the humanized/dehumanized continuum of health care takes varied forms, an important one of which was a national symposium on humanizing health care held in December, 1972, in San Francisco, in which forty persons participated, representing more than a dozen disciplines within the health professions and behavioral sciences. The fundamental issues dealt with at that meeting had no clear guidelines at that time, but scholars who attended paved the way for furthering future understanding of humanized and dehumanized health care.

Concern is shown in other forms, such as medical and nursing audit committees established within health care institutions, peer review committees, consumer advocate representatives in health care settings, patients' bill of rights, standards for practice, and continuing education programs to update professionals' knowledge and expertise. Consumer input is increasingly being sought in dealing with numerous health care issues and concerns.

In closing, it is important to point out that any type of health care intervention attempted during a family's developmental cycle will fall upon deaf ears, and positive outcomes will not come to fruition if clients perceive they are receiving dehumanized health care. Each of us is responsible for defining variables peculiar to those families with whom we work through which they filter and ultimately judge whether the care received is humanized or dehumanized. It is not enough for us to define these variables from *our* frame of reference; what may seem humanizing to us as health professionals may very well be dehumanizing from the client's perspective. Understanding the importance of these variables can only be accomplished by being fully open to the client's point of view, which is based on his or her culturally prescribed way of life and the physical and psychological milieu therein.

REFERENCES

Andreoli, K. G., & Thompson, C. E. The nature of science in nursing. *Image,* 1977, *9*(2), 32–37.

Barnett, C. R., Leiderman, P. H., Grobstein, R., & Klaus, M. Neonatal separation: The maternal side of interactional deprivation. *Pediatrics,* 1970, *45,* 197–205.

Clausen, J. P. The natural experiment: A method for studying conflict resolution between health professionals and clients. (Unpublished doctoral dissertation, University of Colorado, 1977).

Howard, J., & Strauss, A. *Humanizing health care.* New York: John Wiley and Sons, 1975.

William, C. P. S., & Oliver, T. K. Nursery routines and staphylococcal colonization of the newborn. *Pediatrics,* 1969, *44,* 640–646.

CHAPTER EIGHTEEN

COMMUNITY HEALTH FAMILY NURSING

BEVERLY HENRY BOWNS

This chapter provides a backdrop of information to better understand why the practitioner of primary health care nursing came to be and is likely to continue to exist in modern-day nursing. For some, clarification of who is a practitioner of primary health care nursing is to be preoccupied with professional territorialism, as these individuals believe it does not make much difference who is providing the service to the client, it is only important that it gets done. The fact that there is an overlap in the functional services provided by several professional disciplines seems to support that position. Still others believe that it is an oversimplification of a complex network of transactional exchanges within the health care industry between consumer and the professional providers of health care. Those who support the latter position believe that the consumer, as a member of the health care team, has the need and the right to know, who is doing what for or with whom and the qualifications of those practitioners who assume that responsibility. Accountability and quality assurance have become watchwords of the health care marketplace, and primary health care nursing is no exception to this requirement.

The primary objective of exploring this issue in nursing is to present a structural model of the systems approach to primary health care nursing, more specifically the clinical specialty of Community Health Family Nursing (CHFN). The general systems model used is an expansion of the paradigm presented in the previous edition of *Family Health Care*

(Bowns, 1973). A select group of faculty[1] in a state college of nursing was responsible for the development of the design. It evolved over a 5-year period of implementation and systematic evaluation of an educational-service program of primary health care nursing. The structural model is an outcome of that experience.

Chapter limitations control the amount of detail that can be presented, and the intricacies of the system's subsystems are not presented. However, the structural design is a pragmatic one adaptable to almost any community-university complex. Research is critical to the design, but is not discussed as a separate subsystem, because it is considered an integral part of both education and service as the two components of the nursing care system. Evaluative research will document program outcomes according to a standard of quality. Clinical research identifies what nursing care actions make a difference in the health status of individuals, families, and/or communities whom they serve.

Finally, the key thrust of the chapter is to challenge the traditional academic approach to education in the health professions, which tends to insulate the teaching institution from the realities of the community. This has meant that professionals enter practice unable to comprehend the complexity of health care systems so they can function as a member of that system across the health care spectrum of preventive, promotive, curative, restorative, and maintenance interventions.

A PERSPECTIVE

The relatively rapid rate at which community health family nurse practitioners appear to be evolving is in some ways deceiving. One could consider that community health nursing, primary health care nursing, or public health nursing had its beginning in the United States in the New York Mission in 1877, when nurses provided their services in the home, unsupervised, and collected fees for those services under the auspices of a lay group. Not too different a method from those of the 1970s, when Carolyn Whitaker of Red Boiling Springs and Sue Schweer of Briceville, two Community Health Family Nurse Clinical Specialists, were hired by consumers to provide health care services to remote areas of Tennessee. The key difference between the two eras is that the modern-day nurse prac-

[1]Assistant Professor Patricia Brisley, R.N., M.P.H., a CHFN Clinical Specialist, and Barbara Reid, R.N., M.P.H., Administrative Assistant, were responsible for much of the implementation of the basic project directed by Professor B. H. Bowns and funded by DHEW grant no. 5-DIO-NU-01071-03 "Community Health Family Clinician," 1974–1977, University of Tennessee, Memphis.

titioner finds that the scientific knowledge base and technological advancements have expanded at an astronomical rate. This phenomenon has had a universal effect on the health care professional and it has propelled nurses into a level of service at which they are required to make high-level, life-and-death decisions for which they are directly accountable. It is this change in circumstance that has made us painfully aware of the need for research to document what is the character and the quality of nursing care we wish to consider as adequate for all consumers of our service.

A basic assumption has been that quality education would produce quality nurses who would provide quality services. In the real world this does not seem to be the case, as McVicar (1977) of the National League of Nursing pointed out in her confrontation with the American Hospital Association leadership on national television: "Of all health professionals, nurses are in the best position to judge quality care. Yet they have little to say . . . about priorities, enforcing standards, or making changes." In the late 60s and early 70s there was further evidence of this kind of political-social restriction in the health care industry. Community Health Family Nurse clinical specialists, quality nurse practitioners, had difficulty "fitting" into the existing system, a problem shared by many practitioners. Although some were highly successful as change agents, others were able to achieve only minor changes because of problems of underutilization and role deprivation (Bullough, 1974). Nursing care needs were less an expression of needs as nurses knew them to be, but were more often decisions made by non-nurse professionals who selected immediate solutions of political expediency to health care problems. Paradoxically, the "solutions" almost always required nurses to provide the care services being proposed.

Although having the nurse practitioner prepared at a high level of competency is a rather obvious requirement of quality nursing, Michnich, Harris, Willis, and Williams (1976) point out in their publication, *Ambulatory Care Evaluation Primer*, that few in the (health) field have implemented a systematic and ongoing method of achieving quality assessment or quality assurance. This team challenges those who speak for a level of quality care that is acceptable to provider and recipient alike. They ask the questions, "level of what?" and "acceptable to whom?" Since we all see things differently, they suggest nine possible dimensions of quality concern: structural adequacy, access/availability, provider caring, communication skills/attitudes, documentation, coordinational follow-up, patient commitment/adherence to therapeutic plan, patient satisfaction, and patient outcomes. Models specific to evaluation of quality nursing have been developed (Lang, 1977), but application to community health nursing has been problematic. As creditable providers, community health nurses will need to establish criteria for measuring the quality of the care they provide.

In general, quality nursing can be said to be personalized responsive care that is coordinated, continuous, comprehensive; directly available, accessible, and acceptable to consumers of every social class; administered by qualified nurse practitioners by level and across specialties, by setting, by consumer condition, and by law; is health directed, having therapeutic treatments that have predictable outcomes that can be measured. Basic to this statement, we need to look at what is considered therapeutic. Therapy is an educational or reeducational process and is a function of nursing applicable to consumers across the wellness-illness spectrum. The majority of us do not have the serious secondary/tertiary health care problems that require hospitalization, but all of us in our day-to-day activities have everyday health problems to contend with that may or may not be preliminary signals of more serious problems. Nursing in the community considers coping with the common crises of daily living as crucial to a person's state of well-being where preventive and promotive nursing care actions are of high quality.

A SITUATION

In the past few decades, health care has become big business, having promotional methods that focused on the more diagnostic curative (medical) aspects of health, permitting other health care needs to multiply and often go unattended. This created enormous pressures to show quick results to a complex problem, and short-term training was provided for nurses to work as "practitioners" in "expanded" roles in an attempt to plug the gaps in the system. In the hustle and bustle of all the activity, some needs were being met, but not according to an organized plan. Nurses began to take command of their destiny on behalf of themselves and of the clients whom they served. In the rush to meet primary health care needs, nurses were often misguided, if not actually exploited, under the guise of being "educated" for "new roles" for nurses.

Any substantive plan for change will surely depend upon the consumer, who will need to learn how the health care system works for and against one's best interests. Although consumers are better educated today and more informed about health matters than ever before, they still have little knowledge of the inside politics of the health care industry that controls health services. Nor do they have a standard for knowing whether the care received is good or even appropriate. A system of nursing care takes this into account where staff (service), faculty (education), and consumer share the same interests and share the responsibility for effecting the desired change.

In the system, the consumer is accepted as a constant on the health care team where the team goal is to bring the consumer to a point of self-direction and being able to cope with crisis and adapt to change, seeking assistance from others as needed. This places the consumer as a functional part of the system in the business of health care. This approach means faculty and staff need to be properly prepared to help the consumer assume this responsibility.

The Family Health Nurse Practitioner is a clinical specialist with public health or community health plus primary care preparation in nursing at a master's or doctoral level. Experience has shown that faculty must be in active practice if they are to maintain their expertise in their clinical specialty. The premise is you cannot practice what you do not know, nor can you teach what you do not practice. Knowledge of practice and management of care is ever-evolving and ever-changing, leaving active practice as a practical way, perhaps the only way, for a teacher to keep abreast of the realities of the profession—a practice that is challenged by some education administrators as too expensive in an already expensive enterprise. However, expenses can be offset by reimbursement to individual or institution for services provided.

Education and service are reciprocal, and the quality of one is indigenous to the other. It has been shown that when learning experiences are kept close to the realities of practice, the service expectations of education are better understood and the quality of practice improves. A free exchange of staff and faculty who also share responsibilities of service and education begins to create a climate of respect for each other's capabilities, and a colleague relationship builds that is as essential to nurse-nurse relationships as it is to nurse-other team relationships.

A SYSTEM APPROACH

The system is an *ecosystem* and considers people and their environment at each level of the system. It is a system that attends to a host of variables affecting one's state of health, whether from the viewpoint of a consumer, a provider, or an educator. The nurse health care provider is expected to change and sustain the system at all nurse-consumer points of contact to assure the quality of nursing care is the best that can be offered in each situation.

Landmarks of the system are: (1) quality nursing care can be defined; (2) professional nursing care is a subsystem of the health care system, having unique identifiable characteristics and structure; (3) primary health care is the area of practice for the family health nurse; (4) community health nursing (CHN) is a clinical specialty of nursing *in* the community concerned with health care *of* the community; (5) family health nursing has the family unit as the focus of services; it is a subspecialty of Community Health Nursing based on the knowledge and skills intrinsic to that specialty; (6) primary health care nursing is care provided at the point of entry to the health care system and is preventive, promotive, restorative, curative, and maintenance in kind; (7) health is the focus and is not considered the reciprocal of disease; (8) nursing education and nursing service are the *warp* and *woof* of the same cloth; (9) growth in service depends on the marriage of the ideal with the real; (10) behaviors of a "nurse carer" are integral to the nurse's life-style.

Faculty and staff share the same philosophy and commitment to the system and utilize the same concepts in their professional lives that produce the behaviors they expect students to acquire and utilize as practitioners. This attitude of "what I expect of you, I expect of me" helps to develop the sense of equality needed in therapeutic transactions and colleague relationships of professionals. To learn this on a nurse-to-nurse basis helps in transference to the other team members. Because the nurse is a role model in therapeutic encounters, the consumer takes on behaviors that verify achievement of team goals.

In this design, education and service constitute the *nursing care system* within the ecosystem. Each subsystem has external suprasystems and internal subsystems that create the conditions that support or disturb the balances of well-being. Nursing is in juxtaposition as a suprasystem and to health care as a subsystem. Both teaching methods and practices in nursing need to reflect this structure.

Blum's (1976) homo sapiens hierarchy of natural systems adapted from Brody's (1973) model provides a framework for understanding the relationship of suprasystems and subsystems of a universe. The paradigm has "person" in central position with suprasystems external to the individual: person + families + communities + nations + cultures + homo sapiens + biospheres. All internal parts are subsystems of the individual: person-body-systems-organs-tissue-cells-molecules-atoms-subatomic particles. Health of the system is a composite of three interacting and hierarchically related person levels termed as "somatic" (subsystems level), "psychic" (integrating junction) and "social" (suprasystems level) (Blum, 1976, Chapter 3).

In his book *Expanding Health Care Horizons*, Blum (1976) utilizes the paradigm to develop a schema for promoting effective health care. As the system is developed, "primary," "secondary," and "tertiary" are designated as levels of care. Primary care is concerned with populations of 10,000 or less; in local community clinical settings (including physicians' offices); having a family or general practitioner who is patient-care oriented; high level skills in general technology, ambulatory care of common diseases, emergency and preventive types of care, continuous care; major quantity of care that costs least. At the secondary level the care is located subregional, with a population of 100,000 plus, greater specialization at a higher cost. Tertiary care is located in regions (population 1 million plus), highly specialized specific care for a small number of patients at greater cost.

Patterns of employment have led society to believe nurses also follow this medical model; however, this is not quite true. For this reason the comparison is an important one to make, as nursing does not fall neatly into the medical care scheme of things. This may help to clarify why professional nursing is a separate entity rather than an extension of another profession. In nursing, primary, secondary, and tertiary are *areas* of practice with levels of nursing care within an area.

Primary care subsumes that the total population is the consumer, as each person has a real or potential need for the *health* care services of providers. This would mean primary care is concerned with all three areas of care, but not all to the same degree.

Primary care nursing is *majority care* and predominantly practiced in the community setting in private and official agencies other than hospitals. For example, family nurse clinical specialists practice in neighborhood clinics, private physician's offices, home health agencies, primary care centers, satellite clinics, health maintenance organizations, visiting nurses' associations, public health agencies, schools, industries, skilled nursing homes, outpatient services, family practice clinics, and their own offices. Although family health nurses are essentially community based, they do function in hospitals as coordinators, consultants, liaisons, and as practitioners in the hospital primary care settings of emergency and outpatient services.

It is this curative component of the health care system that identifies one of the main differences in focus and preparation of nurses and physicians. Curative functions are less often initiated by the nurse, but when they are, it is generally initiated by the primary care nurses. As an example, common conditions such as pediculosis, scabies, abrasions, impetigo, small cuts, and identification of communicable disease are part of the nurse practitioner's responsibility. This area of overlap in functions merits mentioning.

The concept of team provides for overlap of services to prevent losing the client in the system of care. Though outcomes may be similar in these instances, they are achieved through the special knowledge and skills of each professional. This is to say, a nursing care service, when similar to that of a physician's service, remains a nursing care service, not a medical one, although these are functions physicians have traditionally provided.

As an example, a nurse who diagnoses and treats otitis media in a child, educates the mother in its care and the prevention of recurrence, and prescribes a course of action for follow-up is performing a nursing care service. By the same token, a doctor who treats an adolescent youth for acne, writes up a treatment plan, discusses the plan in detail with the patient, then counsels him via a discussion of the embarrassment the condition causes him when trying to date girls, and offers to discuss the treatment regimen with his mother, is providing a medical care service. Most of these functions are traditionally functions of a nurse, but physicians may provide such service. Both providers could do both things well; *neither will do them in the same way*. Their knowledge base for making the judgments leading to the same high-level decisions are dissimilar and come from different disciplinary backgrounds. Neither service should be denied the client merely because one or the other is not available.

Unlike the physician in Blum's medical model, the highly specialized family health nurse is equally if not more critically needed for the practice of nursing, in rural areas, core city, and suburbia where health care support systems are less adequate. Ideally, all three levels of nurse practitioners are required. Statistics indicate that the mix of nurses in any one of the three areas is skewed toward less prepared than highly prepared nurses (ANA *Facts about Nursing,* 1975). Since this is the case, it might be important to have the better prepared in the less structured, more deprived locales, where sophisticated health care support systems are less accessible and available. As more nurses become prepared at the more advanced levels, the distribution could be directed to adequately covering nursing care needs at all levels.

Another difference between Blum's medical model and the nursing model proposed here is a monetary one. Reimbursement for nursing services would be the same across the continuum of health care whether primary, secondary, or tertiary and would vary only by level of preparation. This means cost of health care would be consistent with services received, whether the same service is provided by physicians or nurses functioning in either primary, secondary, or tertiary care facilities. The fee for a service would be the same. Identification of costs for services would help the consumer to know what a dollar could buy in the health care marketplace. It has been shown that a high-level nursing service is less costly and when appropriately utilized it is economical (Funkhauser, 1976).

Continuity of services in medicine and in nursing has similarities and differences. Two major differences are that (1) nursing care is 24-hour care, often 7 days a week, and (2) continuous care is generally recognized as a responsibility of nurses. The community health family nurse takes the service to the home and from the home to other areas of the health care system. It requires collaboration between and among professional disciplines. For Community Health Nursing it is more broadly defined where the client may be the individual, family, and/or community. The emphasis on health expands and extends services of nursing across the multiple dimensions of health care and includes planning, developing, and implementing health care within and between communities. The education of community health family nurses prepares them to assume this role. This conceptual interpretation has some interesting implications for the education of teams and team relationships. These implications are discussed later in this chapter.

Whether family health nursing is a clinical subspecialty of community health nursing is a moot question. If community health nursing is care *of* a community rather than *in* a community, then all nurse practitioners who function in the community should have some fundamental knowledge of the community whether community health nurse specialists or not. If that sounds like the riddle of the year, then this may be also: A nurse who is in primary care nursing is in an area of practice that transcends all of the nurse clinical specialists functioning in the community, and all should have some knowledge of the philosophy and the basic concepts of primary care. If one agrees that primary care is the supraordinate term, then community health nursing takes its place as a specialized field of primary care practice among all other nurse clinical specialities practiced in the community setting. In this context it is a clinical specialty with numerous subspecialties: adult health nursing, school health nursing, industrial health nursing, women's health nursing, and family health nursing. The community health nurse specialist would have the broad concept of nursing care of a specified community and be concerned with planning, developing, and implementing nursing care actions that would affect the health status of the aggregate and more indirectly affect the individual and the family.

Some areas of specialization have attempted to attend to this problem by having the generalist a clinical specialist, as in psychiatric nursing, with subspecialties such as child psychiatry and adult psychiatry. Other areas of nursing have not adopted that schema and this chapter offers another alternative for consideration. In community health, no clear structure has evolved; however, a group of nurse educators from community health and public health programs are deliberating the problem of how community health nursing is to evolve in the future (Ohlson, 1977). Whatever decisions are made, it will have a ripple effect throughout community health/public health nursing service and educational programs.

In this model, the nursing care system evolved as one of the subsystems of the health care system and the structure appears as follows:

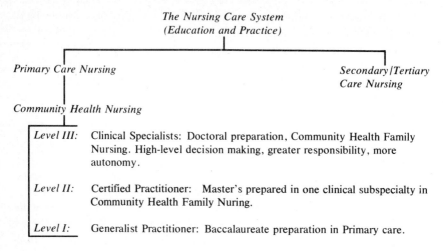

Figure 18-1 Diagram of the health care system.

The Nursing Care System
(Education and Practice)

Primary Care Nursing   *Secondary/Tertiary*
                                                          Care Nursing

Community Health Nursing

Level III: Clinical Specialists: Doctoral preparation, Community Health Family Nursing. High-level decision making, greater responsibility, more autonomy.

Level II: Certified Practitioner: Master's prepared in one clinical subspecialty in Community Health Family Nuring.

Level I: Generalist Practitioner: Baccalaureate preparation in Primary care.

Nursing provides coordinated, comprehensive, continuous care that adapts well to the general systems approach. It means there are no sharp territorial demarcations, but multiples of interlacing junctures where one, two, or more nurse functionaries are prepared to provide care. Overlap prevails within nursing disciplines and across professional disciplines. Figure 18-2 shows how the nursing care system is designed to consider the nursing care needs of society through preparation and practice.

To elaborate, the nurse in the community would have both primary care and community care preparation. The health components of the educational process would cover the content appropriate to community related to the somatic, psychic, and social health of humankind. For example, mental health would be a part of every nurse's repertoire and the subspecialty in community mental health would focus on nursing the psyche as the problem and the somatic-social disruptions as they affect or are affected by the psyche. However, emphasis would be at the wellness end of the health spectrum and prevention of entry and reentry to institutionalized care would be appropriate. Working with identified high-risk groups prior to onset of illness would be one way the mental health nurse would function. Space does not permit full development of all or any one of the subspecialties, but to put another small piece in place the psychiatric nurse as a subspecialty of secondary/tertiary care would be prepared to attend to the institutionalized person with more episodic disturbances of psychic origin and somatic conditions strongly affected by the state of the psyche. Continuous, coordinated, and comprehensive nursing care between and among nurses improves through the use of this

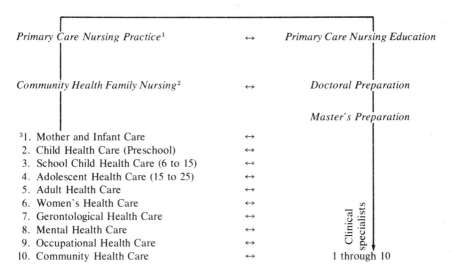

Primary Care is the area of specialization.

[1] Primary Care is the area of specialization.
[2] Community Health Family Nursing (CHFN) is the clinical specialty.
[3] Subspecialties of CHFN.

Figure 18-2 The nursing care system (theory and practice).

schema. Nurse-to-nurse referrals become more effective. When that oc-curs, nurses are able to assure a better quality of nursing care.

In summary, nursing care has the characteristics of a general system with feedback mechanisms (communication), linkages that relate verti-cally and horizontally. It is a system that maintains dynamic equilibrium through its natural resources (faculty, staff, and student practitioners), and the feedback mechanisms transmit energies which have a cause-effect relationship between persons or organizations of persons.

A SYSTEMS MODEL

Nursing education and service, like a helix, share elements and feedback chains with energy exchanges that strive for a dynamic equilibrium and comprise the nursing care system. When linkages fail to connect, energy is dissipated, the system malfunctions, and the quality of nursing care suffers. There are those who might argue that education should not be-come involved in the practice of nursing lest they risk losing their academic objectivity, an objectivity essential to research and theory building. Further, these educators believe that education would be en-cumbered by assuming responsibility for the problems of service in addition to those they must address in education. The counterargument is that health is a broad field of human problems within a complex network of interrelated systems. Therefore, experiments and study cannot be achieved in isolation from the realities of community life and apart from disciplines in other subsystems of the health care system. Nursing research will require a setting appropriate to the clinical area being studied whether it is conducted as a collaborative effort or an independent investigation.

For primary care nursing it is appropriate that the educational experiences be in the community setting rather than the hospital's acute care setting. Nursing care linkages are important to span the interface between primary and secondary/tertiary care just as it is important to span the education-practice interface. Nursing education and service needs to maintain a balance between objectivity and total involvement in delivery of services. The communication process of shared feedback loops is such that faculty are involved in education for the purpose of maintaining and improving the quality of their practice.

The *Nurse Practitioner* (NP) is an independent health care professional; licensed under a State Nurse's Practice Act; certified by the American Nurses Association (ANA); prepared in a National League of Nursing accredited program of study, at the baccalaureate, master's, or doctoral levels (adapted from ANA, 1974 definition). Presently credentialing assures a minimum level of knowledge for practice. Credentialing is also intended to verify that the Nurse Practitioner (NP) is in active practice a reasonable number of hours a week to maintain competency, and the NP has continued education to keep abreast of new research, knowledge, and technology.

The *nurse practitioner in primary care* is formally prepared to give comprehensive, continuous, personalized care to consumers at the point of entry to the health care system. As independent functionaries, they are accountable within solo, group, or agency practice to make sound judgments while providing care to the consumer in ambulatory settings (ANA, A-FNP, Scope of Practice, 1976).

Care given in *ambulatory settings* refers to care on an outpatient basis, and includes care of home-bound clients and/or clinical or emergency situations where the direct course of service is in a primary care setting. *Home* may designate a substitute residence: half-way house, nursing home, home for the handicapped, or facility external to in-hospital episodic services. It is majority care (ANA guidelines for short-term educational programs).

Primary care includes: (1) the care the consumer receives at the entry to the health care system and, (2) the continued care of the individual as a client (ambulatory). The continued care is two-dimensional: (1) the identification, management, and/or referral of the health problem, and (2) the maintenance of the consumer's health, when symptomatic illness is not apparent, by means of preventive and promotive health care actions (ANA 1976).

The *Family Health Nurse Clinical Specialist* is a legally licensed practitioner, prepared in a formal and accredited program of graduate study, as a diversified primary care provider in the discipline of community health nursing, prepared to give comprehensive, continuous personalized care to persons of all age groups within a family constellation (ANA *Scope of Practice,* 1975).

Health in the context of primary health care cannot be considered the reciprocal of disease when the emphasis is on the healthy state and maintenance of that state. For this reason, Freymann's (1974, p. 211) definition seems appropriate. It is derived from an earlier definition by Duhl (1969): "Health is a state of competence—of emotional, mental, and physical strength—enabling a person to set goals, investigate alternatives, make decisions, and take action to control his environment within the sphere for which by nature and circumstances he has been fitted." In his definition, Freymann includes the entire population and bases his definition on twin concepts: "1) Health is a positive state, and 2) a healthy human being controls his environment at a level commensurate with his own society's expectations of him." Examples of a healthy state are exemplified by an infant's smile of recognition or an older person's ability to chew food.

As Freymann points out, an individual who is unable to control the environment at a level commensurate with one's own and society's expectations is *not healthy,* yet from a medical standpoint that individual could be diagnosed as *healthy.* An example of this is the divorced woman who, prior to her hysterectomy, was socially active and contemplating remarriage, but then became introverted and focused her energies totally on herself and her children and activities of the home. The physician has pronounced her completely recovered from an uncomplicated successful surgical experience.

Levels of nursing care are a reality of the practice world that generally are defined by preparation and experience, complexity of decision making, degree of responsibility, and amount of autonomy. *Level I* is the baccalaureate practitioner, a generalist, prepared in the area of primary care. The preparation includes knowledge of primary and community health nursing. *Level II* is prepared as a subspecialist of CHFN. This person has a master's degree with knowledge of primary-community health nursing and the family. There is content in depth, about one age group within a family constellation. *Level III* is the post-master's doctorally prepared nurse or Community Health Family Nurse with knowledge of primary health care across all age groups of a family or community. Presently, the nurse with ANA certification is the Level I and II nurse in our schema of community health nursing care and the nurse carries the initials R.N.C. following the other identifying qualifications such as R.N.C., B.S., or R.N.C., M.S. (see Figure 18-1).

Pioneers in nursing are as important today as they ever were, but it is one thing to send change agents out into the system and another to have a planned system of nursing care for future practice; both are needed. (See Figure 18-3.)

The nursing education component includes degree programs of study, continuing education, and in-service learning. Nursing education would be provided by nurses to other health professionals, not just education on interdisciplinary team basis, but faculty role models in team practice with other professionals. Team is not always a nurse-physician-consumer team, but can be a combination of health care providers who are available and appropriate to meeting consumer needs such as other nurse specialists, dentists, social workers, health planners. Interdisciplinary education also means student learners should be a mix of disciplines in the classroom and clinical settings.

Home care when complex and/or where the service is remote would require a clinical nurse specialist (Level II and III) for management care. Level I nurses are required for supplementing and complementing the team care in any site. Health education of patients with both cardiovascular disease and arthritis would require the special advanced knowledge of the Level II and III nurse. Antepartal health education of the uncomplicated pregnant woman is an example of Level I health teaching. In the more complex cases the Level I nurse provides educational assistance, but the overall management of care would be provided by the Level II or III nurse.

Outreach facilities are satellite to larger facilities either by design or by circumstance. City and county health departments are an example of an outreach resource. Family nurse clinical specialists are more critical to the remote (rural) and isolated (core city and suburbia) segments of society, where the health care support system is weakest, than to regional centers. However, as the faculty and staff work to build a system's network of qualified nurse providers the focus should be on *all* levels of nursing within the nation's *regionalized health planning:* the regional center, intermediate care by population, and sophistication of health resources and the remote areas with small population and common health care needs, so as to demonstrate continuity across areas of practice.

The interface of hospital (secondary/tertiary care) with community (primary care) is the business of the specialists from both areas. The secondary nurse clinical specialist can assist in the transition of patients from hospital to home and the primary nurse clinical specialist from home to hospital. Hospital privileges are required for both to achieve this interchange.

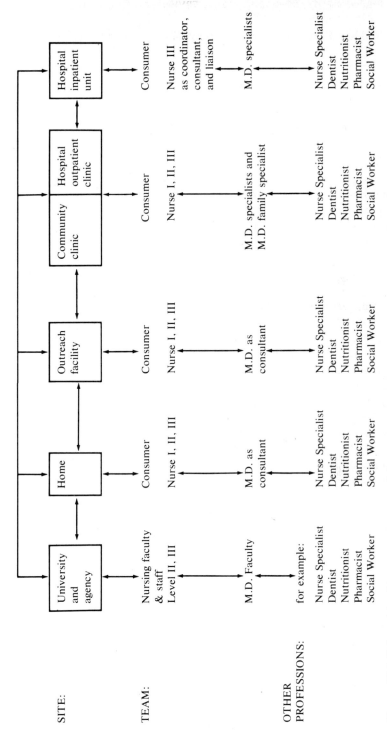

Figure 18-3 Primary health care systems model.

A NURSING EDUCATION—SUBSYSTEM MODEL

Each part, education and service, of the nursing care system can be considered subsystems of the whole; much as Laszlo (1972) has expressed it, evolution has superimposed encompassing systems upon systems. From a social-political sense, service and education have coexisted as separate social systems of community (town) and academia (gown). In nursing care, the position of separate and apart is not justifiable when the quality of human life might be compromised.

As an example of one subsystem, education will be explored as the area the system's capacity to replace and replenish its energy resources (nurses) in order to "survive." It can be considered the reproduction component of the nursing care system.

The educational plan is for entry at three levels: (1) baccalaureate honors study in community health family nursing, (2) master's clinical subspecialty study, and (3) doctoral study in the area of primary health care, namely, community health family nursing. Curriculum content and learning experiences would be delineated by level of outcome expectations for practice.

The baccalaureate program of study already includes the primary care technical skills of a nurse practitioner, and the honors courses would enhance the basic preparation by offering graduate courses as honors courses for undergraduate students, such as nursing theory, philosophy and patterns of practice in primary care, social systems studies, family systems approach to care, and role resocialization. These courses could carry both graduate and baccalaureate credits to facilitate matriculation from one level to the next. Graduate credit could be contingent upon subsequent course work in each of the courses taken, and so these courses become a part of the "vertical core."

The master's and doctoral levels of study would have additional vertical core courses such as social systems that deal with the natural history of the health care system, pathophysiology, laboratory diagnostic methods, role resocialization, and family therapy as some examples.

Horizontal core applies to the master's and doctoral levels of the educational continuum. In addition to vertical and horizontal core courses, there are required courses specific to the requirements of the subspecialties and the doctoral program for community health family nurses. Articulation of curriculum content is facilitated across levels of nursing education. The grid design of the curriculum is tri-level and multidimensional. The articulation is by learning experience and course work with three linkages, (1) vertical core, (2) horizontal core, and (3) specific content by subspecialty and specialty. These are defined as:

Vertical core is required content and experiences relevant to two or three of the levels of study. Course credits are transferable from level to level.

Horizontal core is required content and experiences relevant to one level only; several options are available at that level. For example, a student may wish to combine two subspecialties.

Specific content is required content and experiences related to a single option and at only one level.

Figure 18-4 helps to clarify the structure of the educational subsystem.

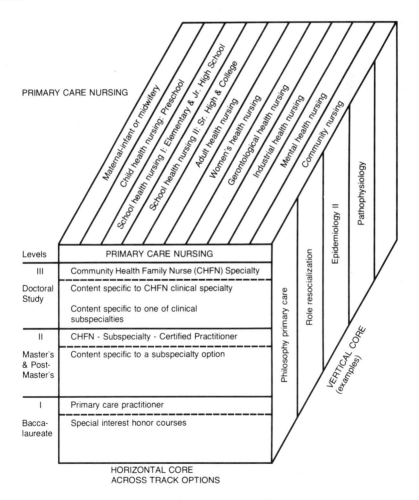

Figure 18-4 Diagram of the educational program subsystem.

CONCEPTS OF FAMILY NURSING

A network of key concepts and processes traverses the areas of special study and form a construct of eclectic theory. Since some knowledge of family health is basic to all the subspecialties, the processes and concepts inherent in that area are discussed to exemplify how this might work.

The family as a system and the focus of community health family nursing is not new. However, it was relatively recently that a community health nurse educator (Bowns, 1969) elected to abandon the "family oriented" approach for the more complex family therapy method of therapeutic practice. Selected concepts, strategies, and techniques appropriate to community health family nursing became part of the curriculum design. In this way family nursing becomes the trunk from which all other nursing concepts branch out.

A *family* as a system is an interacting entity with mutually reinforcing *functions,* transmitted by dynamic *processes,* which provides a setting for the satisfaction and *growth* of the emotional, social, and biophysical requirements of its individual members. Ackerman (1958), an early leader of the field, points out, "There are critical turning points in the life of the family that tend to strengthen or weaken the bonds of the family." One could perceive the crises of daily living as events that repeatedly put these bonds to test. Both Satir and Ackerman conceptualize family growth as an essential element of its healthy state. Ackerman speaks of it as continuity over the family's lifetime from the time a family begins (germination) through the slow decline to dissolution of the old into the new. Satir (1967) believes the family that is growth oriented has a natural, honest, constructive approach to life that accepts differences, negotiates and compromises, and is reality oriented. She calls this the "open system" family in contrast to the "closed system," where differences are treated as dangerous deviations and suspect.

Processes help to integrate and synthesize the knowledge and skills common to family nursing practice. In this model, education, therapy, communication, socialization, management, and growth are the processes emphasized. *Education* is the one process considered critical to all others, as it is an element of the other five. *Maturation, functional adaptation, integrity* (self-esteem), *autonomy, responsibility,* and *accountability* are the key concepts developed in the clinical practice of community health family therapy. Satir (1967) suggests that *maturation* is the most important of these concepts, because it is the touchstone for all the rest. In pursuit of Satir's impression, it suggests a person who is fully in charge of "self," who can make choices and decisions based on accurate perceptions and can accept the responsibility for the outcomes of one's actions is a mature human being.

The family nurse students, in their formal preparation, will develop behaviors that reflect the integration of these concepts and utilization of key processes in their practice. They are inherent to all of the learning experiences and are integrals of the theoretical framework of the program. The family nurse faculty, as role models, are expected to demonstrate those same competencies in their practice and in their professional interactions with nurses, other professionals, consumers, and systems personnel. Since the behavioral performance of the community health family nursing staff in the service setting are also utilizing these behaviors in their interactions with consumers, other staff, faculty, students, and agency personnel, a unified direction of effort emerges. The linkages seem to weld and the system achieves continuity.

To achieve system cohesiveness, faculty role models need to practice in the same clinical settings where students receive their learning experiences, whether the learning experience is part of the clinical course work or the field experience in residence. Field placements need to be selected by an evaluation team, and the physician and nurse clinical specialist in that agency must be qualified academically to meet the criteria of appointment to the university and be philosophically committed to the systems approach to quality care.

Arrangements for joint appointments vary. In some instances, the agency and university would each pay a portion of the faculty person's salary. In these instances, the monies from the agency's budget can be transferred to the community health nursing department budget at the university. In some situations, the reverse may be true and the agency would pay full salary and the university pay the agency for faculty functions. Having one source of payment protects the faculty or staff person's rights to fringe benefits provided by the university or the agency. Within a university the arrangements may be between several departments in the medical school and the community health nursing department where the program is housed.

Appointments may be negotiated to provide clinical teaching to nursing students and medical students in the same setting. Faculty who provide lectures only need not have joint appointments; these can be volunteer or "trade-offs." Whatever the arrangements, the nurses, whether faculty or staff or both, need to be placed strategically where previously linkages seemed weak or were absent. In this manner a system of nursing care delivery is developed as a part of the existing system.

CONCLUSION

Nursing care has the characteristics of a system and is a continuous one of learning and practice. It is a system of interdependent relationships that cannot be altered without affecting the function and viability of the whole system. It is a self-repairing and self-maintaining system, as it has the capacity to replace its energy sources (nurses) and to maintain balances (equilibrium). As a subsystem with feedback mechanisms it relates vertically and horizontally to other subsystems and the suprasystem. As a system, nursing care can complement and support the health care delivery system or, unfortunately, can fail to and thus quality of care is affected. True nursing is an essential component of the health care system and holds the key to its successful functioning.

Having these characteristics, the nursing care system with family health nursing as one part of the whole has a network like a system and in this system the cognate parts are education and service. This effort provides one approach for giving direction to nursing actions and professional relationships that can attain a common goal: quality care for the consumer.

REFERENCES

Ackerman, N. W. *The psychodynamics of family life.* New York: Basic Books, 1958, Chapters 16 and 17.

American Nurses' Association. *Facts about nursing.* Kansas City, 1975, 74–75.

———. *Definitions: Nurse practitioner, nurse clinician, and clinical nurse specialist.* Congress for Nursing Practice, Kansas City, 1974.

———. *Guidelines for short term continuing education programs for adults and family nurses.* Kansas City, 1974.

———. *Scope of practice: Primary nursing care practice for adults and families.* Kansas City, 1976.

Blum, H. L. *Expanding health care horizons.* Oakland: Third Party Associates, 1976.

Bowns, B. H. The family nurse clinician. In D. P. Hymovich and M. U. Barnard (Eds.), *Family health care.* New York, McGraw-Hill, 1973.

Brody, H. The systems view of man: Implications for medicine, science and ethics, *Perspectives in Biology and Medicine,* 1973, *17* (1), 71–92.

Bullough, B. Is the nurse practitioner role a source of increased work satisfaction? *Nursing Research,* 1974, *23,* 14–19.

Duhl, L. J. Health research and the university. *American Journal of Public Health,* Washington, D.C., 1969, *59,* 21–28.

Freymann, J. G. *The American health care system: Its genesis and trajectory.* New York: Medcom Press, 1974, 1–398.

Lang, N. *A model for quality assurance in nursing.* American Nurses' Association, Kansas City, 1976.

MacVicar, J. Are hospitals safe? N.L.N., A.H.A., face the issue. *National League of Nursing News,* 1977, *25,* 3.

Michnich, M. E., Harris, J., Willis, R., & Williams, J. *Ambulatory care evalua-*

tion: A primer for quality review. Los Angeles: University of California Press, 1976.

Ohlson, V. (convener). Meeting of Nurse Educators in Community Health Nursing Programs in Institutions of Higher Education, American Public Health Association, Nurses' Section, Chicago, 1977.

Satir, V. *Conjoint family therapy*. Palo Alto, Cal.: Science and Behavior Books, 1967.

CHAPTER NINETEEN

FAMILY ASSESSMENT GUIDELINES

CAROLYN E. EDISON

Family assessment, to be effective and meaningful, must be regarded as a process that includes the collection of data about family functioning in terms of habits and behavior. The approach to family assessment must be systematic, thorough, and ongoing. Analysis of the data collected should lead to the setting of mutually acceptable immediate, intermediate, and long-term goals. The goals are arrived at, ideally, by interaction of both the family and interviewer in order to be valid and meaningful. Developmental tasks are anticipated and planned for in the assessment process, as the very heart of nursing involves anticipatory guidance.

Knowledge about families and their ways of obtaining or maintaining health cannot be achieved in depth without giving systematic attention to the multiplicity of factors involved in family assessment. Every area of family functioning must be explored, even those areas that we frequently tend to ignore for a number of reasons, some known and others unknown. Experience clearly reveals that nurses often skip over questions about finances, religion, and sexuality either because we are too personally uncomfortable with these topics or because we do not know what to do with the information once we have it. The Family Assessment Tool (see Appendix, page 273) presented in this chapter makes it easier for the interviewer to obtain information about topics we have a tendency to shun.

Basic to the understanding of families and individuals is some knowledge of their respective places in the community setting, their expectations of themselves and others, and their concepts of health and health problems. An assessment tool that is open-ended, comprehensive, and applicable to a wide variety of family constellations is required. Information that will identify the particular strengths and coping mechanisms, as well as weaknesses and potential problems, must be elicited in the complete family assessment. The Family Assessment Tool developed by this writer over a period of several months is being used extensively in her private practice. It is open-ended and constructed in such a way as to allow completion or addition at any time.

Before the assessment process is initiated, the nurse and family members need to establish a relationship that will permit collection and verification of data. This may be done by helping the family understand that you have a sincere and professional interest in them and that you do, indeed, possess the qualities and resources for dealing with their needs.

At all times, while remaining systematic and thorough, flexibility must be inherent in the relationship. A delicate balance is vital between being systematic and flexible and should result in a constantly fluid and ongoing process. This ideal balance is most difficult to achieve, but when it is approached, genuine assessment is then drawing on all the interpersonal and intellectual skills the professional nurse possesses.

The reader will recognize that material presented in this chapter refers to the ideal family assessment process and that many factors may enter into the relationship that render the actual situation less than ideal. The following guidelines are intended to be used in a wide range of assessment settings and adapted to meet specific needs.

FAMILY CONSTELLATION

Identifying data is initiated by determining the family name and the given names of all individual members. The relationship among persons living in the home is vital information in this time of diverse family styles. Whether the adults are married, divorced, separated, single, common-law, or of some other relationship is needed information. Learning that the parents are separated may lead to a discussion of reasons for the separation and provide an avenue for intervention. Early in this time of information-seeking, name and ordinal position of each child are elicited, including whether any miscarriages have occurred, and if so, when and at what stage of gestation. Particularly significant to the maternal-child health professional is information about past pregnancies; however, further discussion of any miscarriages or neonatal deaths is usually reserved for a later time in the interview when a trust relationship has begun to develop. A great deal may be learned by obtaining the age, sex, and relationship of any other persons who may be living in the home as well as significant family relatives and/or friends who may not occupy the immediate residence but who may frequently have close contact with family members.

Significant, culturally divergent child-rearing practices may be uncovered by asking nationality of origin. Some common variations in personality are better understood in light of ethnic differences and cultural backgrounds (Clark, 1959; Whiting, 1973). This writer remembers the Mexican-American mother who became extremely upset because the nurse looked at her 8-month-old son for a few moments without touching him. The mother was able to verbalize her belief that looking at her child without first having touched him meant an evil spell was being cast. Nationality of origin should be included for immediate members of the family and for both maternal and paternal grandparents. Hall describes culture as the "link between human beings and the means they have of interacting with others" (Hall, 1966, p. 213).

EDUCATION

Early in the interview nonthreatening information is more easily obtained and most people seem eager to talk about educational levels and experiences of family members. A question such as, "What does each of the children like best in school?" will often uncover problems at the same time positive information is being given about strengths of family members. General feelings about the significance of education may be arrived at by asking about long-term goals and aspirations for the children and parents. This writer rarely encounters an adult who is reluctant to respond to "If you could have any education you want, what would it be?"

OCCUPATION

From education one can move quite easily into a discussion of occupation. To paint a complete picture it is necessary to learn which family members are working and where, as well as the type of work and hours of work. If specific questions are not asked relative to satisfaction with work and/or problems with employer or co-workers, the interviewer runs the risk of missing possible stressors that may impact heavily on the wellness level of the family. For example, 22-year-old Larry B. accompanied his wife, Judy, age 21, and their children, 3-year-old Jill and 14-month-old Jeffrey, to the well-baby clinic for their regular monthly check-up. The nurse recalled that on a previous visit Judy had been hesitant about discussing her husband's employment and had decided to defer questioning for a later visit. This time the atmosphere was friendly and open so Larry was asked, "Are you satisfied with your work?" Much to Judy's surprise, and perhaps to his own, he began to relate a most unsatisfactory work relationship and stated he never talked about it at home because he "did not want to upset Judy." He had been carrying the heavy load of a most stressful employment situation. Two months later Judy reported that Larry was much happier, not because he had changed jobs, but because he was able to "talk out his frustrations." Judy also stated their marriage was much improved "because we talk about more things now."

COMMUNICATION PATTERNS

Simply asking, "Do you and your husband/wife really talk with each other?" will sometimes elicit very real stressors that need attention. Much has been written about the role of communication in family functioning. Satir states that "without communication we, as humans, would not be able to survive" (Satir, 1967, p. 63). The importance of real communication to the general well-being of a family is obvious and is an area that must be addressed if our assessment is to be complete. Often a breakdown in communication patterns is the first signal of deep emotional problems.

FINANCES

Source of family finances is necessary information that is frequently omitted either because the interviewer is uncomfortable with the subject or because the client is reluctant to disclose this information. Adequacy of resources to meet daily needs, approximate monthly payments, insurance, pension plan, and security for future education all need to be discussed. The young single mother may not have resources available to adequately feed herself and her baby and may not know that assistance is available for meeting her needs. Information gathered at this juncture in the assessment interview should provide a baseline for discussing alternatives and options.

RESIDENCE

Open-ended questions such as, "What does your family like or dislike about where you live?" will provide an opportunity for learning about the family residence and identify possible stressors in the living environment.

Questions about the type of residence, adequacy of space, lighting, and ventilation will possibly assist in the identification of health and safety hazards or inadequacies.

TRANSPORTATION

Assisting the family to make appropriate contacts to meet their health care needs is an accepted part of primary health care. Too often, however, we fail to go one step further and inquire about their ability to keep appointments, especially in view of inadequate transportation resources. For example, Loretta had not kept her last three prenatal visits because she "had no way to get to the clinic." Public transportation is available in her neighborhood and is within her financial means; however, she "just never did ride the bus." The inability to use available resources, as in this instance, is an important bit of information for the health care provider and will sometimes be discovered only by using a comprehensive family assessment.

While transportation needs are being discussed, the health professional should determine whether the family needs teaching about the use of seat belts for adults and safe car seats for infants and children.

FAMILY GOALS AND FUNCTIONING

What are the family goals in terms of housing, car, vacation, job, furniture, etc.? Do individual family members have specific goals, and, if so, are those goals appropriate within the family being assessed?

Many families have not actually thought in terms of how they function and who is the dominant family member, if indeed there is one. Questions about family roles often initiate the self-evaluation process and serve as catalysts in the formulation of a philosophy of family living.

ACTIVITIES OF A TYPICAL DAY

Asking the client to describe a typical day in their family functioning will often expose some very real concerns, enabling the perceptive interviewer to zero in on weaknesses as well as strengths and resources. As clients describe a typical day, they may also be giving information about a number of other areas the interviewer tends to explore with them. This is also the kind of question that makes the one being interviewed feel free to discuss any subject. Frequent comments such as, "Wow, I didn't know you were interested in what I do at home!'' provide an opportunity for discussing the holistic approach to health care and for assisting the client to learn that every area of life has an effect on other aspects, just as the health or illness of one family member has great impact on the family as a whole.

RELIGIOUS PREFERENCE

The spiritual component of wellness has been, by our own admission, too often ignored or only briefly addressed by health team members; however, unless we have an idea of the role that religion plays in the lives of our clients, we are not able to relate fully to the whole person or whole family. Again, using the open-ended question approach, the client is given permission to share the religious orientation. In addition to asking just about "religious preference," this writer asks about religious practices such as grace at mealtime, evening prayers, confirmation practices, and Bible study groups. "What special religious practices does your family observe?" usually provides the nurse with helpful information and adds to a better understanding of the family as a whole.

AVOCATION AND RECREATIONAL INTERESTS

Seeking information about a person's avocation implies that diverse interests and involvements are healthy and that the well-rounded individual or family will perhaps be involved in a number of activities. A complete lack of any hobbies or interests may be a clue to look for signs of depression or other stressors. Whether or not mates have free time together, alone, with friends, relatives, or outside the family circle are all significant elements of family assessment.

HEALTH HISTORY

After determining data relative to the family constellation and functioning, the next major area addressed is that of the health history of each family member and, thus, of the family unit. Beginning with the parents and following through with each child in the family, an attempt is made to elicit a complete health history, including the strengths and coping mechanisms of each member as well as the illnesses or weaknesses. The question, "What does illness do to your family?" will often uncover subtle areas of stress.

If any other person lives in the home, the health history of that person is equally important. An obvious example may be the elderly aunt with a history of tuberculosis who may have a direct influence on the health of other family members. Always included, along with the usual history concerns, is information related to suicide or attempted suicide, use of drugs, accident proneness, and mental health.

Many of the areas covered in the health history are addressed at other times in the interview, but are included in more than one place as a double-check. Often a client will remember significant events or information when questioned in a different way. Generalized reactions such as weakness, tiredness, anxiety, nervousness, depression, moodiness, tantrums, fainting spells, and convulsions are significant and the extra time required to ask these specific questions is well spent.

SPECIAL SENSES

Inquiring whether any family member has vision difficulties, hearing problems, problems with walking, or learning difficulties uncovers potential or real weaknesses. The nurse may be the first to determine that a child has learning difficulties and is in an excellent position to begin searching for reasons for the difficulty and mobilizing family strengths to face the problem.

DENTAL CARE

One of the most important questions to ask parents of young children is, "What does your family do to have healthy teeth?" Because early dental assessment can prevent possible serious conditions such as "bottle-mouth syndrome" (Rabinowitz, 1974, pp. 18–20) and rheumatic fever, the health professional who fails to assess adequately this area is remiss indeed.

FOOD AND EATING PATTERNS

Nutritional status of the family may be assessed by questioning about food and eating patterns, common likes and dislikes, weight problems, meal schedules, smoking, drinking, exercising, sleep, and rest. Although some of this information will have been elicited in the discussion of a typical day earlier in the interview, experience has shown over and over again that restating the question at this point usually leads to more data that are significant.

SEXUALITY

Sexuality is probably the most often ignored or inadequately covered subject in the assessment process. Only recently have we begun to deal with our own comfort levels regarding sexuality and are recognizing the responsibility we have for dealing with this area as a necessary element of family health care (Adams, 1976, pp. 166–169). Beginning with the least threatening aspect of sexuality, usually menstrual patterns or difficulties, one can then move to the subject of male/female roles and how each partner views his or her role. Ideally, this is done with both partners present, but in reality this is not usually the case.

CHILD-REARING PRACTICES

Child-rearing practices are frequently cited as sources of frustration. Learning what role each mate plays in the discipline of the children provides valuable information and insight into stressors that might otherwise be overlooked. This is one of the most crucial areas to be covered in the assessment of any family, particularly the family with young children. Subtle clues pointing to potential or actual child abuse are all too often present (Hopkins, 1970, pp. 589–598). This writer now frequently asks very bluntly, and with much compassion, "Are you ever afraid you might abuse your child?" The response to this question sometimes produces a sigh of relief and an outpouring of concerns and fears. The problem of child abuse is a grave one, indeed, and probably much more widespread than we dare permit ourselves to believe. Never, never fail to give parents the opportunity to talk about their child-rearing practices.

HEALTH RESOURCES

To determine the family's role in obtaining health care, a question about health resources utilized by the family is asked. At this point options and guidance are frequently indicated so that there is an increased awareness of available resources along with assistance in plugging into those resources.

STRENGTHS AND COPING MECHANISMS

Identifying family strengths and coping mechanisms is as much a part of family assessment as the more traditional role of identifying weaknesses and problem areas. Otto has provided us with an "Outline of Marriage Strengths" that may be used as an excellent guideline for helping families identify their own strengths (Otto, 1969). By addressing the positive aspects first, the stage is set for then mutually identifying problem areas.

WEAKNESSES AND PROBLEMS

Identifying the areas of concern that require intervention and assistance must be a cooperative effort between the family and the health care provider. Unilateral decisions on the part of the nurse are not appropriate in the meaningful family assessment and have no place in modern nursing practice. An example of the futility of such action involved Sandra W., a 24-year-old woman with below-normal intelligence, obesity, and epilepsy. She has two sons, 17-month-old Anthony and 7-month-old Lewis, and is supported by aid to dependent children. Her husband is an alcoholic and periodically hospitalized to "dry out." All attempts by the clincial nurse specialist to persuade Sandra to obtain a tubal ligation have been failures because the decision is a unilateral one. Until Sandra has a desire to limit the number of children she bears, the weakness of "ineffective means of birth control" is not appropriate.

GOALS

Goal setting, much like identifying strengths and weaknesses, is a mutual effort between nurse and client. Goals should be realistic, attainable, and viewed as guidelines for functioning. The section on goals in the Family Assessment Tool is meant to serve as a quick reference or summary of the interaction.

REFERENCES

Adams, G. Recognizing the range of human sexual needs and behavior. *MCN—The Journal of Maternal Child Nursing*, 1976, *1*, 166–169.

Clark, M. *Health in the Mexican American culture*. Berkeley, Cal.: University of California Press, 1959.

Hall. E. *The hidden dimension*. New York: Doubleday, 1966.

Hopkins, J. The nurse and the abused child. *Nursing Clinics of North America*. 1970, *5*, 589–598.

Otto, H. A. *More joy in your marriage*. New York: Hawthorn Books, 1969.

Rabinowitz, M. Why didn't anyone tell me about bottle-mouth syndrome? *Children Today*, 1974, *3*, 18–20.

Satir, V. *Conjoint family therapy*. Palo Alto, Cal.: Science and Behavior Books, 1967.

Whiting, B. E. *Six cultures: Studies of childrearing*. New York: John Wiley and Sons, 1973.

APPENDIX: FAMILY ASSESSMENT TOOL

FAMILY CONSTELLATION

Family name: _____

Other names used:_____

Woman: _____ Mate: _____

Relationship:_____
(married, divorced, separated, single, common-law)

Names of children   Ages   Ordinal position (include miscarriages)

_____

_____

_____

_____

Others living in the home: _____
(age, sex, relationship)

_____

Significant family relatives and/or friends who may not occupy immediate
residence (name, etc.): _____

_____

Nationality origin (significant culturally divergent child-rearing practices,
variations in personality with ethnic differences)

Woman: _____

Mate: _____

Maternal parents: _____

Paternal parents: _____

EDUCATION

Woman: _____ Mate: _____ Children: _____

_____

What each liked best in school: _____

_____

Problems in school: _____

General feelings of significance of education: _____

Goals and aspirations for children: _____

Goals for self: _____ Mate: _____

OCCUPATION

Who is working? _____

Where? _____ Type of work? _____

Hours of work? _____ Relationship with boss? _____

Satisfied with work? _____ Problems? _____

Goals and aspirations: _____

COMMUNICATION PATTERNS

Do husband and wife talk with each other? _____

Hear each other out? _____ Verbally or physically battle? _____

Degree of united front with children? _____

Whose voice is final? _____ Whom do children go to? _____

Do children "play games" with parents? _____

Who listens to the stories of happenings at school, job, games? _____

How does each express joy, love, anger, sadness, frustration? _____

_____

FINANCES

Source: _____ Salary: _____ Pension: _____

Public assistance: _____ Earnings: _____ Approximate amount

available to meet daily needs: _____ Approximate monthly

payments: _____ Adequacy of funds: _____

Insurance: _____ Security for future education, retirement,

catastrophes? _____

RESIDENCE

Neighborhood: _____ What does the family like

about where it lives? _____ Dislike? _____

Goals for the future? _____

Type of residence? _____
_____(room, apartment house, mobile home,

_____
_____renting, buying, own, etc.)

Adequacy of room space: _____ Lighting: _____

Ventilation: _____ Heating: _____

Refrigeration: _____ Water and waste disposal: _____

Laundry: _____ Cooking facilities: _____

Architectural barriers: _____ Degree of repair: _____

Safety factors: _____ Recreation and play needs: _____

_____ Comfort needs for privacy and esthetic needs: _____

_____

Who does housekeeping? _____ Likes and dislikes: _____

_____ Shared duties? _____

Problems? _____

Attitudes toward cleanliness and orderliness: _____

TRANSPORTATION

Private vehicle? _____ Adequacy to meet family demands? _____

_____ Public transportation? _____ Monthly costs? _____

Who uses seat belts? _____

_____

FAMILY FUNCTIONING

Goals: _____

(housing, car, vacation, job, furniture, education)

Specific goals for individual members: _____

Who is "teacher" of health practices? _____

Who is the family's best helper and counselor? _____

Do you talk things out together? _____

Anyone dictate and give orders? _____

Believe what will happen will happen? _____

Activities of a typical day   Describe: _____

_____

_____

_____

RELIGIOUS PREFERENCE

Woman: _____ Mate: _____ Grandparents: _____

General feeling of significance of church/synagogue: _____

Religious practices at holiday times: _____

Marriage: _____ Confirmation: _____

Grace at mealtime: _____ Evening prayers: _____

Sunday School or other Bible study groups: _____

AVOCATION

Interests and creative talents: _____

Degree of achievement: _____ Barriers? _____

RECREATIONAL INTERESTS

Do mates have free time together? _____

Alone?_____ Likes and dislikes?_____

Activities of family members together:_____

With relatives?_____ With friends?_____

_____ Amount of time with TV?_____

Participation outside family circle. Woman: _____

Mate:_____ Children:_____

_____
        (including school, PTA, Scouts, church, political and social groups)

Use of telephone with neighbors, friends, relatives?_____

_____

HEALTH HISTORY

Anyone in immediate family or grandparents with heart trouble? _____

_____ Diabetes? _____ Cancer? _____

Tuberculosis? _____ Hypertension? _____ Kidney trouble? _____

Suicide? _____ Excessive use of drugs? _____ Accident prone?_____

_____ If yes, on any of the above, comment below—who,

when, etc. . . . _____

_____

Who has been the sickest in family? _____

Who is sought out for help first when ill? _____

What common nonprescription drugs are kept on hand?_____

_____

Headaches, colds, upset stomachs frequently?_____

What medical people has family used? _____
                                          (doctors, nurses, etc.)

_____

Community health services? _____

What does illness do to family?   _____

Acute? _____ Long-term? _____

Anyone experiencing weakness? _____ Tiredness? _____

Anxiety? _____ Nervousness? _____ Depression? _____
Moodiness? _____ Tantrums? _____ Fainting spells? _____
Convulsions? _____ Effect on family members and family
harmony? _____

SPECIAL SENSES

Anyone complain of eye strain? _____ Earaches? _____ Slow or
unclear speech? _____ Learning difficulties in school? _____
Anyone with glasses or contact lenses? _____
Vision checked recently? _____ Does TV have to be loud? _____
Any problems with walking? _____ Special shoes worn? _____

DENTAL CARE

Do children brush teeth? _____ Frequency? _____ Anyone wear
dentures? _____ Regular dental care? _____ When children first
taken to a dentist? _____

FOODS AND EATING PATTERNS

Common food likes and dislikes: _____
_____

When are children started on baby foods? _____
Concern about neatness and manners? _____
Meals eaten together as a family during the week? _____
Weekend meal schedules? _____ Who plans meals? _____
Who helps prepare? _____ Weight problems? _____
Special diet? _____ Allergies? _____ Who does marketing?
_____ Daily? _____ Weekly? _____ Types of stores
used? _____ Storage facilities? _____ Garden? _____
Canning? _____ Average food costs per week? _____
Schedule of meals on a typical day:
      Breakfast _____ Lunch _____ Dinner _____
Smoking? _____ Drinking? _____ Exercising? _____
Sleep? _____ Rest? _____

SEXUALITY

What find most pleasing about mate? _____
_____ Least pleasing? _____
_____ How is role as a wife or husband viewed? _____

_____ Any specific sexual concerns? _____
Menstrual difficulties? _____ Birth control methods? _____
Family planning and spacing? _____ Marital problems? _____
_____ Compatible? _____ Particular pleasures? _____
_____ Impotency? _____ Physical problems? _____
Any adolescent or other young adult in family making a sexual adjustment?

_____

CHILD-REARING PRACTICES

Roles mates play? _____ Who dominates? _____
Do grandparents or in-laws interfere? _____ How is this
handled? _____ Is anyone picked on or blamed a lot in
the family or school and just never seems to do anything right? _____
Who complains a lot? _____ How is toilet training handled? _____
_____ Expectation of perfection in children? _____
_____ Fear might abuse child? _____
_____ Who gives care during the night? _____
How are bouts of imagination and "wild tales" handled? _____
Effect of awkwardness, secrecy, or moodiness of child on parents and
siblings? _____ Degree of perfection expected
for "little man" or "lady"? _____
Who sets discipline limits? _____ How? _____
How are issues, such as use of family car handled? _____
Dating? _____ Length of hair or skirt? _____
Assignment of household tasks? _____ How are children
rewarded? _____ Parents think children respect
them? _____ How does attachment to separate affect parents?
_____ Who goes to whom for comfort? _____
Conversation, freedom, and creativity encouraged? _____

HEALTH RESOURCES

How does family obtain health services? _____
Community agencies? _____ Private physician? _____
Nurse? _____ Satisfactions? _____
Strengths and coping mechanisms: _____

_____
_____

Weaknesses and problems _____

_____

_____

GOALS

Short-term:_____

_____

Intermediate:_____

_____

Long-term: _____

_____

_____

_____

_____

CHAPTER TWENTY

ASSESSMENT OF THE CHRONICALLY ILL CHILD AND FAMILY

DEBRA P. HYMOVICH

The incidence of chronic childhood disorders is estimated to be somewhere between 5 and 10 percent of the population under 16 years of age (Pless and Pinkerton, 1975). These chronically disabled children and their families can be considered at risk for psychosocial sequelae and/or management problems. As professionals, we have the ability to play a major role in assessing and intervening with these children and their families to minimize these potential problems. To be effective, a comprehensive, consistent, and systematic approach is necessary. Comprehensive care of the chronically ill child implies including the total family and focusing on normal aspects of development as well as on the illness or disability itself (Hymovich, 1976a). Consistent care means providing continuity and coordination of services, often over a prolonged period of time; while systematic assessment and intervention denotes carrying out activities in an organized, orderly manner.

Since there is an interdependence of family members on each other for satisfaction of their sociological, psychological, and economic needs, all family members need to be included when assessing, implementing, and evaluting care. Erikson (1963) indicates that illness can be viewed as a situational crisis superimposed on the normal crises of development. This concept can also be extended to family development. It is suggested, therefore, that chronic illness be viewed in relation to its effects on the development of individuals within the family and the family as a unit, specifically as it relates to their developmental tasks. Comprehensive,

280

consistent, and systematic care of chronically ill children and their families could be expected to result in increasing their capacity to cope with the illness as evidenced by an ability to master their individual and collective developmental tasks. This approach also provides opportunities to predict the developmental expectations of individuals and family units at any point in their life cycle.

The relationship of developmental tasks to the care of chronically ill children and their families is illustrated in Figure 20-1. The stresses of chronic illness (i.e., social, emotional, physical, financial) affect all members of the family, not just the disabled individual. The ability of each family member and the family as a unit to cope with the problems is defined as their ability to accomplish the developmental tasks arising at each phase in the life cycle. Their ability to cope (master tasks) can be viewed as falling along a continuum from poor to good. An example of poor mastery would be the inability of a parent to become attached to a disabled infant. Intervention strategies, such as therapeutic procedures, counseling, and education would be expected to influence the coping ability of the family and its members.

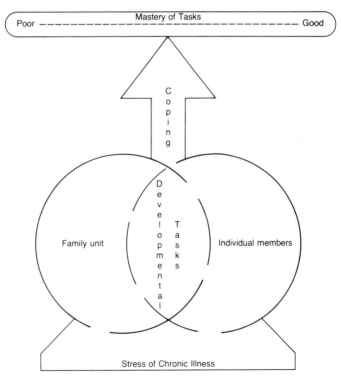

Figure 20-1 Coping with stress of chronic illness.

This chapter presents guidelines for assessing family development and functioning. The same principles can be applied to assessment of individual family members at each stage in their life cycle; however, it is beyond the scope of this presentation to include all of these individual tasks.

Nursing assessment and intervention can only be effective if it is based on a sound theoretical background. Consequently, the first step in developing an overall plan of care for chronically ill children and their families is to base it on a conceptual framework. This framework should meet the following criteria: It should be broad enough to include each individual member as well as the entire unit; it needs to allow for synthesis of numerous disciplines, including human development, the biological and behavioral sciences, and nursing; and it should focus on all aspects of individual and family development (biological, cognitive, emotional, social). The framework needs to be wellness as well as illness oriented (Hymovich, 1976a). It should include the multiple variables affecting the impact of the condition on the individual and family as well as their ability to manage (cope with) their life situation. The major components of the assessment model (see Figure 20-2) described in this chapter are the *developmental tasks* of individuals and families and the *impact variables* of perceptions, resources, and coping abilities. The third dimension of the model is the *intervention needed* by the family as a result of having a chronically ill youngster.

DEVELOPMENTAL TASKS

Developmental tasks have been defined as tasks that arise at a critical time in an individual's or a family's life. If each of these tasks is achieved successfully, then happiness and success with future tasks will result. Unsuccessful achievement results in unhappiness, difficulty in accomplishing later tasks, and disapproval by society (Duvall, 1977).

Individual developmental tasks originate from physical maturation, cultural expectations, and personal values and aspirations (Havighurst, 1972). Individual tasks have been identified for infants, children, adolescents, adults, pregnant women, and parents. Examples of individual tasks are: learning one's sex role, achieving appropriate independence-dependence patterns, and accepting and adjusting to one's changing body.

The developmental approach to the family attempts to synthesize compatible concepts of other frameworks in order to view the family as it changes over time. Conceptually, the family can be viewed as a "unity" of interacting personalities (Burgess, 1926) and as a semi-closed system (Rodgers, 1973).

Family tasks parallel individual tasks and must satisfy the family's

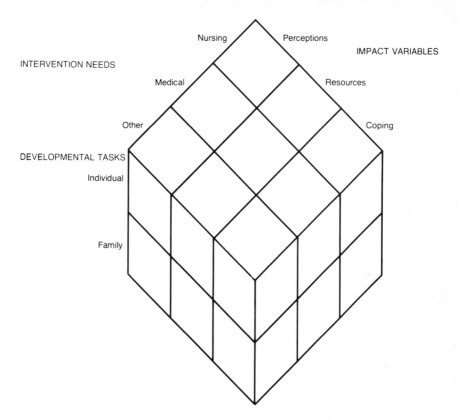

Figure 20-2 Framework for assessing chronically disabled children and their families.

biological and cultural needs, along with the personal aspirations and values of each of its members. Duvall (1971) lists eight family developmental tasks believed to be basic to all American families regardless of social class and subculture. These tasks are related to the physical maintenance and allocation of physical and psychosocial resources within the family. They also include socialization of family members; placing them in the larger society; division of labor; maintenance of order, motivation, and morale; and the reproduction, recruitment, and release of family members. Duvall delineates certain stage-critical tasks that occur when the family is assuming new responsibilities growing out of rapid changes at given points in the life cycle. For example, a stage-critical task of the school-age family is to encourage the child's educational achievement.

Hymovich and Chamberlin have synthesized Duvall's tasks into five clinically relevant tasks: (1) meeting the basic physical needs of the family, (2) assisting each family member in meeting his or her individual developmental tasks, (3) meeting the emotional needs of all family members, (4) maintaining and adapting family organization and management to meet family needs, and (5) functioning within the community. These tasks form the basis for assessing the family's mastery of a child's chronic illness.

IMPACT VARIABLES

The specific variables to look at in relation to each of these five tasks are individual and family perceptions, resources, and coping abilities. The extent to which each family is able to master their developmental tasks depends upon how they perceive each of these tasks, the resources available to them, and their individual and collective means of coping with problems.

Perceptions

The family's *perceptions* of each of their developmental tasks are particularly important, because it is their perceptions that are basic to their behavior. Combs and Snygg (1949, p. 17) stress this relationship between perceptions and behavior:

> People do not behave according to the facts as *others* see them. They behave according to the facts as *they* see them. What governs behavior from the point of view of the individual himself are his unique perceptions of himself and the world in which he lives, the meanings things have for him.

Perceptions are selective and individual and are influenced by the internal state of the perceiver (Allport, 1961; Bruner and Tagiuri, 1954). Individuals who are fearful or insecure will perceive events differently than those who are in a relaxed and secure state. Combs (1952) identified the following factors as limiting one's perceptions: environmental opportunities, self-concept, individual goals and values, time, cultural background, threat, and physiological states. Among the physiological factors influencing perceptions are hormonal secretions, oxygenation, drugs, alcohol, diet, and metabolic dysfunctions (Beach, 1951).

Because perceptions are selective and individual, it becomes our responsibility to gain insight into the perceptions of the family members with whom we are interacting. By understanding their particular frame of reference, we will be able to plan more effective intervention strategies that will be mutually acceptable to both our clients and ourselves. Since perceptions differ from person to person, we need to assess each family member to determine each one's idiosyncratic perceptions. Assessing each family member has the additional advantage of enabling the family and the professional to see where similarities and differences exist within each family unit.

Table 20-1 illustrates the perceptual areas to be considered in relation to each of Hymovich and Chamberlin's five developmental tasks. Of particular importance is the degree of satisfaction expressed in relation to each task. Knowledge of satisfaction can provide some measure of the importance that possible suggestions regarding intervention may have. For example, the family that indicates little involvement in community activities and is satisfied with their involvement has different needs than the family that is actively involved in many community activities but is dissatisfied with the extent of their involvement.

A second major component of assessment is the family's perceptions of their strengths and weaknesses. This is useful in helping the family to identify not only their problems, but also their strengths, for it is these strengths that form the foundation for their growth. Herbert Otto (1963, 1973) has identified a framework for assessing family strengths. The dimensions of his framework are consistent with the developmental task framework presented here. This framework is useful for the family as well as for the professional, because we can use it to identify strengths in relation to each of the family tasks. Specific strengths in relation to each task are as follows:

Task: Meeting the basic physical needs of the family.
 Strength: Ability to provide for physical needs of family.
Task: Assisting each family member in meeting his or her individual developmental tasks.
 Strengths: Being sensitive to needs of family members.
 Initiate or maintain growth-producing relationships and experiences within and outside the family.
 Grow with and through children.
Task: Meeting the emotional needs of all family members.
 Strengths: Communicate effectively.
 Provide support, security, and encouragment.
 Provide for emotional and spiritual needs.
 Have mutual respect for individuality of family members.
Task: Maintaining and adapting family organization and management to meet family needs.
 Strengths: Perform family roles flexibly.
 Show concern for family unity, loyalty, and interfamily cooperation.
Task: Functioning within the community.
 Strength: Maintain and create constructive and responsible community relationships.

Table 20-1 Assessment guide for families of chronically ill children

Impact variable : Perceptions				
Family developmental tasks				
Meet basic physical needs	Assist with individual tasks	Meet needs for emotional support	Adapt organization and management	Function in community
Satisfaction with: housing, health care, financial situation, nutritional needs, community resources	Satisfaction with each member's development	Satisfaction with relationships	Satisfaction with organization and management	Leisure activities outside home: where frequency
Changes in basic needs since diagnosis	Extent to which each is accomplishing tasks (assess each member using appropriate individual tasks)	How decisions are made	Daily schedule change since diagnosis	Satisfaction with activities
Strengths and weaknesses in meeting needs	Strengths and weaknesses of each member	How members get along with one another	Who helps with tasks	Contact with neighbors
		Limit setting/discipline	Sacrifices necessary	Contacts with extended family
		Vulnerable child	Feeling re sacrifices	Availability of community resources
		Stability of marriage	Expectations of each member	Satisfaction with community resources
		Communication patterns	Strengths and weaknesses in organization and management	Attitudes toward child and family of friends, neighbors etc.
		Strengths and weaknesses in relationships		Expectations of community re disabled child
		Relationships with extended family		Strengths and weaknesses in community
		Religious beliefs		
		Ability to organize after crisis		

Impact variable: Resources

Family developmental tasks

Meet basic physical needs	Assist with individual tasks	Meet needs for emotional support	Adapt organization and management	Function in community
Home structure, location, outdoor play area, sleeping arrangements, adaptations for ill child	Appropriate for: developmental needs, extent of child's disability (specific resources will depend upon develop- mental needs of each member)	Individual family member's: temperament, personality, cognitive level, self-concept	Household membership number, age, sex, relationship	Organizations belong to, i.e.: PTA, church/synagogue, volunteer, parent groups, children's groups, other
Health care where, for whom, for what, prevention crisis	What parents do with each child (i.e., recreation, hobbies)	Relationship between family members	Role of each member Role flexibility	Specific resources necessitated by child's condition
obtain needed equipment, medications etc. for child general health of each family member	Development prior to illness	Development prior to illness	Availability of external supports	Resources used, i.e., medical, recreational, educational, vocational, transportation, other
Finances income: sources stability who contributes who supported insurance, major expenses, cost of illness	Past experiences Support systems	Past experiences Support systems		Day care/babysitting arrangements
Clothing appropriate for: weather individual needs	Preexisting family functioning communication patterns decision making feelings of closeness	Preexisting family functioning communication patterns, decision making, feelings of closeness		Attitudes of community
Food basic four special diets	Family values and goals	Family values and goals		

Table 20-1 Assessment guide for families of chronically ill children

Impact variable: Coping				
Family developmental tasks				
Meet basic physical needs	Assist with individual tasks	Meet needs for emotional support	Adapt organization and management	Function in community
Previous coping abilities	Previous coping abilities	Previous coping abilities	Previous coping abilities	Previous coping abilities
Knowledge of: child's condition and therapy available resources	Parental understanding of child(ren)'s developmental levels	Communicate at developmental level of child(ren)	Adjust roles as needed	Become involved in meaningful activities outside the home
Seek relevant information	Understand needs of each family member spouse, child, parent, others in household	Provide appropriate limits and discipline	Use external supports as needed	Work with parent groups
Learn specific illness-related procedures	Provide resources to meet tasks	Express and share feelings	Level of organization	Know available community resources
Use family strengths	Seek relevant information	Use of psychological defenses		Seek relevant information
Adapt family resources	Adapt approaches to developmental level	Stage of reaction to condition (i.e., shock, despair, guilt, denial, anger, depression)		Use community resources
Seek and accept help when needed		Motor activities		
		Seek relevant information		
		Request reassurance and support		

There are two additional strengths that should be assessed in relation to each of the family developmental tasks. These strengths are the family's ability for self-help and for accepting help when it is appropriate and their ability to use crisis as a growth-promoting event. In the case of families of children with chronic illnesses, there is a variety of developmental and situational crises with which they must cope. With appropriate intervention for these crises, it is anticipated that the family will become stronger and better able to cope with subsequent crises.

Resources

The internal and external *resources* available to the family serve as a foundation for understanding the impact of chronic childhood illness on each family and the problems or potential problems with which they need to cope. Resources include the human resources, such as one's temperament, personality, and health as well as the physical resources, such as finances, clothing, and food. To meet the needs of all family members successfully, parents need to maintain their own health and strength. Their relationship with one another may be either a strong or a weak resource. Studies of parents of chronically ill children indicate that parental relationships may be either strengthened or weakened by the demands imposed by their child's illness.

Suggestions for assessment of resources needed to meet each of the family developmental tasks are in Table 20-1. Although it is beyond the scope of this chapter, it is important to point out that for the resource component of the assessment to be complete, it is necessary to assess the needed and available community resources. This knowledge is necessary not only to make appropriate use of these resources for families, but also to help families become advocates for the services they need but are not yet available.

Coping

Coping has been defined in a variety of ways. For example, Murphy (1962, p. 273) defines it as "a matter of strategy, of flexible management of different devices for dealing with the challenges from the environment," while Lazarus and Launier (in press) indicate that coping consists "of efforts, both action-oriented and intrapsychic, to manage (i.e., master, tolerate, reduce, minimize) environmental and internal demands, and conflicts among them, which tax or exceed a person's resources." There is, as yet, no workable theory or taxonomy of coping; therefore, our assessment of this dimension is currently sketchy.

Whether individual or family coping is the focus, certain commonalities in coping strategies have been noted across illness conditions.

Moos and Tsu (1977) have developed a crisis-oriented framework for coping with serious illness. They defined seven categories of adaptive tasks and an equal number of categories of coping skills they believe are abilities that can be taught and used flexibly over situations. They emphasize that specific coping techniques are either adaptive or maladaptive, depending upon the appropriateness of the situation in which they are used. These coping skills are: (1) denying or minimizing the seriousness of the condition, (2) seeking relevant information, (3) requesting reassurance and support, (4) learning specific illness-related procedures, (5) setting concrete limited goals, (6) rehearsing alternative outcomes, and (7) finding a general purpose or pattern of meaning.

Coping serves to maintain self-esteem and interpersonal relationships as well as meeting environmental conditions and containing stress within tolerable limits. Coelho, Hamburg, and Adams (1974) indicate the need for learning what coping strategies are useful in which situations and then being able to identify new coping strategies for individuals that are closest to that person's available repertoire. Hamburg (1974) also emphasized the importance of social support systems in the coping process across the life span, indicating that family support can effect a smoother transition. The significance of strong familial relationships in coping with chronic illness has been found in a number of studies (Burton, 1975; Kaplan, Smith, Grobstein, and Fischman, 1973; Tropauer, Franz, and Dilgard, 1970). Hymovich (1976b) has suggested that to cope with chronic childhood conditions, parents need (1) trust (in themselves, their children, the health professionals), (2) information, (3) resources (human and physical), and (4) guidance and support.

Moos and Tsu (1977) maintain that family members and friends, as well as the patient, use the same types of coping skills in crises that affect all of them. However, this has not always been supported by the data. For example, Mattsson (1972), in a review of the literature on long-term physical illness in childhood, found contrasts in coping behaviors of children and parents. He delineates the importance of cognitive processes for both groups in mastering distressing emotional reactions caused by illness. Coping strategies for parents of leukemic children were found to include shock and disbelief for some, although intellectual acceptance was more common. Other coping strategies included active seeking for hope-sustaining beliefs, searching for meaning in the tragedy, and anticipatory grief. Most parents found their religious beliefs to be comforting (Friedman, Chodoff, Mason, and Hamburg, 1963).

Kaplan and his colleagues (1973) indicate that coping tasks vary significantly from one illness to another, citing the differences in tasks faced by parents of prematurely born infants and parents of children with leukemia. Their studies show that the coping of parents of children with leukemia may be adaptive, maladaptive, or discrepant. Discrepant coping occurs when parents take opposing positions concerning the diagnosis. This discrepancy may lead to poor communications, interruption or prohibition of collective grieving, and weakened family relationships. This is similar to the model proposed by Drotar and colleagues (1975) to describe the adaptation of parents to the birth of an infant with a congenital malformation. Their study of twenty parents suggested that asynchronous parental reactions often caused temporary emotional separation of the parents. Asynchronous reactions were defined as parents having different time durations at each stage of the grieving process.

Assessment of each family member's coping patterns is necessary prior to intervention in order to establish a baseline from which to suggest strategies for enhancing coping. It is important to determine each person's stage of coping with the child's chronic illness as well as their usual coping strategies in a variety of situations.

USE OF THE ASSESSMENT GUIDE

The value of any assessment guide lies in its ability to help us identify areas where functioning is adequate and those where intervention is needed. Once these areas have been pinpointed and intervention implemented, we should be able to use the same assessment guide to measure the outcome of such intervention.

The framework for assessment suggested in this chapter has two major dimensions: family developmental tasks and the impact variables of perceptions, resources, and coping. A variety of direct and indirect measures is available for use in assessing these dimensions as they pertain to disabled children and their families. Selection and interpretation of appropriate measures can be enhanced by considering them in terms of this framework.

There is currently no consensus as to whether one should measure overt behavior or obtain subjective measures of underlying determinants of behavior. Objective measures, based on more overt than covert behavior, are useful when the child's or family's disturbance is sufficient to attract outside attention. Subjective measures are of value in helping to identify those who may be at risk before their disturbance becomes manifest. If one plans to intervene only after manifestations have become overt, then objective measures can be used for obtaining information; however, if preventive intervention is the goal, then subjective measures such as self-concept scales and personality inventories are useful in identifying potential problems.

The developmental task framework allows us to anticipate individual and family development and behavior throughout the life cycle. How well the family is achieving its individual and collective tasks can serve as a basis for assessing, planning, implementing, and evaluating care. By focusing on perceptions, resources, and coping related to each of the family developmental tasks, health professionals will have a sound basis for understanding and helping all family members. This framework provides a means whereby we can practice comprehensive, systematic, and consistent care.

REFERENCES

Allport, G. W. *Patterns and growth in personality.* New York: Holt, Rinehart and Winston, 1961.

Beach, F. A. Body chemistry and perception. In R. R. Blake & G. V. Ramsey (Eds.), *Perception—An approach to personality.* New York: Ronald Press, 1951.

Bruner, J. S., & Tagiuri, R. The perception of people. In G. Lindzey (Ed.), *Handbook of social psychology.* Reading, Mass.: Addison-Wesley, 1954.

Burgess, E. W. The family as a unity of interacting personalities. *The Family,* 1926, *7,* 3–9.

Burton, L. *The family life of sick children.* London: Routledge and Kegan Paul, 1975.

Coehlo, G., Hamburg, D., & Adams, J. *Coping and adaptation.* New York: Basic Books, 1974.

Combs, A. W. Intelligence from a perceptual point of view. *Journal of Abnormal and Social Psychology,* 1952, *47,* 662–673.

Combs, A. W., & Snygg, D. *Individual behavior: A perceptual approach to behavior* (Rev. ed.). New York: Harper & Row, 1949.

Drotar, D., Baskiwicz, A., Irvin, N., Kennell, J., & Klaus, M. The adaptation of parents to the birth of an infant with a congenital malformation: A hypothetical model. *Pediatrics,* 1975, *56,* 710–717.

Duvall, E. M. *Family development* (4th Ed.). Philadelphia: J. B. Lippincott, 1971.

———. *Marriage and family development* (5th ed.). Philadelphia: J. B. Lippincott, 1977.

Erikson, E. H. *Childhood and society* (2d ed.). New York: W. W. Norton, 1963.

Friedman, S. B., Chodoff, P., Mason, J. W., & Hamburg, D. A. Behavioral observations of parents anticipating the death of a child. *Pediatrics,* 1963, *32,* 610.

Hamburg, D. A. Coping behavior in life-threatening circumstances. *Psychotherapy and Psychosomatics,* 1974, *23,* 13–25.

Havighurst, R. J. *Developmental tasks and education* (3rd ed.). New York: McKay, 1972.

Hymovich, D. P. A framework for measuring outcomes of intervention with the chronically ill child and his family. In G. D. Grave & I. B. Pless (Eds.), *Chronic childhood illness—Assessment of Outcome.* DHEW No. (NIH) 76–877, 91–93, 1976a.

———. Parents of sick children: Their needs and tasks. *Pediatric Nursing,* 1976b, *2,* 9–13.

Kaplan, D. M., Smith, A., Grobstein, R., & Fischman, S. E. Family mediation of stress. *Social Work,* 1973, *18,* 60–69.

Lazarus, R. S., & Launier, R. Stress-related transactions between person and environment. In L. A. Pervin & M. Lewis (Eds.), *Internal and external determinants of behavior.* New York: Plenum (in press).

Mattsson, A. Long-term physical illness in childhood: A challenge to psychosocial adaptation. *Pediatrics,* 1972, *50,* 801–811.

Moos, R. H., & Tsu, V. D. The crisis of physical illness: An overview. In R. H. Moos (Ed.), *Coping with physical illness.* New York: Plenum, 1977.

Murphy, L. B. *The widening world of childhood.* New York: Basic Books, 1962.

Otto, H. A. Criteria for assessing family strengths. *Family Process,* 1963, *2,* 329–338.

———. A framework for assessing family strengths. In A. Reinhardt & M. Quinn (Eds.), *Family centered community nursing.* St. Louis: C. V. Mosby, 1973, 87–94.

Pless, I. B., & Pinkerton, P. *Chronic childhood disorder—Promoting patterns of adjustment.* Chicago: Year Book Medical Publishers, 1975.

Rodgers, R. H. *Family interaction and transaction—The developmental approach.* Englewood Cliffs, N.J.: Prentice-Hall, 1973.

Tropauer, A., Franz, M. N., & Dilgard, V. W. Psychological aspects of the care of children with cystic fibrosis. *American Journal of Diseases of Children,* 1970, *119,* 424–432.

CHAPTER TWENTY-ONE

PRINCIPLES OF FAMILY COUNSELING

ROSEMARY J. McKEIGHEN

INTRODUCTION

The positive aspect of mental health, *emotional maturity,* is in many ways identical to the concept of good mental health and is actually an ideal state. For too long, too many mental health professionals have focused their attention and effort exclusively on severely ill people who must be hospitalized, losing sight of the fact that all of us have some state of mental health all the time. Each of us has emotional idiosyncrasies and problem areas and can only approach perfect mental health for a few minutes or a few hours or, perhaps, a few days.

Family counseling is one therapeutic approach that can be used to enable individuals to experience emotional maturity more frequently and for longer periods of time. Family counseling is concerned with examination of the intricate play of developmental pressures, family structure, and family communication patterns upon personality development and behavioral enactment.

There are many facets of the personality, including the emotional, intellectual, social, physiological, and others. These aspects are to some degree determined and affected by inherited traits such as intelligence, physical attributes, and genetic structure and by our social and economic environments. Some of these facets, such as our emotions, must be developed and trained. This emotional development and training is primarily determined by the character of our social interactive sphere and the emotional maturity of the individuals within it.

Some mental health professionals such as Rank (1952), Klein (1932), and Janov (1973) place great emphasis on the birth experience as the core from which all future behavioral enactments are molded. They believe that birth is the individual's first encounter with anxiety (fending off death) and first separation from mother (loss of need gratification). They hypothesize that this birth trauma and the initial separation forms the core for later symptomatology such as separation anxiety, which may be triggered by any significant loss in the child's or adult's later life. Most mental health professionals have agreed on recognizing a child's first human relationship as the foundation of personality; however, there is as yet no agreement on the nature and origin of that relationship. Within 12 months almost all infants have developed a strong tie to a mother figure; yet there is no consensus on how quickly this comes about, by what process it is maintained, for how long it persists, or what function it fulfills.

The child has a number of physiological needs that must be met, particularly for food and warmth. A baby becomes interested in and attached to a human figure, especially a mother, as the result of the mother's meeting the baby's physiological needs and the baby's learning in time that she is the source of gratification. A common belief is that children gain an awareness of the emotional climate in which this interaction occurs and the pairing of these feelings states to their cognitive learnings forms the basis for their personality enactment style.

Attachment behavior, a class of social behavior that occurs when certain behavioral systems are activated, has potential for affecting emotionality and dependency behavior. Ainsworth (1963) and Schaffer and Emerson (1964) report the great range of age (4 to 12 months) at which different children first show attachment behavior. The intensity and consistency with which a child displays attachment behavior also varies. The variables responsible for these differences are of two types, organismic and environmental. Hunger, fatigue, illness, and pain are organismic states that would elicit attachment behavior, while alarm is the environmental factor that increases it.

There is agreement regarding the frequency with which attachment behavior is directed toward figures other than the mothering one. Schaffer and Emerson found that during the month after the children first showed attachment behavior, one-fourth of them were directing it toward other members of the family and by the time they reached 18 months, all children were attached to at least one other figure and often to several others.

Although there is abundant evidence to confirm that the kind of care infants receive from their mothers plays a major part in determining the way in which their personality develops, the fact that few humans remain captive to a single interaction style during personality development might explain why individuals exhibit various combinations of degrees of emotional maturity. The pattern of interaction that develops between family members can be understood only as a result of viewing the contributions of each member that influence the behavior of the others.

Society assigns the tasks of growth and maturation with which the individual must struggle; for most, this growth usually occurs within the context of a family.

DEFINING THE PROBLEM

Individual Perspective

The primary goal of the individual organism is to behave in such a manner that one is able to extract from the environment the satisfaction of needs, both immediately and in a sustained manner in the future. Needs provide the motivating force that energizes behavior and sets the goal to be attained. Behavior repertoire can be defined as the total of all behavior responses that the individual is capable of making. Individuals begin with their inherited capacities and through maturation and experience build a behavior repertoire. Thus, *experience* becomes the first element of this developmental process. The unit of experience can be conceived of as being any size objective occurrence external to the "psyche." The second element is *perception*. Perception is the individual's interpretation of the experience. Our perception and our understanding of our environment are very closely intertwined, and this relationship between what we perceive and what we understand is complex, each having the potential to modify the effect of the other. The better we understand the world around us, the more effectively we can gather information about a particular part of it; similarly, the better we perceive our surroundings, the more efficiently we can interpret what is going on around us.

At no time in our lives is this connection between perception and understanding more important than during childhood, because it is then that both undergo the most radical changes. It is during childhood that we lay the basis of our understanding of the rules that govern our environment. However imperfect our grasp of these rules as adults it is nonetheless the product of a very lengthy development. It is also fairly certain that there are greater changes in our perception during childhood than at any other time. Recent research (Kassen, Haith, and Salapatek, 1970) has established that even very young babies possess an impressive range of perceptual abilities. Nevertheless, it is still certain that these capacities change and generally become more effective as children grow older.

The third element is *generalization*. To group perceptions that appear to be similar and draw one rule or generalization from the whole class of events is a natural tendency. We then use this generalization to guide our behavior at any time in the future when we encounter an event perceived to be of the same class of events as those about which the generalization was drawn. For example, if one enters a strange room that is dark and wishes to turn on the light, one gropes for the switch near the door and not the floor. This generalization, based on past experience, guides our behavior in this present situation. Before application of a generalization to a new situation is made, one must determine that the new situation is identical to the class of situations from which this generalization came. Thus, if the dark room mentioned prior was in a log cabin in a remote wooded area, one might suspect there would not be electricity available and would not reach for a switch. Thus, the ability to differentiate accurately is of vital importance.

The constellation of all generalizations developed out of past experience gives direction and selectivity to our behavior in order to satisfy present needs. If this constellation of generalization, which we have labeled behavior repertoire, directs our behavior in such a way that our needs are satisfied, we can consider it adequate.

Behavior inadequacies manifest themselves as problems in living. These inadequacies can be conceptualized as fitting into three general classes: (1) a lack of experience, (2) inaccurate perceptions and, (3) errors in generalization.

A deficient experiential bank needs no elaboration: A void exists. The alteration and correction of the client's inaccurate perceptions form the basis of psychotherapy. Much of psychiatric literature describes prognostic behavioral instances in which patients try to apply generalizations developed from childhood experience to adult situations. Even though the generalizations were valid for the childhood situations, the apparently identical adult situations were in reality not identical. Consequently, the employed behavior repertoire was ineffective in satisfying the patient's needs. Lack of experience or distortion cause erroneous generalizations that would make problems in living more complex.

The intricate play of developmental pressures, family structure, and family communication patterns have added both theoretical and clinical richness to our understanding of personality development. By providing insight into the basis of some of these pressures, family counseling/therapy promotes conditions for behavioral change. An individual's delay in seeking medical aid reinforces the notion that "something critical" must ordinarily happen to make a family seek help. The statistical norm for any population is to delay, perhaps indefinitely for many, and there is often an enormous discrepancy between the declared intention and the actual act. Families have their symptoms for a long period of time before ever seeking therapeutic help, conceptualizing general kinds of disturbance in interpersonal behavior and social living as being transient.

Most striking is the lack of any increase in the objective seriousness of the disorder as a factor in seeking help. If anything, there is a kind of normalization in the family, an accommodation to the problem behavior. The treatment occurs not when the disturbance becomes greater, but when the accommodation of the family, of the surrounding social context, breaks down. There are varying accommodations, physical, personal, and social, to the "symptoms" and when this adaptation becomes ineffectual, the family seeks, or is forced to seek, help.

Reflection on the part of an individual family member is the common internal pressure that brings families into treatment; however, frequently, some serious repercussion of the family symptom that has come to the attention of a community authority exerts the motivating force. Thus, the "illness" for which the family seeks help may only in part be a physical relief from symptoms.

Family Perspective

The family is a product of evolution. It is a flexible unit that adapts subtly to both exterior and interior influences. Family function is mainly vested in two broad functions, that of providing nurturance and insuring physical survival, and that of socializing the individual by building essential humanness.

The family is made up of a number of individuals of varying ages who share a common living arrangement. It may be viewed as a contemporary, ongoing system with circular networks of interaction between members. It can be defined as the operating process when people, drawn together by common needs and interests become warmly, intimately, and personally interrelated by responding to each other's needs. Family dynamics cannot be understood by studying each individual member of the family in isolation. Family dynamics have an existence of their own that depends upon how parents relate to each other, how parents relate to children, and how children relate to parents and each other. Whenever family disruption occurs, it is common for one member of the family to be designated as the "sick" individual. This is the person for whom help is sought, despite the fact that intensive studies of the family would indicate that there are perhaps other members of the family who are much "sicker." The subtle interaction of the various members of the family can both produce and preserve pathological behavior. An understanding of these interactions is essential to the effectiveness of counseling/therapy and to the successful delivery of health care. Dramatic illustrations of family dysfunction are seen in the abused child syndrome and in well-documented cases of what can be for some children a life-threatening psychosomatic disorder, asthma.

The problem of cause and effect still draws the attention of clinicians in their attempt to answer whether family members behave in a certain way because one member is "disturbed," or is that member disturbed because the other family members are the way they are, and presumably were when the identified client or patient was born?

This is an essentially pointless and irresolvable debate when it is couched in such terms, because study of ongoing families reveals that it is comprised of a reciprocally causative system, whose complementary communication reinforces the nature of the interactions between members. It matters little how this originated, because once it is under way (by the time a clinician sees them), this pattern of interaction tends to be self-perpetuating and reciprocally causative. The responses that each person makes are the only ones available to him and the longer the process continues, the more rigidly such responses will be made, thus inevitably triggering the sequence. Individual psychiatric symptoms, then, can be seen as functional, adaptive, even appropriate, in terms of the particular family system within which the individual operates.

INITIATING INVOLVEMENT

The essence of family counseling/therapy is a clear conceptualization of emotional disorders and/or dysfunction within the family context and active participation in the struggle toward change. Most persons are ambivalent toward the idea of change. They may be dissatisfied with how things are, but frightened of how they might be if changed.

The requirements for increasing the potential for change to occur within a family system are: (1) a fairly high degree of dissatisfaction on the part of two or more members, (2) awareness of how one behaves within the system in relation to identification of problems and provision of opportunity for feedback, and (3) a person who is external to the system (counselor/therapist) to resolve the central issue. Persons who are being asked to change must have an opportunity to "save face." The responsibility rests with the therapist to facilitate conditions in which this occurs. Family systems are very resilient and, in fact, hard to change (Wynne, 1965). The therapist must take the active role of being both participant-observer and active member, even though it will take some time to "get a feel" for the family. The family-oriented therapies attempt to arrange interventions that will accomplish family alterations in order to further family growth, flexibility, and effective communication. This process is complex. In many ways it is a more difficult skill to master than individual therapy, since it requires greater activity on the part of the therapist and is therefore more susceptible to errors. These errors stem from both the ease with which subtle verbal and nonverbal cues can be missed in the turmoil of an active family session, and the fact that the content may call up feelings, attitudes, and bias for the therapist that may impede the process.

The therapist proceeds methodically through several steps in approaching the family. First, the therapist works to obtain acceptance as a temporary and yet very important member of the family group. Minuchin (1974) refers to this crucial step as "joining." Its successful accomplishment is prerequisite to the next step of redefining the "emotional illness" from an individual family member to a family problem—a problem in family functioning that is partly manifested through the symptomatic behavior of the designated patient. This can be difficult in some families. The family must be shown, not told, that the family system, not the symptomatic member, is in need of help by change.

Parents can react with resentment and resistance if they are directly confronted with the family conflicts that the child is expressing. This parental behavior may pose a hazard to the therapist, as it carries the potential for disrupting focus. The therapist needs to be sensitive to these behaviors but must realize that an interference in focus could destroy the therapeutic mission. This interference may cause the therapist to entertain the idea that the fault lies within the child and offer advice accordingly. Advice offered by someone who does not blame the parents because of a feeling that the child has an internal problem leads the parents to accept directions and respond in new ways with less resistance. However, there are two main disadvantages to this action. Both have serious implications for the family's communicative growth. The first handicap is the idea that the problem is within the child. If this theory persuades the therapist that there must be an attempt to change something within the child, the therapist will not communicate with the parents through the child, encouraging healthy interactions and open communication, but will focus upon the child and risk the possibility that no change will take place. The second danger is based upon the therapist's lack of understanding of the ways the child is responding to the interpersonal context. If the nurse therapist interprets the child's communicative behavior as a statement about his or her inner self rather than a determination about the social situation as well, the therapist will have difficulty in directing energy to influence the social situation to effect change in the child's behavior. Frequently, the child expressing some behavior has drawn attention to the family, has earned the label of "sick," and with "his problem" has legitimatized therapy for the family. By not recognizing that the child is responding to a conflictual family structure, the therapist will be unable to indirectly influence that structure in any systematic way.

Reports of the child's problematic behavior generally dominate the initial session. This fact should alert the therapist to the necessity to monitor content, making sure each member's perspective of the problem is presented, including a self report by the "identified patient." A climate must also be maintained of openness, fairness, and support for each member as the family process begins to yield data. Certain environmental contingencies can cause a child to distort the verbal report when asked to describe personal behavior. Admittedly, the presence of an observer in an environment, particularly the family, alters the situation and may affect the behavior of the child and those in attendance. Nevertheless, most often the information given under these circumstances is less biased and more useful for establishing a climate for change than the data obtained from individual members' retrospective accounts apart from the family. It is then natural and no longer important to begin therapy with "Why the delay?" rather than "Why now?"

This topic focus allows for the family to move quickly to the "heart of the matter" and forces a demonstration of their interaction patterns and communication style. This limitation also exerts an inhibiting effect upon those members who might have a propensity to overreact, overexplain, or present an historical accounting of every problematic behavior of the identified patient.

The knowledge that the scheduling of family therapy tends to increase the guilt and defensiveness in family members (Rabiner et al., 1962) should be kept in mind and serve to keep the goals of therapy in focus.

Psychotherapeutic Approaches

The therapist should have a clear idea of the differences between various approaches of psychotherapeutic intervention and be knowledgeable enough to suit technique to situation rather than to require that all families conform to the same methodology. The therapist who can use a variety of methods is much more likely to be capable of helping families with a broad range of problems than is the one who takes a singular approach to psychotherapy. Regardless of approach, the usefulness of supportive measures cannot be overstated. This unconditional sustainment is vital, particularly in the early phases of therapy. This can be maintained by gathering data through facilitating the family's telling of its own story and being unobtrusively supportive and avoiding premature commitment to a therapeutic strategy. In some cases, it may take four or five sessions to make the family feel ready to enter the problem-solving phase. Beginning therapists frequently fail to appreciate the fact that trying to understand what a family is saying and to help them clarify their own thoughts and feelings is therapy in itself. Generally, elements from several approaches will be employed.

Both *facilitation* and *confrontation* are useful in helping the family tell their story and to become aware of their feelings through self-discovery. This creates a different therapy atmosphere than does *questioning,* yet it accomplishes the same purpose. Even though in each instance family members will give similar information, obtaining it through *direct questioning* reduces their sense of responsibility for their own feelings.

FAMILY ASSESSMENT

The therapist must assess *family functioning* in a number of interlocking dimensions. The first of these is the definition of the family boundaries. The therapist tries to determine if there are clear generational boundaries, boundaries between individuals in the family, clear boundaries between the family and the surrounding society, and clear sex-role boundaries. Dysfunction or problems in living may result from boundary definitions that are excessively rigid, vague, or capriciously changeable.

The second structural feature of the family is the nature of the *subgroups* within the larger family. For example, a common dysfunctional subgrouping consists of mother and children allied against the father. The result is that the father is rendered ineffective in the parenting role and is lost to the wife as a gratifying husband. In normal families subgrouping occurs in a variety of patterns determined by the emotional or practical issues that occupy the family at the moment. In normal families, there is flexibility in that alliance patterns shift without strong family efforts to resist the change.

The third area for scrutiny is the family *patterns of communication* in order to note both the conceptual clarity and the affective range of messages. Normal families have relatively open communication, which tends to be clear as well as being determined by present needs rather than defensive maintenance of family myths or the need to deny particular affective states. Some disturbed families cannot permit the expression of angry feelings. When these threaten to emerge, communication may be blocked by irrelevant expressions of mutual concern or warmth. Other families block expressions of tender feelings.

Other dimensions of assessment that need to be delineated are the *parenting skills* and styles in the family. The questions to be answered are: Do the parents provide adequate nurture? Are they able to set limits? Can they provide information in a form that is usable and accurate? Can they deal openly with husband-wife conflict or do they utilize the parenting function to fight one another? Have they relegated parenting partially or wholly to one of the children as evidenced in role reversal?

The fourth area of assessment is the family's style of *problem solving.*

The therapist must see whether the family allows wide involvement in reaching decisions and planning actions or whether it depends on one autocratic leader. If there is a single leader, is this person supported or is there implied rebellion and contempt behind the apparent passivity of the other family members? Some families seem incapable of reaching a decision. In these families either there is no leadership or the process of problem solving is so contaminated by rage affecting conflicts that it becomes chaotic and inconclusive.

The therapist cannot deny or ignore the impact that *cultural heritage* exudes upon family life in the expressing of its function. Time and again anthropologists have called attention to the practice of designating certain behaviors as abnormal in one cultural situation that would be considered quite normal and even ignored in another. They explained this phenomenon in terms of value orientations: Culturally, the Irish convey a concern for something specific, something that has gone wrong, or been impaired, whereas Italians describe their complaints in a more diffuse way (The Committee on the Family, 1970).

Stress tolerance and a family's response to noxious stimuli is another measure that is modulated by their value system. This orientation should be considered when evaluating family stress. The family's source of stress can be traced to two primary areas—the family as an institution and as a social context.

Stressors in the family vary in form, severity, and degree of continuity. Some are brief crises, yet others are long term and persist in contributing to situations of conflict. Many are clearly delineated events; others are more subtle, such as structural arrangements in the family or long-term patterns of interpersonal conflict seldom verbalized and perhaps infrequently recognized. A particular family phenomenon may be a source of stress and it may also generate a response to stress. It carries the potential of being an independent and dependent variable at the same time. It may also operate as a mediating variable. In these conditions, the problem of identification and clear definition of stressor source may be a difficult one.

Two problems occur in the case of social phenomena that cause stress. One is the difficulty of delineation of the stressor element and the other is the assessment of the level of force the stress carries. The variables that should be considered when assessing an individual member's reaction to stress within the family context are marital conflict, sibling rivalry, child-rearing practices, family structure, behavioral attributes of the home, family priorities, communication forms, power, and authority.

Mechanisms of suppression of conflict may serve to disguise the nature of stressors operating within the family, thus hampering their measurement. Hostilities that arise between members frequently are expressed to other persons in situations outside the family system. The conflict may emerge at work or school, in peer groups, or during illness. This displacement serves to maintain a situation of apparent peace within the family.

Family stressors differ from family to family—an element that may generate stress in one family context may not do so in another. Thus, stressor elements within the same family do not operate equally on all members. Hence, to identify stressors, it is often necessary to do so in terms of their effects. Stressors should be traced to determine if the elements are either external to the family or peripherally related. This ascertains whether or not it is the family itself that is a source of stress for the member. Stresses that appear to be centered in the family may actually be a displacement of emotions, with the stresses arising from situations or developmental factors outside the family. For example, a situation of interpersonal conflict in a marriage may be described at one level as a source of stress for the children of the family. However, the problem of marital incompatibility may have its origins in personality problems of the individuals involved, thus predating the marriage relationship.

The family counselor/therapist appreciates the fact that direct therapy contacts with individuals or subgroups of the family have great effects on the entire family structure, i.e., the therapist makes a strong statement supporting the importance of legitimacy of the husband-wife relationship apart from the couple's parenting function merely by scheduling an interview that will focus exclusively on this subgroup and role relationship within the family. This message will reverberate throughout the family, influencing or perhaps threatening previous configurations of family priorities, alliances, and status distributions.

The marital assessment should demonstrate a basic understanding of the primary forces that impinge on and determine the course and quality of married life. Some of these forces stem from the historically evolving problems and values of our society, some from the basic biological differences between the sexes, and still others derive from psychological factors, often subconscious, molded by past experiences and by the vicissitudes inherent in an intensely intimate relationship.

Causes become complicated by interrelationship of elements within a social system. The nature of interpersonal relationships may frequently be a reflection of the level of integration or disintegration of the social system within which subunits such as the family exist. Child-rearing practices are the most obvious examples that are linked to norms and values outside the family system itself. They may be associated with such elements as economic institutions, religious systems, and other areas of social structure. In defining the nature of a problem for action, it is important to consider the relationship of the stress factors between the family and external sources.

Comprehensive *environmental assessment* is a direct method that can be employed for recognizing the significance of everyday physical environment for human experience and behavior. This information reveals the ambience in which process occurs and provides a diagram for understanding family members' interactions.

The criteria used for comparison is knowledge that any stable activity pattern that tends to occur in a place contributes importantly to the overall character of that place. The initial and primary place to be evaluated is the home; however, any place that family members, individually or collectively, spend an abundance of their time needs to be incorporated into the informational system. Five levels of analysis must be considered when assessing places. One must take into account information regarding their physical and spatial proprieties, their organization of entities and activities, their environmental traits, their behavioral attitudes, and their institutional characteristics. Each of these levels has some influence upon the autonomy and unique expression of family members.

The counselor/therapist, while gathering this data, must be mindful that it is to be integrated into a pattern and must resist the urge to make interpretations and base actions on one specific item. It remains critical to view these places in the perspective of how they relate to each member, their perception of them, and what impact they have for their relationships and interactions.

The physical attributes of the home are usually determined by the parental dyad and influenced by their value system. One or both members determine how space, form, and structural units are to be utilized, and this arrangement provides the general atmosphere in which family process evolves. The decisions that are made to specify the use of these units convey the climate of the home. Collaboratively these factors covertly stipulate the degree of autonomy and individual expression that will be permitted.

The physical and spatial proprieties are self-evident and observable. This set of attributes directly affects the level of activity and autonomy of family members. These conditions may also be conducive to provoking emotional expression between family members. Some social scientists suggest conditions of childhood that thwart and inhibit the child's attempts at establishing a sense of identity is the spawning ground for the motivation for future aggressive, noxious, or pathological behavior.

The organization of entities and activities category speaks to such things as time that is allotted to various activities (i.e., lunch, sleep) and the spatial distribution of ongoing activities. This form of control has influence upon one's tolerance for routine and socializing and recreational behavior. It serves to regulate present behavior and to predispose future socialization and recreation attitudes. It is necessary that each member's perception of these actions interfacing with their own personal goals be compatible and clear. Distortions have power to disrupt family process. If a member perceives any incongruence with a personal view, the cost is a sense of not belonging and low self-worth for the individual and unbalance for the family system.

By examining the institutional attributes of places, the counselor/ therapist can know and experience the climate in which family members interact, the roles each member enacts, and the risk-taking behavior that is tolerated. The atmosphere reflects the family's enduring norms, values, patterns of communication, expectations, rules, routines, and styles of personal relations. This is an important level of analysis, because treatment outcome is related to the therapist's ability to comprehend accurately the environment in which family members interact and to select interventions that are justifiable within that system. Ideally, family process should be carried on in an atmosphere of honest, mutual respect, sensitive listening, and caring love. The family should provide a safe place to release frustration, to ventilate hostility, and to express deep feelings. Open communication should help to make the family a center for personal problem solving and a perpetual fortress of emotional security. The counselor/therapist is committed to activating the family to attain this state of being.

WORKING PHASE

Once the presenting problem has been evaluated and the family perspective redirected, family action must be taken to work toward change. Acceptance of the notion that problems in living in families is exhibited by a problem behavior on the part of some member of the family signifies change of perspective. The clinician should not take for granted that recognition of reality is the equivalent of adaption to reality. The most rational attitude does not necessarily carry with it a desire or motivation to consider change. The counselor/therapist must wait for the family to initiate the therapeutic alliance. This alliance implies a contractual agreement stating that the clinician will work to maximize the possibility of improvement. It also gives the family power to terminate the alliance at any time. The hazards of not waiting for this alliance to be negotiated by the family is that psychological seduction allows for the family to avoid responsibility and sets the stage for sabotage through passivity. The counselor/therapist should be viligant for both overt and covert bribery behavior on the part of family members. Statements such as "Tell me everything will be all right" and "You will solve our problems" are signals that the process has not been successfully completed.

Problems of living call for two di coveries to be made—the first being to determine the error and the second to learn a way to correct the error.

The critical issue to be resolved is who is to make these discoveries: the counselor or the family? Will the method adhere to facilitating the family's self-discovery or will it be counselor/therapist discovery followed by interpretation? Although there has been much discussion regarding which approach is more effective, many have come to the conclusion that both types are equally cogent. This suggests that each operates from the belief that behavior can be changed and features common to both are the essential rudiments of the process.

One commonality between the two approaches is the exposure to models whose patterns of behavior can be imitated, whether or not intentionally. That social learning and consequent personal growth can take place more readily after intense or strong feeling states have been reduced is another commonality. The concept of learning new social behavior through modeling can be mediated very effectively by concentrating upon the family's style of communication. Through such learning from models and observing the consequences of others' behavior, people can learn to control their behavior to varying degrees. As people change their behavior, the response of others toward them is likely to change. Behavior that evokes positive and rewarding responses is likely to be perpetuated. Naturally, genetic endowment and constitutional factors may limit the range of behavior that a given person can develop and the rate at which behavior can change. The clinician clearly can and does serve as a model for the family by making deliberate efforts to utilize the learning processes and to present new models of behavior for the family to internalize.

The system of family rules, conveyed through the nonverbal signaling system, imputes social control of members by conveying the rules about what may or may not be communicated in the verbal mode. An inability to translate the nonverbal mode into the verbal crucially contributes to perpetuating problems in living for some families. When this is so, the nonverbal components of interactions need to be recognized and translated into the verbal mode for everyone. Frequently, the nonverbal denotes a breakdown of the verbal method of communication. The latter may be restored more readily when special support and sanction for expressing content verbally is provided. The possibility of communicating about communication makes it acceptable for the family to stand back from, observe problems in, and improve their communication processes. The clinician is outside the system, with a base not in the family conflicts, but in theories about family conflicts and is therefore helpful. The therapist's communications are on a different level from those of the family.

Insight or dynamics into the interactions of what is going on between oneself and others is another essential feature of behavioral change and relates to the therapeutic process. Insight includes dynamics into the factors presumed to have caused the "symptom" as well as insight into the interactions of what is going on between oneself and others. The clinician helps family members to translate their private unconscious nonverbal interaction into the verbal mode, where it cannot only be said, but also talked about. The best-prepared therapy regime will not produce change in the family unless they are motivated to respond as required. Hence, this necessitates that the clinician be visually attentive and continually assess which objects, events, and conditions will serve as effective reinforcers for a particular family.

Yet another item of similarity of therapeutic approaches, that of social or psychological manipulation, is reflected in the use of therapeutic strategies such as suggestion, direction, structuring the environment, role playing, and selected techniques of behavior modification. These are representative of the tools the clinician uses in the working phase. Discussion of interactions and experimentation with new forms of relating increases the possibility of objectivity. The clinician's accumulated knowledge of others' behavior in like situations can be shared, providing an opportunity for modifying the family's established pattern or developing a more adaptive reaction to the same stimulus.

Information about the family's repertoire of behavior and the circumstances in which they occur provides the basis for the interventions during the working phase. This interaction yields a systematic ordering of content-exposing actions, interactions, relationships, interrelationships and feelings of family members from which alternative problem-solving methods evolve. The work of this phase begins with a report of behaviors that are of concern. It then moves to relating these examples to the family's earlier development, including parental rules, regulations, and any other situations or conditions for necessary identification of specific environmental circumstances both past and present when these behaviors occurred to present emotional and behavioral expression. It concludes with the family postulating, experiencing, and experimenting with alternative forms of behaving and interacting.

Setting Priorities

Which problem should be selected as the initial target? Should treatment begin with individual growth or skill acquisition? Or should it be a training in cognitive, social, or emotional behavior, or perhaps a combination of these? The decision is generally based upon the severity of the problem, i.e., its aversiveness to society, its debilitating effect on an individual member, or its possible causal relationship to the family's other problems. The clinician forms a mental set that influences perception of the family and listens for those communications that best afford the opportunity to take the kind of action considered helpful.

Intervention Strategies

The choice of interventions is guided by a tentative diagnosis of the family pattern and pathology, a conceptual framework that is constantly revised and refined to include the data that are related by the family's response to those interventions the counselor/therapist attempts. Clearly, the nature of the interaction will be strongly influenced by the clinician's theoretical grounding and view of what is therapeutic. Insight-oriented and process-oriented derivatives of psychoanalytic methods are types of therapy techniques frequently used, although there has been increased use of communication minilabs, some behavior therapy methods, social learning modeling, and gestalt exercises.

Using confrontation in an empathic way is difficult. Skill in its use requires practice with a clear understanding of what it is. Even though support and reassurance each have a different effect upon the family and dissimilar conditions warrant their expression, many clinicians confuse the two and this confusion results in nontherapeutic sessions. Understanding the differences between various psychotherapeutic techniques and knowing which of them one is using at a given point of interaction helps to clarify one's communication, thereby increasing its therapeutic effect. Some clinicians err in giving the family too many messages in the same communication. This action places the level of trust that the clinician has established in jeopardy, because the communication style has become unclear. It also disrupts the focus of the session. Another negative consequence is the production of ambiguity for the family—ambiguity in the sense that family members have to guess the hierarchical value of the messages and the expected response pattern. Even experienced counselor/therapists should continue to scrutinize their response to each family member and their professional behavior in each session.

The process is interactive and as the clinician intervenes to facilitate change in the family, the approach must repeatedly respond to the countermeasures the family mobilizes to obstruct change. These resistances reflect the individual family member's concerns of power, competence, legal and administrative considerations, information, participation, energy, and belief systems. Their questions are: How will my status within the family influence the change and be affected by it? Will change allow me to demonstrate my ability? How will change be related to mandates or restrictions given me? How will I participate in change or will I be helpless to officially resist it? What is the time, money, and amount of work that will be involved in change? Will my beliefs, values, and norms be supported or undermined by change?

Their position usually is to remain benevolently skeptical of all methods until the challenge to construct and maintain a process-oriented system is integrated. When this occurs, change is expected, anticipated, and desired.

Throughout the working phase, the focus is primarily upon family strengths and skills and a general expectation that family members will help one another. The value position that mutual support is the function of the family is clearly enunciated.

The content focus of this phase is with current interactions, except when the family brings up the past to reveal a family secret to the clinician. This is clear indication of a successful opening up of family interactions. This form of past occurrences continues to have a strong impact on the entire family in the present and knowledge of them serves to clarify current issues and conflicts.

Another exception tends to occur late in this stage when an individual family member has shed defensiveness and accepts personal responsibility for a role in the family's problems. This member may focus on experiences from the past that serve to distort appropriate responses to present family reality. Such a member may need some extended interaction with the clinician, since persons who have little capacity to effect changes in their life situation are most vulnerable. The primary aim remains to mobilize a rational and effective communication system between family members, one that brings to awareness the hidden and distorted expressions of emotion that pervade the family. Generally, the clinician must resist any ploys of being sought as an ally against other family members. Throughout this phase the clinician is viligant (1) to detect subtle changes of behavior of family members as expressed through entry into the room and spontaneous seating arrangements; (2) needs to determine whether previous repetitive patterns of association and communication that have existed between particular family members have changed; (3) intervenes to change patterns of those who formerly dominated the commentary, those who interrupted, coerced, denied, or expressed their reactions through nonverbal behavior or withdrawal by structuring the environment and planning an interventive strategy.

By the use of clarifying questions and interpretations of behavior, the therapist assists the family in becoming more open in their communication, to reassay and reorganize their patterns of coercion and misappropriate alliances, and to resolve conflicts by exposing their emotional responses to the real and unreal differences they perceive amongst themselves. Some clinicians elect to have family members express their transference perception. Some may be questioning, yet remain supportive of, those members who bear the brunt of family attack in the course of the sessions. The hope is to bring about a change in the family as an ongoing social institution. The interactions focus upon developing trust in the family's potential for competence, caring, and intuitive judgment in their interactive process.

Some decision-making process is required that will permit both mutual consultation and discussion to find compromises most satisfactory to all. An agreed-upon procedure allowing for controversies unresolvable by these means to be settled is also necessary. This pattern should change with time, responsibility and control becoming more asymmetrical as new members are incorporated into the system. Most marital partners share responsibility according to their attitudes and interests, often gender related. They share decisions following discussion and enjoy giving way to gratifying each other. Ultimately, effective responsibility and dominance patterns in healthy families are always by agreement and cannot be imposed or arbitrary.

The internalized model of the parents as a couple, rather than separate individuals, will have a deep influence on the quality of the marriages of their children. To understand the relationship of models in a marriage, it is important to remember that each partner may at times enact either role of an early relationship that has been witnessed. Because of this the clinician may become confused and need help in identifying the positions each is taking at a given time.

Aggression and sexuality are commonly expressed in families. Just as there has been a growing awareness of the extent of physical abuse of infants and children, sexual abuse has also been reported more frequently. Such assaults may occur in infancy: The adult masturbating the infant to pacify it, or in a more covert way, persistently and repetitively taking the child's rectal temperature, inserting suppositories, hitting the child's naked buttocks, or sleeping in the same bed. Overt sexual attempts of an incestual nature may also occur. If it is not evidenced within the system, it may be expressed in a disguised form or be expressed elsewhere. Within the family system, these feelings may be expressed as meaningless symptoms in one or more members. If denied expression, they may be evidenced through the member who acts as a safety valve for the total group, but has to be excluded from the family system or self-exiled from it to make this possible.

The family problem needs to be examined in view of the marital relationship. Many times the mirror image of the family constellations in the family of origin is reenacted. The role of learning and readiness guarantees the repetitiveness with which models of human functioning are transmitted from one generation to the next. Parental abuse of children is one manifestation that clearly indicates the efficacy of this process while clear and explicit linking of different levels of developmental arrest in children with corresponding immaturities in the marital relationship of parents is another. By demonstrating that one is not upset with intense, emotional experience and that one can contain such impulses, the clinician grants permission to family members to acknowledge similar feelings in themselves.

There is general agreement among clinicians that a clear and unambiguous differentiation of the two gender roles within a marriage is required for children to develop without a harmful degree of confusion and conflict. Money and Ehrhardt (1972) suggest, "Cultural and historical variations of the masculine and feminine social and vocational roles are acceptable so long as there are clear boundaries delineating at a minimum, the reproductive and erotic roles of the sexes. The traditional content of the masculine and feminine roles is of less importance than the clarity and lack of ambiguity with which the tradition is transmitted to a child" (p. 164).

Every family system's structure defines the limits that must be maintained. Sometimes the source for antisocial behaviors such as fire setting, truancy, stealing, and unacceptable sexuality is believed to stem from the parents' unwilling sanction or indirect encouragement of this behavior. In these cases, the child is not deprived emotionally or exposed to cultural patterns that encourage the pattern—but the parent appears overtly to interdict the act that is the source of complaint. Study of the parent-child interaction reveals that through unconsiously driven behavior, the parent or both parents communicate their permissiveness to the child. The approval is often expressed in nonverbal forms by undue attention to the child's disturbing behavior, by the lack of consistent firmness, or in its management through unwilling and sometimes suggestive remarks or encouragement. To effect a change, the therapist must help the permissive parent to see that vicarious gratification is obtained from the child's misbehavior that acts out the parents' repressed impulses. The need for boundary constancy becomes greater when the stability of a situation increases. Boundary conditions should be given particular emphasis, with the time, place, duration, and characteristics of the situations kept as contained as possible when a change in growth is being facilitated.

Changes in family members' behavior can be categorized as changes in communication style, life-style, interpersonal relations, and interpersonal transactions. Basic to each of these is that family members be helped to perceive each other more objectively, to communicate more effectively, and to negotiate more satisfying forms of interactions.

Interpretive analytic methods sometimes achieve far-reaching changes and are necessary where problems are more complex and motivation more conflicted. Modeling and interpretative approaches need to be used selectively. Facilitating open and honest communication, assisting the family toward an attitude of mutual respect and concern, giving each other room to move, change, and grow appear more important than any other single quality to be undertaken.

INDICATIONS FOR COUNSELING/THERAPY

Counseling/therapy as a treatment form for individuals whose emotional origin of physical disorder has been clearly established, such as those with asthma, duodenal ulcer, or ulcerative colitis, is a common practice. Inclusion of the family into the counseling session is a more recent practice. Counseling/therapy has also become the treatment of choice for such conditions as deviancy, crisis, or severe, inhibiting emotionality. A counselor/psychotherapist may be a member of any of the helping professions, and may engage in brief or extended efforts to improve the state of "health" or well-being of the family. This form of therapeutic intervention may be employed as the sole effort or as part of an overall treatment plan.

Sessions with the entire family seem to be the treatment of choice in most situations and for certain kinds of emotional disorders. This is true particularly in those instances where interpersonal boundaries of individual members and family boundary diffusion are of long duration and will require long-term efforts.

The majority of individuals labeled as "overinhibited" are reared in families where punitive or critical suppression of activity is the general mode of transaction. Many of these, as children, had some physical deficiency or inadequacy. Their affective life is one of shame or guilt for presumed failures in meeting their own needs or parental expectations. They indulge in daydreaming and have few or no close friendships. They seem to have an inability for affective relations of any kind. In their deprivation they have turned to fantasy and social isolation. If withdrawal continues, their capacity to evaluate reality effectively will be impaired.

The briefer insight-oriented therapies are more focused and more limited in their goals. They entail conjoint examination of current problems by clinician and family, looking to the past only to clarify present-day difficulties. Interpretation is used primarily for clarifying troublesome aspects of the family's life rather than uncovering deeply buried memories with their associated feelings. The clinician is generally supportive, asking questions chiefly for clarification or to get information for an interpretation or confrontation. Working through involves the family's acceptance and incorporating what it is beginning to learn about itself.

Many clinicians, when working with families, prefer to work conjointly, utilizing an approach based on modeling and identification processes where the model provided is a relationship between therapists rather than the behavior of an individual therapist. The general approach is a conscious attempt to alter behavior by presenting different models for the family to internalize.

Crisis situations in adolescence, runaways, suicide attempts, and illegitimate pregnancies often are best approached through brief family counseling. Sessions focus upon the family's finding adaptive ways of responding to the immediate problem, and in revealing the enduring family patterns that resulted in the eruption of symptomatic behavior. An underlying excessive closeness of the child to one or more family members may be the cause of the delinquent action, which represents an attempt at emancipation. Although the greatest amount of change occurs early in the therapy regimen, Morrison and Collier (1969) found that families do not seem motivated to continue with therapy once the immediate crisis is solved.

Apart from crisis, the adolescent whose difficulties seem primarily related to problems in separating from parents is best treated in long-term family therapy. Frequently, external agencies such as the school detect the child's social immaturity and recommend counseling/therapy. These youngsters express clear developmental immaturities, including social anxiety, academic difficulties, and overt clinging, childish behavior. They may disguise their excessive dependence, with the family's collusion, as psychosomatic illness and complaints of illness. This family pattern may be precipitated and potentiated by the presence of actual physical disease, particularly a chronic illness, in the child. An unsatisfactory marital relationship leading to inappropriate utilization of the child to satisfy parental affectional needs or to provide a buffer between the parents is generally the basic problem. Therapy efforts are directed to strengthening the husband-wife dyad. If this is unattainable, the dissatisfactions can be made explicit and the parents helped to meet their needs elsewhere. The adolescent's intent to separate is encouraged and supported. The clinician needs honest empathy for the parent who is resisting this posture to safeguard the family's remaining in treatment and permit extrication of the child. Overidentification with the youngster on the part of the clinician frequently leads to blaming the parent and lecturing about the child's right to its own life. This misguided action of advocacy on the part of the clinician results in increasing anxiety and perpetuating the frightened, clinging pattern in the family. Many of these parents have some level of awareness of what they are "doing wrong," but cannot come to grips with the feelings of abandonment they portend they will experience if relationships change. They need help in discovering alternatives.

Forms of family structure that tend to prevent individualization and separation continue to be regressive and contribute to the development of depressive phenomena. These include the symbiotic survival patterns. Symbiotic family survival patterns operate in a cycle (Haley, 1963). Parents did not trust their own parents to be responsive to their needs, and therefore they need to control the "other" to overcome the sense of separateness. Each member of the family feels omnipotent and overtly responsible for the other, as well as helpless, and extremely controlled by others. The child in this situation has difficulty in achieving autonomy and a separate identity, feels responsible for the self-esteem of parents, and needs the familial symbiosis to sustain self-definition.

When interpersonal ownership is denied the child, its effect is transacted on the family level in symbiotic relationships. Differentiating the self from other bodies, thoughts, perceptions, and ideas is most apt to break down when an individual emphasizes and establishes closeness with another. Ambivalence, a normal constituent of an individual's make-up, may cause difficulty in feeling whole if tied to another's identity. Schizophrenics, existing at the lower limits of inner ownership, feel fragmented, depersonalized, and disembodied. On the other hand, certain adolescents with extremely developed moral judgment and sensibility exist at the upper limits of inner ownership.

Family relations affect the extent and manner of owning and disowning one's inner life and property. Overowning parents damage their child's capacity to tolerate ambivalence and violate both integrity and age-appropriate separation and individuation. We can only hope to own ourselves when we have been owned. History records the lives of those who have been psychologically exploited by a parent. In these instances, the exploitation ruined the persons' life, yet at the same time gave meaning and power to it. While withdrawing from the world socially, the person had become satisfyingly important to mother and family. Their purpose in life was to let parents live through the child. Moral credits were amassed and got the upper hand in operating the guilt lever on mother and father.

Youngsters whose predominant behaviors reflect persistent anxiety, excessive or overdetermined fears, and nightmares are often described by their parents as being sensitive, shy, and aspiring. They admit to feeling inferior, are submissive to others, and their major drive is to maintain security through pleasing. Generally, the parental injunction is to meet high standards of achievement and social expectations. Ambitious middle-class families frequently create such a situation for the child. These children soon come to recognize that their acceptance within the family is contingent upon continued outstanding performances. This results in repeated attempts to enact a life-style that calls for extraordinary expectations and excessive demands upon themselves. Hence, self-destructive acts are a common form of expression. Long-term treatment postcrisis is required as the sources of the child's anxiety and rage in relation to the parental figures needs to be uncovered and worked through.

Families who externalize problems can be helped in family counseling. In these families, each member is preoccupied with the shortcomings of various other family members and expresses the belief that whatever unhappiness and adjustment problems one is having actually results from the shortcomings of another family member. There is virtually no intro-spection and the capacity for self-observation seems limited while the skill in finding fault in other family members is highly refined.

Diagnostically, adolescents from these families often are identified as having behavior or personality disorders. Individuals who depend upon external approval and are sensitive to external criticism or the absence of praise have never adequately developed a mature capacity for internal self-esteem. With patience and perseverance, it is possible to gradually require these families to communicate in ways that diminish the need for cycles of recrimination and blame. An effective method is to consistently point out conflicting messages or instructions that prevent the individuals receiving them from either finding a solution or escaping from the conflict. This phenomenon is known as the "double bind" within family systems and is a common form of communication in such family situations. Another style of communicating frequently seen is that of mystification, a systematic provocation of confusion and bewilderment generated by vague or incompatible information with hostile and destructive intent on the part of the sender. In these instances, the clinician may elect to use some behavior modification techniques or employ role play to facilitate change of communication style. Another way to accomplish this is by establishing the ground rule that prohibits critical statements between family members to be made. Instead, all communication must be trans-lated into personal requests and statements of personal need. For exam-ple, if mother wishes to complain that her husband is not affectionate, she must say, "I feel lonely and I need affection. Is there any way I can help you show me more warmth?" This clinician may also request the parents to hold hands to graft new behaviors and to block previous stereotyped in-teractions that serve to avoid awareness of internal feelings by displacing them onto other family members. Many other techniques can be used to change destructive relationship patterns. Clinicians whose primary aim is to reduce fears and improve the family members' self-control emphasize anxiety-reducing interventions. They use emotional arousal either at the beginning of therapy, followed by systematic reinforcement of newly de-veloped attitudes, or in the latter sessions crystallizing gains of preceding therapeutic sessions. It is critical that the initially induced emotional arousal be followed by cognitive learning.

A neurotic family homeostasis is maintained within the family by scapegoating a particular child or by producing a youngster whose be-havior typifies an absence or low level of conscious development (Haley, 1963). The scapegoat child serves to reduce tension between the paren-tal dyad. By accepting the brunt of their tensions, this child reduces the contact they have with each other, minimizing the expression of negative feelings toward each other. The child selected generally is available, is in a powerless position, and the cost of such dysfunction is low compared to the gains for the family. Although this role is functional within the family, it is dysfunctional for the individual child's emotional well-being and societal adjustment. Frequently, the child chosen for this role has symbolic significance for the family and/or is conceptualized as different.

At times, it is necessary to provide individual therapy to raise the scapegoated child's status in the family group and to discover and activate personal goals that are external to the family. Without this special assistance, the scapegoat is often unmotivated to give up this central role in the family, feeling the role is uncomfortable but more of an honor than a burden.

The family's expectation of effective treatment may greatly enhance therapeutic effects. Also, the encouragement or approval given by the clinician to the family as they learn new behavior may be very important in eliminating old, incompatible behaviors.

The aim of treatment of those who act out in antisocial ways is primarily to help them achieve inner controls over their behavior by changing the family environment and utilizing it as a source of support. The clinician must assist the family to set realistic goals, work flexibly, and build awareness insight with considerable caution. The clinician works to enhance the family's ability to tolerate anxiety and guilt while teaching them to avoid manipulation, reinforce desirable change, and fully utilize other resources.

Children whose predominant feature is running away from home come from environments where family transactions have led them to feel rejected because of unusual severity or inconsistency. Their growth is associated with a derogatory self-image and a deep lack of self-confidence and esteem. They seem incapable of developing an aggressive adaptation to living. The entire family needs to be immersed in the process of change.

Rejecting parents provide limited opportunities for association and fail to offer the needed warmth and support through indifference for healthy identification and development. They need to be helped to reformulate attitudes and rechannel their energies for change to begin.

Sometimes the key to the family problem needs to be searched for explicitly in the unconscious internalized models of dead or absent figures, as in family myths. Here, the clinician seeks to bring back to awareness the past experiences that underlie present projections and distortions. If this is not done, the repressed content will continue to interfere with the emotional development of the children or interfere with the therapeutic process of parenting.

Many times a loss is casually dismissed and grieving interrupted or not allowed—yet each loss has its effect upon the mourner. Mourning is both natural and necessary and if repressed will reassert its claims in other areas of the survivor's life. Those who refuse or are not allowed to grieve may find themselves years later affected and disabled in some measure by the loss.

CONCLUSION

With the expanding awareness of the importance of the interactions between family members in shaping and maintaining behavioral patterns of the individual family, counseling therapy has emerged within recent decades as an important therapeutic technique.

With an understanding of the interplay of social, psychological, and biological forces, the clinician will be better equipped to evolve a therapeutic approach shaped to the unique needs of the family seeking aid and counsel.

The clinician does not need to have solutions to all problems, but it is vital that he or she guide the family toward a clearer perception of their problems and engage them in the effort toward change.

REFERENCES

Ainsworth, M. D. The development of infant-mother interaction among the Ganda. In B. M. Foss (Ed.), *Determinants of infant behavior* (Vol. 2). New York: John Wiley and Sons, 1963.

Attwell, T. H. Self awareness, self responsibility and self esteem: A treatment plan. *Transactional Analysis Journal,* 1974, *4,* 25–26.

Bandura A. *Principles of behavior modification.* New York: Holt, Rinehart and Winston, 1969.

Berkowitz, L., & Green, J. A. The stimulus qualities of the scapegoat. *Journal of Abnormal Psychology,* 1964, *64,* 293–301.

Bowlby, J. *Attachment and loss.* New York: Basic Books, 1969.

Burk, P. J. Scapegoating: An alternative to role differentiation. *Sociometry,* 1969, *32,* 159–167.

Clark M. *Health in the Mexican American culture.* Los Angeles and Berkeley: University of California Press, 1970.

The Committee on the Family, Group for the Advancement of Psychiatry. *Treatment of families in conflict.* New York: Science House, 1970, 269–280.

Engel G. L., & Schmale, A. H. Psychoanalytic theory of somatic disorders. *Journal of American Psycho-Analytic Association,* 1967, *15,* 344–365.

Ferreira, A. J. Family myth and homeostasis. *Archives General Psychiatry,* 1963, *9,* 457–463.

———. Psychosis and family myth. *American Journal of Psychotherapy,* 1967, *21,* 186.

Franks, V., & Burtle, V. (Eds.). *Women in therapy.* New York: Brunner/Mazel, 1974.

Freud, S. *Collected Papers* (Vol. 2 & Vol. 5). New York: Basic Books, 1959.

Haley J. *Strategies of psychotherapy.* New York: Grune & Stratton, 1963.

Hazzard, M.E. An overview of systems theory. *Nursing Clinics of North America,* 1971, *6*(3), 385–389.

Heaton, R. C. & Duerfeldt, P. H. The relationship between self esteem, self reinforcement and the internal extra personality dimension. *The Journal of Genetic Psychology*, 1973, *123*, 3–13.

Henry, W. E., Sunis, J. H., and Spray, S. L. *The fifth profession: Becoming a psychotherapist*. San Francisco: Jossey-Bass, 1971.

Jackson, D. D., and Yalom, I. Family research on the problem of ulcerative colitis. *Archives General Psychiatry*, 1966, *15*, 410–418.

Janov, A. *The feeling child*. New York: Simon and Schuster, 1973.

Kaplan, H. I., & Sadock, B. J. *Comprehensive group therapy*. Baltimore: Williams and Wilkins, 1971.

Kassen, W., Haith, M. M., and Salapatek, P. H. Infancy. In P. H. Mussen (Ed.), *Carmichael's manual of child psychology* (Vol. 1). New York: John Wiley and Sons, 1970.

Kirchner, E. P., & Vondracek, S. I. Perceived sources of esteem in early childhood. *The Journal of Genetic Psychology*, 1975, *126*, 169-176.

Klein, M. *The psycho-analysis of children*. London: Hogarth, 1932.

———. *Envy and gratitude*. New York: Delacorte Press, 1975.

Krantz, B. & Clancy. Drives, differences and deviations. *Human sexuality for health professionals* (1st Ed.), Chapter 12. Philadelphia: W. B. Saunders, 1977.

Laing, R. D. Mystification, confusion and conflict. In F. Nagy and Framo (Eds.), *Intensive Family Therapy*. New York: Hoeber, 1965.

Lennard, N. D., & Bernstein, A. *Patterns in human interaction*, San Francisco: Jossey-Bass, 1969.

Masuda, M., & Holmes, J. H. Magnitude estimation of social readjustments. *Journal of Psychosomatic Research*, 1967, *11*, 219–255.

Matteson, R. Adolescent self esteem family communication and marital satisfaction. *The Journal of Psychology*, 1974, *86*, 35–40.

McKeighen, R. J. Basic counseling of children. *Issues in Comprehensive Pediatric Nursing*, November/December 1976/1977, McGraw-Hill.

Miller, T. Effects of maternal age, education and employment status on the self esteem of the child. *The Journal of Social Psychology*, 1975, *95*, 141–142.

Minuchin, S. *Families and family therapy*. Cambridge, Mass.: Harvard University Press, 1974.

Money, J., & Ehrhardt, A. A. *Man and woman, boy and girl: The differentiation and dimorphism of gender identity from conception to maturity*. Baltimore: Johns Hopkins University Press, 1972.

Morrison, G. C., & Collier, J. G. Family treatment approaches to suicidal children and adolescents. *Journal of the American Academy of Child Psychiatry*, 1969, *8*, 140–153.

Moss, G. E. *Illness, immunity, and social interaction*. New York: Wiley, Interscience, 1973.

Parks, C. M., & Brown, J., Jr., Health after bereavement. *Psychosomatic Medicine*, 1972, *34* (5), 449–461.

Paul, N., & Grosser, G. H. Operational mourning and its role in cojoint family therapy. *Community Mental Health Journal*, 1965, *1*, 339–345.

Perls, I. *Gestalt therapy verbatim*. Lafayette, Cal.: Real People Press, 1969.

Rabiner, E. L., Molinski, H., & Gralnick, A. Cojoint family therapy in the impatient setting. *International Journal of Social Psychiatry*, 1962, *5*, 131.

Rank, O. *The trauma of birth*. New York: Brunner/Mazel, 1952.

Rokeach, M. *The nature of human values*. New York: Free Press, 1973.

Rubin, R. Body image and self esteem. *Nursing Outlook*, 1968, *16*, 20–23.

Ryckman, R. M., & Sherman, M. F. Relationship between self esteem and internal-external control for men and women. *Psychological Reports*, 1973, *32*, 1106.

Schaffer, H. R., & Emerson, P. E. The development of social attachments in infancy. *Monographs Society for Research in Child Development* 1964, *29*(3), 1–77.

Schneider, D. & Turkat, D. Self presentation following success or failure defensive self esteem models. *Journal of Personality*, 1975, *43*, 127–135.

Schonbar, R. A. Group co-therapists and sex role identification. *American Journal of Psychotherapy*, 1973, *27*, 539–547.

Schwartz, S. Are you one of your favorite people? *The Journal of School Health*, January 1977, *44*, 30–32.

Sherman, B. The adolescent in family therapy. *Family Therapy*, 1972, *11*, 35–40.

Spiegel, J. P. The resolution of role conflict within the family. *Psychiatry*, 1957, *20*, 1–16.

Stoller, R. J. *Sex and gender*. New York: Jason Aronson, 1974.

Szasz, T. S. Illness and indignity. *Journal of the American Medical Association*, February 4, 1974, *227*,543–545.

Vogel, E., & Bell, N. W. The emotionally disturbed child as a family scapegoat. In L. V. Rabkin & J. Carr (Eds.), *Sourcebook in Abnormal Psychology*. Boston: Houghton Mifflin, 1967.

Weigert, E. Loneliness and trust: Basic factors of human existence. *Psychiatry*, 1960, *23*, 121–131.

Wynne, L., et al. Pseudo-mutuality in the family relations of schizophrenics. *Psychiatry*, 1958, *21*, 205.

Wynne, L. Some indications and contra-indications for exploratory family therapy. In N. I. Bozzormenijr & J. L. Frame (Eds.), *Intensive Family Therapy: Theoretical Practical Aspects*. New York: Harper & Row, 1965.

Zborowski, M. *People in pain*. San Francisco: Jossey-Bass, 1969.

CHAPTER TWENTY-TWO

GENETIC COUNSELING AND THE FAMILY

MIRA L. LESSICK AND PETER T. ROWLEY

Genetic counseling as a clinical service is a relative newcomer to the health care scene. Until the 1940s, the domain of genetics was primarily basic scientific research. Subsequent advances in the understanding of the genetic basis of human disease, improved techniques for examination and detection of chromosomal aberrations, the ability to diagnose certain disorders during fetal life, and the advent of screening programs has resulted in increased interest in genetics and expanded clinical practice.

Birth defects, in general, are the primary reason for genetic counseling. They include all structural and metabolic abnormalities evident at birth as well as inherited disorders not obvious until later in life. They have become an important health concern in the United States today. They are relatively frequent, do not necessarily result in early death, and a growing number are preventable. Birth defects have many causes: genetic factors (e.g., PKU, Down's syndrome), environmental factors (e.g., viruses and drugs) and combinations thereof (e.g., myelomeningocele, cleft lip/palate).

According to figures from the National Institutes of Health (DHEW Publication No. NIH74-370), more than 15 million Americans have some genetic or congenital disorder. A significant portion of this prevalence involves infants and children. It has been estimated that approximately 30 percent of pediatric hospital patients manifest a gene-related disorder (Clow, Fraser, Laberge, and Scriver, 1973); these include chromosomal aberrations, with a newborn incidence of 0.5 percent and major congenital malformations, with an incidence of 4 to 6 percent. For many of these disorders, more effective therapy—surgical, medical, dietary—has reduced morbidity and mortality.

At the same time contributions from the fields of biochemistry and cytology have clearly established a genetic basis for an increasing number of diseases. Biochemists in the past decade have furthered understanding of the structure and properties of DNA, RNA, and proteins. Thus, the mechanisms involved in the synthesis of abnormal protein, such as abnormal hemoglobins, have been well-defined. In many other genetic diseases, the abnormal protein is presumed to be an enzyme, but, for the majority, the actual enzyme defect has not been identified. The increased knowledge in biochemical genetics has led to the development of various screening tests for detecting individuals who may be carriers of a gene for a particular genetic disease (e.g., Tay-Sachs disease, sickle-cell anemia, galactosemia).

The year 1956 was a milestone in human cytology, for it was then that the number of human chromosomes was correctly established, 46 total or 23 pairs. Three years later, it was discovered that Down's syndrome was, in most instances, the result of an extra chromosome 21. With the advent of prenatal diagnosis through amniocentesis, it is now possible to detect prenatally all chromosomal abnormalities detectable after birth, and an increasing number of inborn metabolic disorders. In the majority of X-linked disorders, one can demonstrate fetal sex through amniocentesis. Amniocentesis for prenatal diagnosis is generally done between the fourteenth and sixteenth week of pregnancy. At this time there is approximately 150 ml of amniotic fluid surrounding the fetus. The fluid contains cells that have been shed by the fetus. These cells are then cultured, and the status of the fetus can be ascertained. Tay-Sachs disease, a rapidly progressive fatal neurological disorder of infancy, illustrates the impact prenatal diagnosis has had on counseling. Previously, one could only explain to the parents of such a child that the disorder was inherited as an autosomal recessive trait and that subsequent children would have one chance in four of developing the disorder. We now know that Tay-Sachs disease stems from the absence of an enzyme, hexosaminidase A, and if this enzyme has normal activity in fetal cells, the fetus is free of the disorder. The diseases to which prenatal detection is directed are severe and chronic. Therefore, prenatal diagnosis, coupled with the alternative of selective abortion, provides an important option to couples at risk.

GENETICS AND FAMILY HEALTH

The clinical application of genetic knowledge through genetic counseling has become an important and effective means of providing information to families at risk. Parents need information that will help them to make rational decisions about further reproduction. This information concerns the origin of the disorder, the risk of recurrence, the probability of carrier states among unaffected siblings, risks for collateral relatives, family planning options, and future prospects for intervention.

There are two common situations in which genetic counseling may be sought. The most common is that which arises when a child is born with an inherited or congenital abnormality. The parents need to know whether the condition is likely to recur in subsequent children. The second common situation is the occurrence of a heritable disorder in one member of the couple or one of their relatives.

GENETIC COUNSELING

The primary task of genetic counseling is to answer the questions: "Why did it happen?" and "Will it happen again?" Through genetic counseling facts are not merely presented, but attempts are made to enhance their usefulness for the family.

Genetic counseling is a communication process that deals with the human problems associated with the occurrence of a genetic disorder or congenital defect in a family. This process involves an attempt by a trained health professional to aid the individual or family to (1) comprehend the medical facts, including the diagnosis, nature, and course of the disorder, and available treatment; (2) understand the genetic or nongenetic aspects of the disorder, as the case may be, and the risk of recurrence; (3) understand the alternatives available for potential or future family planning (e.g., prenatal diagnosis, artificial insemination, adoption, or taking the specified risk); (4) choose the course of action that is best suited to their family needs and goals; and (5) make the best possible adjustment to the disorder in an affected family member and/or to the risk of recurrence of that disorder (Fraser, 1974).

The medical, psychological, social, and religious background of the parents, their relationship with each other, their concerns and feelings regarding the disorder, and the nature and history of the disease all need to be considered in counseling couples. The genetic counselor must accept both the responsibility to explore the significance of genetic factors in disease and to help families to deal with the emotional stress that this knowledge may bring. Insight into the psychodynamics of the family unit is essential in establishing an atmosphere conducive to alleviating these stresses.

CAUSES OF BIRTH DEFECTS

Known causes of birth defects include genetic and environmental factors.

Genetic Factors

Characteristic of genetic counseling is the assignment of a risk to individual family members. Risk assignment requires accurate diagnosis and knowledge of the inheritance pattern of the condition diagnosed.

The classification of genetic disease falls into three main categories, Mendelian or single-factor inheritance, polygenic inheritance, and chromosomal aberrations.

Mendelian or single-factor inheritance Mendelian patterns are principally of three types, autosomal dominant, autosomal recessive, and X-linked recessive.

Autosomal dominant In an autosomal dominant trait, a single copy of a mutant gene is sufficient for the presence of the trait. The chance that a child of an affected individual will inherit the abnormal gene is 50 percent. Both males and females are equally at risk. Multiple generation involvement is characteristic of dominant inheritance. Examples of autosomal disorders include Marfan's syndrome, neurofibromatosis, achondroplasia, polydactyly, and Huntington's chorea.

Autosomal recessive In an autosomal recessive disorder, affected individuals have the abnormal gene in double dose. They have received one dose from each parent, who generally has only a single dose and who is generally well (carrier or heterozygote). The relatives at risk are generally siblings. Both males and females may be equally affected. All individuals are carriers of genes for some recessive disorders; their carrier status remains concealed except in those situations that involve unions between two individuals who happen to be carriers of the same such gene. For the offspring of two carriers, the probability is 25 percent or ¼ for being affected and 50 percent or ½ for being a carrier. Most of the inborn errors of metabolism follow this pattern of inheritance. In rare recessive conditions, there is an increased frequency of consanguineous marriages among the parents of affected individuals. Examples of autosomal recessive disorders include galactosemia, sickle-cell anemia, cystic fibrosis, Tay-Sachs disease, phenylketonuria, and albinism.

X-linked recessive The X-linked recessive disorders are seen principally in males. Affected individuals are generally the progeny of unaffected parents, the mother being a carrier. A female carrier married to a normal male has in any given pregnancy an equal chance of producing an affected male, a normal male, a carrier female, or a normal female. Normal brothers of an affected male cannot transmit the disorder. None of the sons of the affected male will be affected and all of the daughters will be carriers.

As with autosomal recessive disorders, many of the X-linked disorders are associated with considerable morbidity and mortality. It is advantageous to be able to identify carriers or heterozygotes in these conditions. This is especially important with regard to the female relatives of persons with X-linked disorders such as Duchenne muscular dystrophy or hemophilia. The mother or sister of an individual with Duchenne muscular dystrophy, as well as the sisters of the mother, may wish to know the likelihood of carrier status in order to predict the possibility of having affected sons. The patient's mother is not necessarily a carrier, for the affected proband might be the result of a new mutation. In view of a positive family history (e.g., two affected sons or one affected brother and one affected son), the mother can definitely be considered a carrier. A woman with only one affected son and a negative family history may or may not represent a carrier. For some X-linked recessive diseases, a laboratory test for the carrier state is available.

Polygenic inheritance Most human characteristics and many common diseases are determined not by genes at a single locus, but by genes at many loci with small additive effects. Many common malformation syndromes have this type of inheritance. Examples include cleft lip with or without cleft palate, spina bifida, clubfoot, and congenital dislocation of the hip. Risk estimates for polygenic disorders are empirical, i.e., they are determined by observing actual recurrences in similarly constituted families. It has been observed that the more affected relatives there are in the family, the greater is the risk to subsequent siblings. For example, normal parents who have a child with spina bifida can be advised that the incidence is approximately 4 percent for subsequent children. After the birth of two affected children, the risk may increase to 10 percent. In most cases of the common congenital anomalies, the risk of recurrence in subsequent siblings after the birth of one affected child is relatively low, usually 5 percent or less.

Chromosomal aberrations Aberrations of chromosomes are deviations in structure or number. Numerical abnormalities include such disorders as trisomy 21, trisomy D, trisomy E, Klinefelter's syndrome, and Turner's syndrome. They are usually the result of *nondisjunction,* an error in meiosis during gametogenesis. This results in the loss or gain of a chromosome in a daughter cell. The probability of recurrence in subsequent siblings is low, on the order of approximately 1 to 2 percent. In some instances of Down's syndrome, a chromosome is given an extra portion of chromosomal material, while another chromosome is shortened by the loss of a segment. This is known as *translocation.* Translocations may be either balanced or unbalanced. In the balanced state, though numerically lacking one chromosome, the total chromosome mass is normal. The result is a phenotypically normal person, but one at higher risk for producing a child with an unbalanced translocation. In the unbalanced state, there is extra chromosomal material, as in the nontranslocation type.

If the individual has a translocation chromosomal abnormality and the parents have normal karyotypes, the risk of recurrence is low. If the translocation is inherited from one parent, the observed recurrence estimates vary, depending on the type of translocation and the sex of the parent carrying it. Before accurate counseling can be provided, the specific karyotype of the individual must be identified. For example, if a child has usual trisomy 21 with 47 chromosomes and the parents are phenotypically normal, it may be presumed that the parents' karyotypes are normal. If, however, the child has Down's syndrome due to a translocation, the karyotype of the parents must be determined. If a parent has the translocation, the risk to a subsequent child may be much greater than in the nontranslocation type.

Environmental Factors

Birth defects constitute a heterogeneous group of disorders and their etiologies are equally heterogeneous. There are many congenital defects due to nongenetic factors. Environmental agents such as viruses, drugs, and radiation may contribute to some defects. Examples include the rubella virus, cytomegalic inclusion disease virus, toxoplasma, and thalidomide.

THE PROCESS OF GENETIC COUNSELING

The contexts of genetic counseling are varied. For simplicity, we shall deal primarily with the case of parents of a child with a birth defect who seek information about the risk of recurrence.

The first consideration is who should attend the counseling session. In the common situation involving a child with a birth defect, both parents should attend. This will provide more reliable data and aid in mutual understanding of the information.

Identifying Counselee Needs

The usual anticipation during pregnancy of a normal child can be rudely terminated by the delivery of a child with a birth defect. This creates a crisis in the parents' lives that reflects the personalities, relationships, and interactions of every family member. The reactions of parents to their child are influenced not only by the type and severity of the defect, but also by previous sibling and parental experiences, by attitudes of relatives and friends, and by other family circumstances. There may be feelings of loss, disappointment, helplessness, insecurity, or isolation. Underlying these feelings may be anger, guilt, and frustration. Repression, rationalization, and self-condemnation are not uncommon. These processes may arise out of misconceptions about reproduction and the genetic nature of disease and require correction for successful counseling.

The first stage of genetic counseling is identification of the parents' expectations and concerns about the disorder in question. In most situations, these concerns focus on the questions: What is the cause? Why did it happen to us? Will it happen again? Can it be prevented? The parents need an explanation of the child's disorder and prognosis and much emotional support. The interview should be conducted so that family members can express their feelings.

> A 21-year-old college student came to genetics clinic because of hereditary multiple exostoses. He had required nine operations because of benign bony growths on his extremities. His father, paternal grandfather, and all three of his siblings had similar growths.
>
> This patient knew about and accepted the manifestations of his disease. Through genetic counseling we were able to accomplish two points of clarification. First, although he had assumed that all of his children would be affected because all of his siblings were affected, he learned that the chance of any given child of his being affected was only 50 percent. This pleased him. Secondly, his major complaint was depression, because he felt that his inability to excel in sports was a result of his "genetic defect." In this regard he learned that his defect involved only his bones and that he could expect the same improvement in athletic performance by training as anyone else.

FAMILY HISTORY TAKING

A complete family history is an essential component of the counseling process and entails formulation of the family pedigree. In most cases, the family history need only be elicited for the first three degrees of relationship—including parents, siblings, and children, grandparents, aunts, uncles, and first cousins. A meaningful family history should state the age and state of health or age at death and cause of death for each relative. The number of abortions, stillbirths, and nonliving siblings should be noted. Pregnancies should be recorded in chronological order to ensure that perinatal environmental factors such as drugs, radiation, trauma, maternal infection, and anoxia are not overlooked. Inquiry should also be made about parental consanguinity. The ethnic background of the parents should also be recorded, as certain inherited disorders are more common in some populations. It is important to assess the reliability of the informant(s). Additional information may be needed from a relative's physician, a hospital record, or a death certificate.

A 33-year-old man was admitted to the hospital with renal failure. He did not mention that anyone else in his family had a similar problem. Only when directly asked by the intern did he admit that his only two siblings had died at 22 and 24 of renal disease. When other branches of the family not in close touch with the patient were contacted, fourteen other individuals with renal disease, some dead, some ill, and others asymptomatic, were identified. In this case taking an extensive family history was responsible for explaining fatigue and anemia in members in whom renal disease had not been suspected, determining the type of renal disease (medullary cystic disease) that was the cause of renal failure in individuals in whom a cause had not been found, raising the possibility of renal transplant at an early stage in the disease when better therapeutic results could be expected, and avoiding transplantation of a kidney from a related donor who might later turn out to have the same disorder.

ESTABLISHING THE DIAGNOSIS

Estimation of the recurrence risk for a particular disorder is based upon an accurate family history and a precise diagnosis. An accurate diagnosis depends upon a careful history and physical examination of the proband. Examination of other family members is often necessary as well.

Often the diagnosis has already been made by a physician, and the counselee wants to be informed about the implications of the disease for the family. Further diagnostic procedures may be necessary; e.g., chromosome analyses or enzyme assays. For instance, it is important to distinguish microcephaly secondary to degenerative brain disease from idiopathic microcephaly inherited as an autosomal recessive trait. Microcephaly may also be produced by exposure of the fetus to excessive radiation or viral agents (e.g., rubella syndrome). Microcephaly may also occur as part of a syndrome; e.g., Trisomy 13, Seckel's syndrome, or Smith-Lemli-Opitz syndrome.

A 73-year-old man was admitted bcause of anemia. An intern obtained the history of anemia in a sister and a son. As a result a diagnosis of hereditary spherocytosis was made in this man for the first time at the age of 73 and his anemia was corrected by removal of the spleen.

ASSESSMENT OF RISK

In many cases, the information attainable about the family suffices for determining risk of recurrence. In other cases, it is necessary to review current genetic and medical literature. Victor McKusick's catalogue (1975) is an appropriate reference for Mendelian disorders. It also serves as a source for further genetic information from the literature.

DETERMINATION OF COUNSELEE'S UNDERSTANDING

Counseling must be tailored to the needs of the family. Their current understanding of the disorder must be determined. The central question usually concerns the likelihood that a particular disorder that has already occurred in the family will recur in future offspring. Counselees may have been referred to a genetic clinic because their physician thought it desirable without any explanation of the purpose. Some parents may be stunned by the birth of a defective child and still be experiencing shock, guilt, anger, or denial. Counseling should, therefore, not be done too soon after the diagnosis is made, as parents may be too upset to benefit from it.

> A 26-year-old girl, whose father and brother have Marfan's syndrome, came for premarital advice regarding recurrence risks, having been told that it is a genetic disorder and that all her children would be affected. Upon careful examination, she also was found to have this condition. Counseling reassured her that the risk to each child of inheriting the condition was only 50 percent.

PROVISION OF INFORMATION

The actual risk must be placed in proper perspective both in relation to risks for the general population and to the likely burden or degree of handicap. The counselee must understand what the risk means in practical terms in order to decide upon a course of action appropriate to the individual situation.

Charts and other visual aids are helpful in explaining concepts, particularly in relation to genetic transmission of the disorder. It is also important to indicate that recurrence risks are independent of previous events. For example, in recessive inheritance, the risk of occurrence is one-fourth or 25 percent with each pregnancy regardless of whether any affected or unaffected children have already been born. The approach must be adapted to the parents' educational backgrounds and to their ability to understand.

In discussing risks with a family, it may be desirable to present the information in a positive manner. For example, a 5 percent risk of recurrence means that there is a 95 percent chance that the next child will be well.

It is important to understand that reaction to risk is highly individual. While a risk of 5 percent is considered high for some individuals, for others a risk of 50 percent is acceptable. A number of studies have shown that the burden the disorder carries is more important than the numerical magnitude of the risk (Leonard, Chase, and Childs, 1972). The burden is measured by the degree and duration of physical, emotional, social, and financial load on the family.

In discussing genetic factors in disease with the family, it is important to relieve guilt feelings. In recessive conditions, it helps to explain to parents that every individual carries several harmful genes and that this does not mean the parent is unusual in any way.

Beyond assignment of recurrence risks, parents need not only knowledge of the course and prognosis of the disorder in question, but also guidance as to what options are available. The counselor must be prepared to provide information on the pros and cons of future reproduction and various alternatives to it, including adoption, contraception, sterilization, abortion, artificial insemination, present and future prospects for prenatal diagnosis, as well as future improvements in treatment. Counseling should be nondirective. Parents should be given the opportunity to express their feelings and beliefs regarding the disorder and their attitudes about family planning. The actual decision of whether or not to have more children is the choice of the parents.

PSYCHOLOGICAL ADJUSTMENT

Much has been written about parental reactions to the child with a defect and adjustment processes. The operational approach for dealing with parents of a mentally retarded child developed by Olshansky is noteworthy because of its applicability to children with all types of birth defects and its emphasis on long-term care (Olshansky, 1962). He suggests that "chronic sorrow" on the part of parents is a reasonable reaction to having a child with a birth defect, and he urges recognition of the family's need for constructive assistance at various stages of the child's life. Much of the genetic counselor's efforts must be directed toward relieving anxiety and aiding parents to express their feelings. Genetic counseling may, therefore, take several sessions.

> A young couple were referred to a genetic clinic because of Apert's syndrome (bilateral syndactyly, craniostenosis) in their 6-month-old son. In view of a negative family history, the child's condition occurred as a result of a spontaneous change in a gene at the time of conception and their risk for subsequent offspring having the same disorder would be negligible. The mother expressed feelings of guilt and anxiety about why it happened and expressed thoughts regarding difficulty in becoming pregnant and its relationship to the child's disability. Parental concerns were also directed toward whether or not there would be any possibility of mental retardation, future function of the child's hands, limitation of motor skills and possible other physical defects that might occur (e.g., eye and speech abnormalities).
>
> Over a period of approximately 6 months, both parents became increasingly more comfortable in caring for and handling their child. The parents had

decided to limit further reproduction until the child was older. This was decided in view of their financial situation, future surgical procedures, and previous pregnancy history.

FAMILY FOLLOW-UP

Multiple visits with parents help reinforce their understanding of the information given and correct any misinterpretations and apprehensions resulting from such. Not infrequently, follow-up sessions reveal that understanding of the genetic information has been modified. Certainly a significant portion of this is due to the psychological distress and disorientation individuals may experience at the time of counseling. The provision of advice in counseling, from the perspective of the client, includes not only the acquisition of knowledge, but also necessitates adjustment and appropriate utilization of this knowledge over time.

The counselor must also be knowledgeable about community resources for treatment and for financial assistance.

The counselor must also consider who else in the family may be at risk for development of the disorder, or of having a child with the defect in question. Genetic counseling should be available to other family members who may be at high risk for certain conditions.

All information given should be recorded and letters sent to both the physician(s) who referred the patient and to the parents for future reference.

A 70-year-old man was admitted because of persistent bleeding following a prostactectomy requiring 50 units of blood. He was found to be a hemophiliac never previously diagnosed, mild enough not to bleed spontaneously, but severe enough to bleed excessively with surgery. Through him the diagnosis was made in seven male descendants and suspected in nine others. These relatives may now avoid excessive bleeding during surgery by forewarning their surgeons of their diagnosis.

THE TEAM APPROACH

The rapid advances in knowledge of human genetics and of human hereditary disease have provided the opportunity for new services to families with birth defects. The most important service is comprehensive genetic counseling. Genetic counseling can best be provided by a team of health professionals. This includes medical geneticists, nurses, medical social workers, genetic associates, and biomedical scientists. The extent of each member's responsibilities is determined by mutual agreement among the members (McKusick, 1975).

Since accurate diagnosis is a prerequisite for genetic counseling, a medical geneticist with clinical experience is essential. The role of the medical geneticist most often includes diagnosis, consultation, counseling, and education. It may also be necessary for the physician to obtain diagnostic expertise from medical specialists in other fields.

A nurse clinician with additional preparation in medical genetics assumes a collaborative role in the provision of genetic services. Responsibilities may include history taking and data collection, follow-up, supportive counseling, community and hospital consultation, education, case finding, and liaison with health practitioners. The role of the medical social worker may include management of social and financial problems of the family and assistance with implementation of local health resources. The role of the genetic associate is currently being explored in various genetic counseling centers around the country. These individuals can effectively act as the interface between medical geneticists and the patient population, in regards to enhancing communication and assisting patients and families in dealing with their problems (Fraser, 1974).

USEFUL SOURCE BOOKS

In view of the rapid growth in understanding the role of hereditary factors in the etiology of disease, health care providers may wish to become familiar with a few useful references. Several of the most helpful guides include: McKusick, *Mendelian Inheritance in Man* (1975); Smith, *Recognizable Patterns of Human Malformation* (1976); and Bergsma, *Birth Defects Atlas and Compendium* (1973). In addition, the National Foundation–March of Dimes has published an *International Directory* (Lynch, Guirgis, Bergsma, 1977) indicating where families may be referred for specialized diagnostic studies and genetic services.

CONCLUSION

Genetic counseling has been defined, its various genetic, medical, and psychosocial aspects discussed, and its importance for family health care emphasized. In view of the increasing interest in and demand for genetic counseling by large segments of the population as well as the complex psychological and social aspects of hereditary disease, an interdisciplinary team approach is suggested as the most effective method to deliver genetic health services.

REFERENCES

Bergsma, D. *Birth defects atlas and compendium*. National Foundation-March of Dimes, Baltimore: Williams and Wilkins, 1973.

Clow, C. L., Fraser, F. C., LaBerge, C., & Scriver, C. On the application of knowledge to the patient with genetic disease. *Progress in Medical Genetics*, 1973, *9*, 159–213.

Fraser, F. C. Genetic counseling. *American Journal of Human Genetics*, 1974, *26*, 636–659.

———. Genetics as a health-care service. *New England Journal of Medicine*, 1976, *259* (9), 486–488.

Leonard, C., Chase, G. A., & Childs, B. Genetic counseling: A consumer's view. *New England Journal of Medicine*, 1972, *287* (9), 433–439.

Lynch, H., Guirgis, H., Bergsma, D. (Eds.), *International directory of genetic services* (5th ed.). National Foundation-March of Dimes, May, 1977.

McKusick, V. Genetic counseling. *American Journal of Human Genetics*, 1975, *27*, 240–242.

———. *Mendelian inheritance in man* (4th ed.). Baltimore: Johns Hopkins University Press, 1975.

Milunsky, A. *The prevention of genetic disease and mental retardation*. Philadelphia: W. B. Saunders, 1975.

Motulsky, A. G., & Hecht, F. Genetic prognosis and counseling. *American Journal of Obstetrics-Gynecology*, 1964, *90* (7), 1227–1241.

NICHD National Registry for Amniocentesis Study Group. Midtrimester amniocentesis for prenatal diagnosis. *Journal of American Medical Association*, 1976, *236*(13), 1471–1476.

Olshansky, S. Chronic sorrow: A response to having a mentally defective child. *Social Casework*, 1962, *43*, 192.

Smith, D. W. *Recognizable patterns of human malformation*. Philadelphia: W. B. Saunders, 1976.

Thomas, G., & Scott, C. Laboratory diagnosis of genetic disorders. *Pediatric Clinics of North America*, 1973, *20*(1), 105–119.

What are the facts about genetic disease? National Institute of General Medical Sciences, National Institutes of Health, DHEW Publication, No. (NIH 74-370).

CHAPTER TWENTY-THREE

SEXUALITY, EDUCATION, AND THE FAMILY

NANCY L. DIEKELMAN AND MELINDA M. SWENSON

The concept of anticipatory guidance is very important to nurses in providing for the sexuality education needs of the family. It is not sufficient for the nurse merely to know normal sexual development of children and adults; nurses must also be aware of sexual development as it is expressed in the activities and behaviors associated with daily living in a variety of settings and life-styles. This chapter focuses on how the nurse can use these events in providing anticipatory guidance to the family to facilitate coping with the complexities of human sexual behavior.

CHILDHOOD SEXUALITY

Sexual activities are quite normal and natural, and if parents do not make an issue of sex, children will probably develop into normal, sexually healthy adults. Parents can be encouraged to touch their children as much as they wish. Much of the touching, patting, rubbing, or even cleansing may evoke sexual response in the child, but this is a normal part of the child's development.

Infancy

> As a mother is undressing her 6-month-old son, the nurse notices that the child, smiling and happy, has an erection and is trying to touch his penis with his hands. The mother is obviously embarrassed. "I never know what I ought to do when Kevin does that."

A situation like this is an excellent opportunity for the nurse to discuss normal childhood sexuality. Like Kevin's mother, parents are often uncertain how to react to infant genital play. They want their children to grow up as heterosexuals, get married, and have children of their own; but they may also feel that children should not perform any sexual act prematurely.

Most infants manifest some type of genital play during their first year. Masturbation, the deliberate self-stimulation that leads to sexual arousal, is often performed by infants and young children. Masturbation in children can create a state of relaxation and satisfaction comparable to the postorgasmic state. Children usually stimulate their genitals manually, although some use a rhythmic movement of the buttocks while lying face down with their genitals pressed against an object like a blanket or a toy (Reevey, 1973, p. 150).

Some parents may fear that allowing infants to masturbate encourages them to enjoy self-stimulating experiences, perhaps with the result that as adults they will not develop heterosexual relationships and will instead become compulsive masturbators. This fear is not well founded. "It is an error to assume that the meanings given to an activity early in life have any simple or direct connection with what the activity will mean in the future" (Gagnon, 1977, p. 81). Adult sex activity depends upon a whole sequence of experiences. The nurse's role is to be nonjudgmental and informative; to help the parents understand the theories of sexuality and human development so that they will be in a sound position to make their decisions.

Toddler

In our society, direct manipulation of the genitalia is discouraged, and the toddler begins to learn how to channel sexual impulses into socially acceptable ways. Sensual-erotic activities include kissing and hugging family members, friends, and toys, as well as such rhythmic motor activities as riding a toy horse or swinging (Martinson, 1973, p. 143).

During the time between 18 months and 3 years, the issue of gender identity is of great importance. This is the child's psychological sense of "I am male" or "I am female," and we have come to realize today that it is a much more complex affair than the hard-and-fast birth announcements "It's a boy" or It's a girl." Gender identity, the first step in gender development, is pretty well established by age 3 (Money, 1975, p. 121).

There are several theories of gender development. Freud felt gender was developed by biology, cognition, and social learning, and influenced by specific differences such as those of anatomy. In addition, he felt that there were stages of development that influenced how the mother and others related to the child, and thus with whom the child identified. A second view is that men and women, fundamentally different as a function of biology, function with a clear-cut division of labor: men hunt, women gather food, and bear and care for children; men are aggressive and dominant, women passive and submissive (Katchadourian and Lunde, 1972, p.188). According to this theory, as opposed to Freud's, if men and women were raised under identical circumstances they would differ as adults, because even before birth each embryo possesses a mechanism determining whether it is male or female. A third, and more generally held view maintains that gender development is determined by social learning and the continuous construction and maintenance of gender role throughout the life cycle. By watching others, the child will continue to develop and learn what gender means, and with this view the environment is very important (Janis, Mahl, Kagan, and Holt, 1969).

Formerly, little boys were told, "Don't cry; boys don't cry"; and little girls were encourgaged to "Be like a little lady." Many obvious social changes reflect our increasing realization today that men have no monopoly on bravery and women have no monopoly on sensitivity and understanding. We are much more aware of the influence that toys and children's books and television have on children's gender development. In today's children's books, the boy may play with dolls and the girl may climb a tree. However, the changes are still, perhaps, not quite evenly balanced. Many parents who are glad to have their daughter play in Little League are not quite so happy to have their son take ballet lessons.

Moreover, relatives and friends may pose a problem. A grandfather may be so delighted that his first grandchild is a male that he is no sooner in the door than he starts saying, "Where's our football player?" rather to the distress of the parents who see no particular signs of athletic prowess in their little boy. Visitors will tell parents, "Your kid will be a great athlete," or "Your little girl will be a real princess."

The nurse, through problem solving and providing anticipatory guidance, can help the parents see how subtle and complex a process gender development is, and how various and numerous are the facets in the child's environment that can influence it, and thus help them to make intelligent decisions.

Preschooler

Some time between the ages of 3 and 5 years, the child can be expected to exhibit some oedipal or related gender-identifying behavior. Little girls enjoy having a curler in their hair like Mommy or carrying a purse like Mrs. Smith next door. Little boys may insist on helping Dad mow the lawn.

This early identification with the parents of the same sex is reinforced in many ways. While toddlers, boys and girls may be dressed alike in overalls; for preschoolers pants and dresses begin to appear. The identification may lead to identifying with the same parent love object: "I want to be just like Mommy. Mommy loves Daddy, I love Daddy." It is not uncommon for identification to lead to favoritism with the parent of the opposite sex. It is thought "cute" for the child to be "Mommy's little boy" or "Daddy's little girl." But this tends to be a passing phase, and before long the child reidentifies with the parent of the same sex.

> We're really having a bad time with Amy. She wouldn't do anything for me, but will do anything for Gary, so he puts her to bed, and gets her to pick up her toys. But when he tries to talk to me and tell me how his day went, she's a real pest; she won't let me get a word in edgewise. I sure don't know now to handle the situation.

The nurse with a knowledge of normal growth and development can reassure parents going through the experience for the first time. "What should I say if my child says, 'I'm going to marry Mommy when I grow up?' or 'You sleep in my bed tonight and I'll sleep with Daddy?'" "Will it be bad for our child if he or she sees us having intercourse?" The nurse might respond to an anxious parent like this: "There is no real proof that seeing parents having intercourse is harmful to the child. What really is important is how the parent-child relationship affects and interprets the experience. It should be a truthful explanation, however. Perhaps that Mommy and Daddy are loving each other very much and this is one way they can get very close to one another. This is a special way for grownups to love each other." The nurse should not wait for questions of this sort to be brought up, but should assume that the area is of interest to parents, unless parents indicate that this is not an area of concern for them.

Preschool children may also ask questions about pregnancy, and the nurse can help parents in trying to find the right way to answer them. For a child so young, it is often hard to decide how full answers should be. The context in which the question occurs is very important, for it gives an indication as to just what is on the child's mind, and will often furnish the key to the response.

School-Ager

At this time, children actively develop same-sex peer relationships, and have special educational needs related to sexuality. School, teachers, and peers become very important.

Sex play, both same-gender and cross-gender, is common at this age. It may be playing "doctor and nurse," or showing each other the genitals. The play, and not the sex, is probably more important to the child. Children are active and inquisitive, and they may not be erotically aroused by seeing another child's genitals, merely curious.

Preadolescent

In this period, ages 11 to 13, because of conspicuous body changes, most children are very much interested in one another's bodies. The physical changes are very important in their lives, for these are often directly linked to social interaction. For example, height and weight may determine success in sports; breast development may increase a girl's desirability in dating.

These physical changes may or may not be accompanied by social or intellectual changes. Some parents assume that physical changes automatically herald maturity, but this is a fallacy. A child may be physically immature and socially mature, or vice versa. The nurse, therefore, should assess all areas of development, and take great care in determining sex-education needs. Children can be very sensitive as to whether they are developing at the same rate as their peers. Girls may even compete to see who menstruates first. The preadolescent may be knowledgeable factually, but emotionally too immature to discuss implications of the information possessed.

In the area of sexuality, peer learning is very important at this age. In studies going back as far as 1917 (Gagnon, 1977, p. 81), 90 percent of both adults and young people reported they obtained information on sexuality "from friends." This applies regardless of social class, race, religion, or even sex-education courses in schools. Children learn about sex mainly by talking with their friends, for these discussions are immediate, open, and real. Technically, of course, much of this information is inaccurate.

While it is recognized that no time is the "best time" to teach sexuality and that when the child is interested and ready is the best time, certain content areas are best taught at specific times.

Schools and parents face the problem of when to teach the child about sexuality, what and how to teach, and who should do the teaching.

What and how? This is a difficult problem. We tend to focus on the physiology and the facts of sexuality, but what is often not taught, and what the child is often very much interested in, is how sexuality feels, what the consequences are, what people can and can't do. Preadolescent children are often treated as asexual, but this is a mistake. They need this information before puberty.

The nurse should offer information on menstruation, sexually transmitted diseases (especially gonorrhea and syphilis), masturbation, and human reproduction. Since nocturnal emissions ("wet dreams") may also occur during this stage of sexual development, the normal physiological changes of both male and female reproductive systems should be explained in detail to both boys and girls. At this period, before the greater emotional maturity of the adolescent, sex education should focus first of all on providing facts, then on the opportunity to discuss the difficult areas of values and judgments, and finally, of course, on the opportunity to ask any questions.

When? From ages 10 to 13 is the optimal time. Earlier than this, children often forget what they are told. Many schools begin sex education at age 14; but this is too late. By this time many children have already had an abortion or other sexual experiences.

Who? Anyone is is prepared to discuss sexual issues in an interested, nonjudgmental, caring way. It is not automatically the parents or gym teacher; it could be an aunt or uncle, an intimate neighbor, or the school nurse.

ADOLESCENT

> Barb is pregnant at 16, and still attending classes in her third trimester. The school nurse joins in conversation with two of Barb's friends, whose views of pregnancy and motherhood are rather romanticized: "How beautiful Barbara looks!" "What a good mother she will make!" The nurse—not by authoritarian statements, but rather by careful questioning—attempts to help them reach a more realistic view. How must it actually "feel" to be pregnant? What qualities do you really need to be a good mother—for instance, when the baby wakes you up by crying in the middle of the night?

During adolescence, the heterosexual activities associated with dating are very important, and this is an excellent time to discuss the implications and responsibilities of various sexual behaviors. This is a very difficult topic to discuss, since there are great differences in family points of view, but it should not be neglected because of its difficulty. Of the 21 million 15- to 19-year-olds in the United States, an estimated 11 million have had sexual intercourse. The consequences of this sexual activity include adolescent pregnancy and an increase in sexually transmitted diseases (Guttmacher, 1976, p. 9). The nurse can assess the adolescent's understanding of contraception and venereal disease and deal with any existing myths. For example, many teens share the dangerous belief that unprotected intercourse during or right after menstruation presents the greatest risk of resulting pregnancy. The nurse has a responsibility to contribute to helping the adolescent make responsible decisions on the basis of consequences that may follow certain behaviors. This is often a period of conflict between parent and child in our culture, and the nurse should try to keep the lines of communication open, and help each side consider the other's point of view.

In our culture, adolescence is typically a time when all authority figures are threatening and challenged, and the nurse should be careful not to become one, which would automatically jeopardize credibility. Above all, the nurse must be honest, must give information in a nonjudgmental way, must be supportive, must provide confidentiality. In this way, the nurse can give inestimable help to adolescents taking the difficult leap into adulthood.

ADULT SEXUALITY

The Young Adult

Although there is more premarital sexual experience today than formerly (Gagnon, 1977, p. 198), many couples come to marriage with little factual knowledge of their own or their partner's sexuality. Some are informed by reading, and some intuitively respond and communicate; but many are unprepared. Unfortunately, for some the only source of information about human sexuality is the magazine rack and talk with friends in the bar or locker room. But sexuality is far too important in a marriage to ignore.

> When Tom and Chita came to the clinic for a premarital exam, both were sexually inexperienced but anxious for a fulfilling marriage. Since the nurse sensed they were open and comfortable together, the nurse and physician performed both physical exams together. During the breast exam the nurse showed both how normal breast tissue felt. During the male genitalia exam, the physician explained erection and the male sexual response cycle. During the pelvic exam, a mirror was used to show the external female genitalia, particularly the clitoris. Patience and communication were encouraged. Contraception was discussed, and they decided to use foam and condom, which allowed them to share responsibility. When they left after a 90-minute visit, they had learned not only about their own bodies, but also about each other as well. Their marriage was off to a good start.

Sexual response The external manifestations of response to sexual stimulation are obviously different for males and females, but the underlying physiological responses are similar and best understood when compared. Regardless of the source of stimulation (which may be by manual or mechanical masturbation, intercourse, visual or auditory stimulation, or fantasy), the responses are the same. The experience of orgasm, however, differs from person to person, and there is no "right" or "wrong" way to feel. (For a more detailed description of the response cycle, see Masters and Johnson, 1966.)

The nurse may be asked, "Just what does happen during intercourse?" The knowledgeable practitioner, who has studied the sexual response cycle, can explain it to clients in terms the client can comprehend. A good way to start is with technical terms the nurse is most familiar with, then assess the level of understanding of the client and modify or negotiate a mutually comprehensible, nonthreatening terminology. The nurse must become desensitized to "street language" and the use of childhood vocabulary, such as "wee-wee" or similar phrases.

Female clients need to know that their sexual feelings are acceptable and healthy. Many women are not at all aware of their external genital anatomy. The nurse, using illustrations, can give the woman permission to use a mirror to examine her various external structures. Many nurses and physicians are using the mirror technique during the pelvic exam to instruct clients.

Many women have questions about reaching orgasm, largely due to the attention paid this phenomenon by the popular literature. Nurses can explain that women experience orgasm in different ways and that it is largely a learned response to pleasurable stimulation. Several books (e.g., Barbach, 1975) are currently available to assist women to help themselves to reach orgasm. It is important that clients, both male and female, understand that orgasm in the female is clitoral in origin, and can be achieved through intercourse, through self-masturbation, partner masturbation, breast stimulation and, for a few women, fantasy.

Male clients may have questions regarding erection and ejaculation. Many men also worry needlessly that their penis is abnormally small and therefore could not possibly satisfy a woman. Research reported by McCary (1973, p. 66) shows that there is no correlation between the length of a flaccid penis and the length of the same penis when erect. Most erect penises are nearly the same size.

Another common problem is painful intercourse (dyspareunia). This may result from inadequate foreplay prior to intercourse. Vaginal lubrication in the sexually aroused female usually is sufficient for intercourse, but some couples find that additional lubrication is beneficial. The nurse should urge use of a water-soluble lubricant such as K-Y Jelly. Petroleum jelly, though commonly used, is a poor choice because it feels greasy and is "unwettable" (Comfort, 1972, p. 132). Petroleum jelly may also lead to vaginal infections and is reputed to deteriorate the rubber in diaphragms (Boston Women's Health Book Collective, 1976, p. 58).

Sexual behavior Clients often have questions about what is "normal" sexual behavior. The nurse must be aware of a personal value system and should not let this intrude upon the client.

> Shortly after their marriage, Chita came to the clinic reporting that she and Tom were very happy. The nurse discovered, however, that Chita was rather worried about Tom's recent suggestion that they try oral-genital sex. While not trying to force her decision, the nurse indicated that this was a healthy and acceptable form of sexual expression, that vaginal odors are normal, requiring no hygiene beyond a daily bath, that some couples found the experience rewarding, others not, and choice was an individual matter.

Almost any sexual activity is normal and permissible to long as the participants are informed, consenting adults and no coercion is involved.

Autosexuality (self-pleasuring, masturbation) is normal and healthy. Homosexuality is normal and healthy for the person who prefers relationships with a same-sex partner. Heterosexuality is normal and healthy for those who are most comfortable with this pattern. Bisexuality is normal and healthy for the person who enjoys sex with both men and women. Celibacy (abstinence from sex) is normal and healthy for some people.

Sexual practices vary from person to person. There is no evidence to suggest that oral-genital sex, use of a vibrator, anal sex, or any type of fantasy or daydream is dangerous in any way. (Delora and Warren, 1977, p. 63). So long as the client enjoys the activity and is not coerced into it, the activity is probably healthy and acceptable.

Sexually transmitted diseases Since the term "venereal disease" is derived from the name of Venus, goddess of love, and transfer of these conditions often does not involve love at all, "sexually transmitted diseases" is a more precise term and will be used here.

A major epidemic of gonorrhea is currently occurring in the United States, and its incidence is much higher than that of syphilis, though the latter remains a major problem (Catterall, 1974, p. 14). Recently herpes simplex virus type II (herpes genitalis) has increased to, or above, the incidence of gonorrhea. Other diseases commonly transmitted by sexual contact are monilia and trichomonas infections, condylomatoa accriminata (genital warts), *phthirius pubis* (crab lice), and scabies. Table 23-1 summarizes information regarding these conditions.

Education about sexually transmitted diseases should begin whenever sexual activity begins; probably in the junior high school years. Information should be made available concerning how diseases are spread, what the symptoms and treatment are, and where to get examined and treated. The information should be factual, nonthreatening, and nonjudgmental. The examination and treatment should be confidential and affordable (or free).

Myths and fallacies abound regarding sexually transmitted diseases. Gonorrhea and syphilis often are confused, and many people erroneously believe themselves cured when symptoms disappear. Women may try home remedies for vaginal infections or borrow medications from a friend that may temporarily relieve the symptoms but that also lead to the development of resistance in the strain of bacteria involved.

The social stigma attached to any genital infection is still very strong, since having a sexually transmitted disease may mean the admission of sexuality. The embarrassment and shame felt by some clients is acute.

Table 23-1 Summary of sexually transmitted diseases

Condition	Etiology	Diagnosis	Incubation	Symptoms	Complications	Treatment
Candida (yeast infection, monilia)	*Candida albicans* (a fungus)	Gram-stain smear culture		Vaginal discharge, vulval irritation. Discharge is thick, white, cheesy. Frequently itches. May also be asymptomatic. Males may notice itching, soreness of penis.	Underlying conditions include diabetes, pregnancy. Oral contraceptives may increase incidence.	Nystatin per vaginal cream or suppository Triple sulfa Vinegar douche: 1 to 2 tbsp white vinegar in 1 qt warm water
Trichomoniasis	*Trichomonas vaginalis* (a parasite)	Identification of flagellated organism on wet prep slide	4 to 28 days	Vaginal discharge. May be greenish-yellow, frothy, itchy, Dysuria, dyspareunia. Males may be asymptomatic carriers.	Urethritis, cystitis.	Metronidazole (Flagyl) 2 g PO over 1 day period
Condylomatoa acuminatum (genital warts)	Virus	By appearance (firm polyplike growth)		Painful. Look like small "mushrooms," or "cauliflower."	Easily spread by autoinoculation. Transmitted to sexual partners. Spread extensively during pregnancy.	Soap and water. Topical application of 10 or 25% solution of podophyllin in alcohol

Condition	Etiology	Diagnosis	Incubation	Symptoms	Complications	Treatment
Gonorrhea	*Neisseria gonorrhea* Site of infection: urethral, cervix, eyes, rectal area, throat	Gram-positive diplococci (smear; good for males only). Positive culture (for both males and females)	Approximately 1 week	*Male:* Discharge, dysuria. N.B.: 10 percent of males may be asymptomatic. *Female:* Mostly are asymptomatic; may have greenish vaginal discharge.	Ascending infection may lead to pelvic inflammatory disease in females (PID) with possible sterility. Males may also be sterile as a result of ascending infection. Systemic involvement includes joints, septicemia.	1 g probenecid PO 4.8 million units procaine penicillin IM [For allergic patients, may use spectinomycin IM or 9 g tetracycline (total, over 4 days)] Repeat cultures 2 times after treatment (at weekly intervals)
Syphilis	*Treponema pallidum*	VDRL and FTA (blood screening tests). Dark-field smear to look for spirochetes.	9 to 90 days	*Primary:* Lesion is rounded, clean indurated, usually is painless; may be anyplace on skin. Heals in 4 to 12 weeks. *Secondary:* Rash, especially on palms and soles, May itch. Looks like many other conditions. Rash contagious. *Tertiary:* Systemic, involves heart, nervous system.	Brain, cardiac involvement. Congenital syphilis.	Always sensitive to penicillin or tetracycline—never too late to treat. 2.4 million units benzathine penicillin IM

Table 23-1 Summary of sexually transmitted diseases (*continued*)

Condition	Etiology	Diagnosis	Incubation	Symptoms	Complications	Treatment
Herpes genitalis	Herpes simplex virus, type II	By observation of lesion; by history		*Female:* Itching, discomfort. Lesion may be a lump or a blister. Lymph nodes enlarged. Fever. *Males:* Lesion at first blistered, then are eroded leaving multiple superficial erosions.	Acute pain. Danger to newborn if mother has genital herpes.	Sitz baths, pain medication, local application of ether.
Crabs (pediculosis pubis)	*Phthirius pubis* (crab louse)	By observation of lice and/or nits		Intense itching in pubic region.	Excoriation from itching.	Kwell shampoo in two applications.
Scabies	*Sarcoptes scabiei*	By observation		Lesions are usually papular. Burrows are grayish or black irregular lines on the skin. Itching is usually worse at night, or when patient is warm.	Excoriation.	Kwell lotion after bath. Repeat in 1 week.

Sources: R. D. Catterall, *A Short Textbook of Venerology*, Philadelphia, J. B. Lippincott, 1974; Boston Women's Health Book Collective, *Our Bodies, Ourselves*, New York, Simon & Schuster, 1976.

The health professional must be accepting and nonjudgmental while providing initial care and follow-up.

A commonly held myth is that the odor of female genitalia is unpleasant, and discharge is abnormal. In fact, so long as daily bathing takes place, the female genital odor is natural and pleasant. All women experience vaginal discharge, which varies in consistency and amount with the menstrual cycle. The discharge is usually clear to whitish, and has no unpleasant smell. Some women feel that bathing is insufficient, and they douche unnecessarily often. Madison Avenue advertising has convinced many that they are not clean without perfumed douching or the use of "feminine hygiene deodorant spray." Actually, many women are allergic to such products, which may cause serious harm to the genital mucous tissue. No deodorizing is necessary when no disease is present. If the discharge becomes profuse, smelly, or itchy, medical treatment should be sought.

Occasionally in women with chronic vaginal infections (diabetics or women taking oral contraceptives), a douche can be used just before and/or just after the menstrual period to control the vaginal pH and thus the yeast infection. In these cases the nurse should advise using the hanging-bag type rather than the bulb syringe. The douche may be prepared using 1 quart of warm water containing 2 tablespoons of white table vinegar.

Another myth is that a pap smear is not necessary before sexual activity occurs or after a hysterectomy. This technique for the diagnosis of cervical cancer has been invaluable, allowing many cases to be found early enough for complete cure (Boston Women's Health Book Collective, 1976, p. 144). Since cervical cancer has been found in virgins, the yearly pap smear should be routinely recommended to all women over 18, regardless of sexual activity, and to all sexually active teen-agers regardless of age. It is also useful in diagnosing vaginal cancer even if the cervix has been removed by hysterectomy, so certainly these postoperative women should not be excluded from screening.

The Middle Adult

In the years from 30 to 45, social, familial, psychological, and physiological changes occur in both men and women that may affect sexuality. Aging causes changes in the body image, and fewer sexual options are available.

There are indications that women reach their peak in sexual drive about age 35. Men peak much earlier, usually in late adolescence or early manhood (Sheehy, 1976, p. 308). This difference in timing is sometimes the cause of sexual incompatibility in the middle years for couples formerly well matched.

> Frank and Helen, aged 33 and 34 respectively, have been happily married for 15 years, with mutually satisfying intercourse. Helen tells the nurse that Frank now is so busy at the office that he is too tired to make love when he comes home, and she wants more sex. She is not interested in any other man.

The nurse can first explain the difference in sexual interest at this time, and then suggest the possibility of self-pleasuring, that is, masturbation. In the normal course of events, the discrepancy may be temporary, and this might be an acceptable solution to help Helen through this particular time.

It now appears that both men and women experience a menopause that marks a change in their sexual and reproductive lives. Much more information is available on female menopause, although myths and fallacies regarding the "change of life" persist (Weideger, 1976). Some women, from the experiences of their mothers and grandmothers, approach the menopause with great fears of loss of femininity, loss of physical attractiveness, and loss of interest in sex. They anticipate nervousness, depression, and other irreversible psychological problems. In fact, however, only about 10 percent of menopausal women experience symptoms other than cessation of the monthly period. The most common symptoms are vasomotor: "hot flashes" and a reduction of pelvic congestion causing a lessening in vaginal lubrication. Estrogen deficiency also causes the vaginal musculature to atrophy and the vaginal walls to become more fragile (Armbrecht and Futterman, 1977, p. 174).

> Mrs. Nelson has had no particular dread of the menopause. She and her husband have been using the rhythm method of conception control successfully; their last child is now 10, and they do not wish to have any more. When Mrs. Nelson stops having her "monthlies," she thinks, she will no longer need to worry about pregnancy. But when the periods become irregular, it becomes difficult for her to predict her "safe time." When she has missed several periods and goes to her doctor for what she considers "the change of life," he tells her she is three months pregnant.

Many women are not aware of their reproductive capacity during the pre- and intramenopausal periods. The true definition of menopause is twelve consecutive missed periods—no menstruation for a year. Until then, a woman cannot be sure of inability to conceive.

In its current state of development, rhythm is a risky method of conception control. During the pre- and intramenopausal period, it becomes even less reliable. At the same time, as a woman passes the age of 40, the chances of producing a defective child are considerably increased (Luker, 1975, p. 99; Milunsky et al., 1970). Before the menopause, the nurse should provide women with accurate and specific information about contraception and the risks of pregnancy.

The Older Adult

The stress in our society placed on youth and beauty might seem to preclude sexuality in the elderly. But research shows that although the sexual response cycle may slow down for some aging people, it does not stop. Though other factors may affect libido or energy levels, there is no physiological reason why older adults should curtail their sexual activity.

In the aging female, lubrication may occur more slowly and the amount may decrease. Reduction in estrogen levels after menopause may cause a thinning of the vaginal walls and may decrease the size of the clitoris. Topical vaginal estrogen cream is the best solution to these problems, since there is reason to believe that systemic estrogen replacement increases the woman's risk for the development of uterine cancer (*Menopause and Aging*, 1971, p. 4).

Sexual response is essentially the same for an older as a younger woman, though the phases may be shorter. During orgasm, contractions of the uterus may cause some momentary pain, which indicates that the estrogen level is low. The genital area disengorges rapidly after orgasm, but the woman can still achieve one or more additional orgasms if that has been her pattern in the past. "A woman who has regular sexual opportunity tends to maintain her sexual responsiveness; without such opportunity, sexuality declines markedly" (Kaplan, 1974, p. 112).

In the male, erection takes longer to achieve and may be less firm, but once achieved, the erection can be maintained longer than in a younger man. There is increased need for direct genital stimulation, either by the man himself or by his partner. The secretion of the Cowper's gland decreases, creating the need for additional lubrication.

Many men are pleased by an enhanced ability to maintain erection before ejaculation that comes with aging. This phenomenon enables the older man to engage in foreplay and intercourse for a relatively longer time before orgasm. During orgasm, ejaculation may have decreased force and volume, and disengorgement is rapid. For the aging male the period before another ejaculation is possible may be much longer, ranging from an hour or two to several days.

For both elderly men and women, it is important to understand that regularity of sexual release is the most significant factor in the maintenance of sexual response capacity. "If you don't use it, you'll lose it." Nurses can encourage satisfying sexual behavior in elderly clients by continuing to discuss sexual concerns, by helping discussion of feelings and needs between sexual partners, and by explaining to younger family members the normality of maintaining a sexual relationship during old age.

MEDICATION EFFECTS

Medications are clearly the concern of the nurse, either in the hospital or in the home setting. Nurses spend hours of preparation learning side effects of drugs, yet we rarely consider sexual side effects of the medications taken by clients. The belief that clients should be fully informed of the consequences of medical treatment carries with it the responsibility to teach clients and families the sexual side effects of drugs. If a drug increases or decreases sexual interest or affects sexual response capability, the nurse should be able to provide anticipatory guidance to clients in this

Table 23-2 Drug effects on human sexual behavior

Drug or drug category	Effect on sexual response and libido
1. Oral contraceptives (estrogen)	Questionable
2. Antihypertensives	Negative
3. Antidepressants	Negative
4. Antihistamines	Negative
5. Antispasmodics	Negative
6. Sedatives and tranquilizers	Negative
7. Ethyl alcohol	Transiently positive, then negative
8. Narcotics	Transiently positive, then negative
9. L-Dopa	Positive
10. Amyl nitrate	Questionable
11. Adrenal steroids	Negative
12. Amphetamines	Positive
13. Hallucinogens	Questionable
14. Androgen	Positive
15. Vincristine can cause neuropathy and subsequent impotence.	
16. Cytoxin can cause hematuria.	

Sources: N. F. Woods: *Human Sexuality in Health and Illness,* St. Louis, C. V. Mosby, 1975; H. S. Kaplan: *The New Sex Therapy,* New York, Brunner/Mazel, 1974.

regard. The summary in Table 23-2 can serve as a reminder to the nurse about the most commonly used drugs that affect human sexual response. For more information about pharmocologic action, the reader should consult Kaplan (1974).

SUMMING UP

The evaluation of genital health is frequently overlooked by nurses, either because of embarrassment or ignorance. Because we often fail to introduce the subject, clients infer it is taboo and not to be discussed.

It is safe to say, however, that all human beings have sexual concerns. Ideally, nurses should be comfortable with their own sexuality and value systems, and possess skill in nonjudgmental phrasing of questions and answers. We are reliable sources of information and advice. It remains only that we become aware of, and openly acknowledge, the sexuality of our clients.

The easiest way to indicate willingness to discuss genital or sexual concerns is to ask, "What are your questions or concerns about your sexual health or activity?" The client may say none; but the message has been received that the nurse is able and willing to discuss the topic, and sooner or later it may be acted upon. A good opening question for parents is, "What are your questions about your child's sexual health or activity?"

When a client does pose a question, the nurse must be very careful to provide accurate, nonjudgmental information. If nurses are in doubt, it is better to admit it and say they will try to find out. Misinformation is often more damaging to clients than no information. In no field does more popular misinformation and confusion exist; in no field does the nurse have a greater responsibility. The nurse's responsibility is to listen carefully to the concerns of the client, to help the client with terminology, definitions, and cognitive concepts, and to learn about one's own sexuality in order to be comfortable with the sexuality needs of clients.

Effective, perceptive interventions with clients regarding their concerns about sexuality do not happen easily or automatically. Many excellent nurses who have had no formal education in human sexuality manage on intuition alone. However, most nurses, like other people, have difficulty coming to terms with the sexuality of themselves and their clients. Our discomfort, even though covert, is obvious to the people whom we are attempting to assist, and they also become uncomfortable.

Reading is a good beginning, but it rarely is sufficient for building an awareness of sexuality. A few schools of nursing are providing educational experiences for students in the form of courses, workshops, and curriculum integration. Agencies and institutions are beginning to offer in-service education on human sexuality. Students and practitioners alike are urged to take part in these experiences in order to enhance their awareness of the importance of human sexuality in themselves and their clients.

REFERENCES

Alan Guttmacher Institute Publication. *11 million teenagers.* Planned Parenthood Federation of America, 1976.

Ambrecht, C., and Futterman, L. A. Periods of change in the lives of women. In N. A. Lytle (Ed.), *Nursing of women in the age of liberation.* Dubuque, Iowa: William C. Brown, 1977.

Barbach, L. *For yourself: The fulfillment of female sexuality.* New York: Doubleday, 1975.

Boston Women's Health Book Collective. *Our bodies, ourselves.* New York: Simon and Schuster, 1976.

Catterall, R. D. *A short textbook of venereology.* Philadelphia, J. B. Lippincott, 1974.

Comfort, A. *The joy of sex.* New York: Crown Publishers, 1972.

Delora, J. S., & Warren, C. A. B. *Understanding sexual interaction.* Boston: Houghton Mifflin, 1977.

Gadpaille, W. J. *The cycles of sex.* New York: Charles Scribner's Sons, 1975.

Gagnon, J. H. *Human sexualities.* Chicago: Scott, Foresman, 1977.

Gordon, S. *The sexual adolescent.* Belmont, Calif.: Duxbury Press, 1973.

Green, R. *Human sexuality: A health practitioner's text.* Baltimore: Williams and Wilkins, 1975.

Janis, I. L., Mahl, G. F., Kagan, J., & Holt, R. R. *Personality: Dynamics, development, and assessment.* New York: Harcourt Brace Jovanovich, 1969.

Kaplan, H. S. *The new sex therapy.* New York: Brunner/Mazel, 1974.

Katchadourian, H. A., & Lunde, D. T. *Fundamentals of human sexuality.* New York: Holt, Rinehart and Winston, 1972.

Luker, K. *Taking chances: Abortion and the decision not to contracept.* Berkeley, Cal.: University of California Press, 1975.

Martinson, F. M. *Infant and child sexuality.* Privately published, 1973.

Masters, W., & Johnson, V. *Human sexual response.* Boston: Little, Brown, 1966.

McCary, J. L. *Human sexuality.* New York: D. Van Nostrand, 1973.

Menopause and aging, Summary report and selected papers from a research conference on menopause and aging, May 25, 1971, Hot Springs, Arkansas.

Milunsky, A., Littlefield, J. W., Kanfer, J. N., Kolodny, E. H., Shih, V. E., & Atkins, L. *Prenatal genetic diagnosis.* Birth Defects Reprint Series, The National Foundation–March of Dimes, 1970.

Money, J. Sex assignment in anatomically intersexed infants. In R. Green (Ed.), *Human sexuality: A health practitioner's text.* Baltimore: Williams and Wilkins, 1975.

Reevey, W. R. Adolescent sexuality. In A. Ellis and A. Abarbanal (Eds.), *Encyclopedia of sexual behavior*. New York: Jason Aronson, 1973.

Sheehy, G. *Passages—predictable crises of adult life*. New York: E. P. Dutton, 1976.

Weideger, P. *Menstruation and menopause*. New York: Alfred A. Knopf, 1976.

Woods, N. F. *Human sexuality in health and illness*. St. Louis: C. V. Mosby, 1975.

CHAPTER TWENTY-FOUR

BEHAVIORAL PEDIATRICS[1]

EDWARD R. CHRISTOPHERSEN

Behavioral pediatrics is an exciting and fairly recent development in the general area of ambulatory pediatrics. Several recent textbooks have discussed behavioral pediatrics in general terms, supplying a much-needed discussion of and introduction to this area of interest (Kenny and Clemmens, 1975; Friedman, 1975). However, probably one of the few books presently available that provides a practical, problem-oriented approach to the behavior problems frequently manifested by children under the age of four is Spock's *Baby and Child Care* (1976). Owing to the audience to which this book is directed, there are really no guidelines provided for the pediatric clinician to follow.

Friedman (1975) puts behavioral pediatrics within the perspective of general pediatrics with his statement that:

> Behavioral pediatrics maintains the pediatric tradition of emphasizing prevention, with curative and rehabilitative orientation always "second best" to preventing the disease or defect in the first place. Those identified with behavioral pediatrics do not claim expertise in the major psychiatric problems of childhood, but emphasize early intervention and treatment of the less severe problems.

[1]This chapter was adapted, in part, from the book *Little People: Guidelines for Common Sense Child Rearing* by Edward R. Christophersen, Lawrence, Kan.: H & H Enterprises, 1977. Preparation of this manuscript was partially supported by grants (NIMH 26124; NICHD 03144) to the Bureau of Child Research, University of Kansas.

The purpose of the present chapter is to provide the reader with a practical, problem-oriented approach to the prevention of and early detection of behavior problems in families, including suggestions for office management and referral (e.g., Christophersen and Barnard, 1978).

PREVENTION OF BEHAVIOR PROBLEMS

The pediatric clinician can best begin taking the necessary steps to prevent or minimize behavior problems during one or two prenatal office visits. At this time, the clinician can discuss with the parents such things as how the clinician prefers to manage new pediatric patients (immunization schedules, etc.), the mother's choice to breast- or bottle-feed, baby- and child-proofing the home (for safety factors), and, in general, what the new parents can reasonably expect from their baby. The clinician might want to recommend one or two books to the parents (please, never more than two!) that deal with beginning the parenting process (Dudding, 1975). Discussion and reading of this type seems to serve two purposes: It provides the expectant parents with some factual information that can help to reduce anxiety about the forthcoming baby, and it lets the parents know that their clinician acknowledges and understands that there is more to rearing the child than simply meeting physiological needs.

As an integral part of the first and second postnatal visits, the clinician should devote a few minutes to educating the parents about what to expect from their new baby. The parents should be encouraged to develop standard care-giving routines and, within reason, to stick with these routines. For example, it is a good idea to use the same place and the same procedure each time the baby is diapered. This should be a place that is relatively safe for the baby and that has all of the necessary items within easy reach of the care-giver. The reason that establishing a routine is important is twofold. One is that the parent will become proficient more quickly, which in turn will make care-giving less of a chore. The other is that as the baby becomes accustomed to the routine the baby will fuss less during that routine. Crying is one behavior that babies exhibit or engage in a great deal and a behavior that too many professionals tend to underestimate. Most parents, perhaps through instinct, learn to read their baby's signals, and crying is almost always read as a distress signal. Therefore, when a parent has to listen to crying throughout every diaper change, the parents begin to wonder what it is that they are doing wrong, and eventually, through frustration, the parents conclude that their child is just very difficult to take care of. If parents are instructed to use the same routines each time they engage in a care-giving activity, and this results in the baby's crying less, then the parent figures out that they must be doing something right. This notion of using consistent routines was first proposed by Becker and Becker in their book, *Successful Parenthood* (1974). They have an excellent discussion covering a variety of different routines that makes easy, practical reading for new parents.

INFANT CARE-GIVING

There are several simple ideas, in addition to the actual physical acts, involved in taking care of a new baby. One is that parents should be encouraged to talk to the baby while they are taking care of it. By this I mean normal adult speech, not baby talk. Talking to a baby tends to have a soothing effect on the baby, gets the baby used to the mother's and the father's voices, and provides the baby with the first example of how the parent is going to expect the baby to talk many years later. There is no sense in having the majority of speech that is directed to a baby be baby talk. It is not necessary, it is not particularly becoming, and it does not do anything to provide a sound basis for later language development. Along this line, I also recommend that parents begin reading to their child long before the child has any chance of understanding what is being read. This can consist of anything from actually reading children's bedtime stories to reading the evening newspaper out loud. Although the baby does not know the difference, the repetition of adult speech over the first several years can do wonders for the child's own speech.

Another important point to stress to new parents is that they should spend time playing with their new baby. Obviously, this doesn't mean playing catch with the baby—it means encouraging the parents to spend time exploring their new baby. While feeding a baby, the parents should be encouraged to explore the baby's fingers and toes, stroke the hair, simply hold one of the feet, etc. Most parents are fascinated by the intricate detail of their baby's fingers and toes. These gestures, again, have a soothing effect on the baby and also facilitate bonding between parent and baby.

Giving parents suggestions for activities that will be both soothing to the baby and enjoyable to the parents serves one primary function—they make care-giving more enjoyable, and the more enjoyable it is, the more the parents are going to do it—that's just plain human nature. This process, then, tends to have a snowballing effect; the more time parents spend pleasantly interacting with their child, the more pleasant the child will be to interact with.

The most common behavior problem, and one alluded to above, is *crying*. Recent research indicates that young babies spend from 10 to 50 percent of their waking time crying (Quilitch and Risley, 1971; Sostek, Anders, and Sostek, 1976; and Brazelton, 1962). This far exceeds the average parental expectations and leads parents to wonder what they might be doing wrong. In addition to reducing crying during normal care-giving, as described in the preceding section, crying can be reduced at the other two most common times—on wakening and upon being put to bed. When babies first come home from the hospital, they usually go from a sound sleep to a full cry with no transition time whatsoever. One minute they're asleep and the next minute they're crying. There's nothing that can be done to change this, nor would you want to, since this is the only way the baby has, initially, of telling you that he/she is awake and ready to eat. But, after the babies are a month or two old, they do begin to go through a transition phase between sleep and crying. This transition phase is usually indicated by the child gradually awakening and making soft noises and small movements about the crib. Most parents can hear when the baby begins this transition, but, because they don't know any better, the parent just stays in bed until the baby starts to cry. In effect, then, the parent teaches the child that it can wake up, make noises, and move gently about the crib, but if it wants something to eat, then it had better start to cry. What a silly thing to teach a child—particularly when crying gets on parents' nerves the way it does. Instead, instruct your parents to go into the baby's room as soon as they hear that the baby is awake, but *before* the crying starts! In this way, the baby learns (is taught by its parents) that when it wakes up, if it plays quietly for a little while, mommy or daddy will be in to pick it up, change a diaper, and give it something to eat. Using these procedures, most parents can virtually eliminate crying in the morning, and, thus, start the day on a much more pleasant note. After several months of using these procedures, many children will awaken and play in their cribs for 30 to 45 minutes before they begin crying. This allows the parents to get an extra 10 to 20 minutes of sleep and still go in to get baby before the crying starts.

The other common crying time is bedtime. In fact, over the years, crying at bedtime has been the most frequently reported problem. Bedtime problems do not usually start suddenly (with the exception of a child either being sick or just having returned home from being hospitalized—both of which tend to result in increased crying at bedtime). Crying at bedtime begins small and grows ever so gradually until the parent comes in to the clinic to complain about intolerable bedtime crying. The way parents teach their child to cry at bedtime is by putting the child to bed, leaving the room, hearing the child crying, and returning to see what the problem is. Now what problem could have developed? The parent was in the room five minutes earlier and everything was fine. But, the parent goes in anyway, out of legitimate concern, and the teaching process has begun. A week or two after going into the child's room after 5 minutes or so of crying, the parent will decide that the crying is unnecessary and decide to ignore it. Of course, after 15 minutes of crying parents begin to feel guilty about leaving the baby in bed crying, so they go into the bedroom to check on the baby, pick it up and comfort it, and now the baby has learned that it has to cry for at least 15 minutes if it wants to get mom or dad to come back into the room. The obvious solution to preventing this problem from ever occurring is to make sure everything is all right with the baby before putting it to bed, then leave the room, and do not reenter just because the baby cries a little. In this way, the baby learns that when it is placed in the crib, it can cry, play quietly, or just go to sleep (as soon as it is ready), but the parent is not going to come back into the room because of the crying (cf. Williams, 1959; Wright, Woodcock, and Scott, 1970).

These two problem times—waking up and going to bed, when handled properly, can make child-rearing a more enjoyable task, with absolutely no detriment whatsover to the child. In fact, if anything, the baby gains because it learns that the crib is for sleeping and it will probably get a much better night's sleep.

One variation on the bedtime problem that this writer has seen several times recently involves having one of the parents (usually the mother) hold the baby in her arms (sometimes even breast-feeding) until the baby drops off to sleep, at which time the mother tries as skillfully as possible to place the baby into the crib without awakening it. If the baby is awakened, the process begins anew. Parents should be advised that this practice is only going to cause unnecessary problems later on and, thus, is best not started in the first place.

Probably the second most frequent problem that we see in the clinic is mealtime or *feeding problems*. These usually begin at the time when the parents begin to introduce variety into the baby's diet. Usually, as long as the parent just offers (spoon feeds) the white mush (cream of wheat, etc.) the baby accepts it well. But the first time that the parent offers peas or carrots or anything really new, the baby immediately spits it out and the parent concludes that the baby doesn't like peas or carrots. What this teaches the baby, of course, is that it should spit out any new-tasting food and then it will not be offered again. The best procedure to use here is to warn the parent that the baby might spit out foods the first time that they are offered. Suggest that the parent offer, for example, five spoonfuls of cream of wheat, then one of peas (which is spit out), then five of cream of wheat, etc. After five or six spoonfuls of peas, the baby comes to recognize the new taste and, to the parent's amazement, the baby just swallows the peas. As long as the parents are able to get the baby to swallow a reasonable variety of foods, the parents don't need to be concerned over any one food. But, if the parents find that the child comes to exhibit a very strong preference for one or two foods, to the exclusion of everything else, then they have a full-blown mealtime problem that will require a specific intervention program, which is beyond the scope of this chapter.

The clinician who is able to anticipate the parents' needs and is able to offer simple, practical suggestions for minimizing problems generates confidence in the parents while doing so. Heavy intellectual discussions with parents about the "how and why" of children's development cannot and do not take the place of practical advice on child-rearing. Most clinicians do not have the time to do both, so they just offer practical advice and skip the short course on child psychology. An excellent resource book for clinicians is Burton White's *The First Three Years of Life* (1975). This book is practically an encyclopedia detailing the types and ranges of behavior that can be expected to occur during the first 3 years of life. The main reason that I recommend this book for clinicians and not necessarily for parents is that parents have a tendency to read a book like this and become concerned because their child isn't doing what he or she is supposed to at a particular age. This book, when tempered by the experience of a good clinician, can provide an excellent guide in counseling parents.

Before leaving the topic of prevention, there are two additional subject areas that need to be briefly addressed: toilet training and automobile rides. *Toilet training,* if begun before a child is actually ready to be trained, can lead to all kinds of problems, including a really strained relationship between the parents and the child. Probably the major reason that many parents have tried to train their children before the child was ready is that, up to a short time ago, no one had really adequately covered "readiness" for toilet training. Sure, most clinicians would tell parents when they thought that a child was ready to be trained, but unfortunately this advice was usually based entirely on conjecture or personal experience.

The following "readiness" criteria are paraphrased from a recent book by Azrin and Foxx, *Toilet Training in Less Than a Day: How to Do It* (1974). Their four criteria are:

1. Does the child have the manual dexterity to raise and lower his pants by himself? If he doesn't, then he can't be toilet trained.
2. Does the child urinate only a few times a day, completely emptying his bladder or does he still urinate a little bit many times a day? It is much easier to train a child who urinates four times a day than one who urinates seven to ten times.
3. Does the child have sufficient vocabulary to understand the necessary words connected with toilet training? This includes such words as "wet," "dry," "pants," "potty," etc.
4. Does the child understand and follow simple commands like, "Come here, please," "Sit down, please," etc.? This criterion is probably the most important of the four. Many parents think that their child is good at following instructions, but they never ask the child to follow instruc-

tions. The parents do practically everything for the child. This doesn't mean that the child is good at following instructions. If the parents report having problems with temper tantrums, make certain that the parents can manage the tantrums before you suggest that they begin their training efforts.

The rule of thumb that this writer gives to clinicians is that they wait until 3 months after a child meets the four readiness criteria. This provides a safety margin in case the clinician or the parents have overestimated the child's abilities. What this means is that the majority of parents will not be starting to train their child until it is between 24 and 30 months of age. There are no known problems arising from waiting a little too long before training. Besides, some children will train themselves if the parents have waited too long.

After the clinician is confident that a child has met the readiness criteria and has allowed the recommended safety margin of 3 months, the actual method of toilet training is secondary. Many parents seen in the clinic have successfully used some adaptation of the procedures that Azrin and Foxx recommend (if you do suggest these procedures, specifically tell the parents not to expect the training to be complete in one day). However, I think that if parents wait until a child is actually ready to be trained, most of the procedures in the folklore will probably work. Whatever procedures are used, the parents can expect several months to pass before the child is totally accident free.

Automobile rides, for the majority of American families, have become an integral part of their life-style. Much has already been written about the safety aspects of children's car seats or safety restraint seats. In a recent study (Christophersen, 1977a), data were reported that demonstrated that children behave much better on auto trips if they are in a safety car seat. They are much less likely to stand up, hang out of the window, or climb all over the driver. (Of course, it is a little hard to jump around when you're strapped down!) The prevention or reduction of disruptive child behavior during auto rides is an obviously important, but previously unreported, benefit of the use of child restraint seats. This fact might well be used by the pediatric clinician to further encourage or persuade parents to purchase and use child restraint seats. By educating parents in the use of car seats, the clinician can make car rides not only safer, but also much more pleasant.

EARLY DETECTION OF BEHAVIOR PROBLEMS

In addition to counseling parents on how to prevent or minimize behavior problems, the clinician needs to be skilled in assessing the presence of behavior problems as soon as possible in the child's development. The old notion that the clinician could simply ask parents whether or not they are enjoying their child, or what kinds of questions they have, is inadequate. Asking parents if they are having problems with their child is like asking them if their child has otitis media; the shortcoming with doing this is that the clinician is leaving the clinical judgment up to the parents. It would be far better to ask the parents appropriate questions and then have the clinician form a judgment. The type of question depends, of course, on the problem area being explored, but several examples will suffice to show, in principle, how to explore very common problem areas. Instead of asking parents if they are having bedtime problems with their child, ask them what time their child usually starts getting ready for bed, approximately how long it takes, and what time the child is finally down for the night. If the parents say that they usually start at about 8:30 and have the child down by around 9:00, then no problems are evidenced at bedtime. If, however, the parents state that they usually start around 9:30 to 11:00 and that the child is usually finally quiet after an hour or two, then parents are obviously having a problem. Of course, the clinician needs to also explore where the child sleeps, whether or not there are problems with awakening during the night, etc.

The detection of mealtime or feeding problems can be handled in a similar fashion. Instead of asking the parents if they are having feeding problems, ask them questions, such as what the child's favorite or preferred foods are, what foods the child does not like, how long the meals usually last, etc. If the parents can only come up with one or two preferred foods, but can list six or eight foods that the child refuses to eat, then this potential problem area needs to be explored in more detail.

Generally, then, in order to detect possible behavior problems, the clinician should have the parent(s) describe relevant portions of a typical day (Christophersen, Rainey, and Leake, 1975). This concern on the part of the clinician can really serve two purposes. The first, just discussed above, allows for the detection of problems, and the second just makes it clear to the parents that it is all right to discuss or ask questions about behavioral growth and development. Too many clinicians unwittingly discourage discussions about possible problem areas by cutting discussions short, or giving inadequate answers like, "Don't worry about it," or "It's a stage he's going through." Typically, the mother would not have asked about it if she were not already worried about it. Granted, there are some things that children will outgrow, but, for the most part, this does not hold true.

For the skilled clinician, this recommended discussion of relevant portions of a typical day, particularly when spread over several well-child visits, need not even add any time to the length of the average well-child visit.

OFFICE MANAGEMENT OF BEHAVIOR PROBLEMS

In the quote by Friedman at the beginning of this chapter, the point was made that behavioral pediatrics does not deal with severe or psychiatric problems. Fortunately, the majority of children seen in pediatric practice do not present with psychiatric problems such as autism, self-mutilative or self-injurious behaviors, or disorganized thought processes. These problems, and problems similar to them, are clearly beyond the scope of the pediatric clinician. By the same token, problems such as crying at bedtime or mealtime and temper tantrums do not usually necessitate referral to one of the variety of mental health professionals. In fact, most mental health professionals do not have the training to deal with commonly encountered pediatric behavior problems. There are several additional general points that need to be made prior to addressing the theme of management of pediatric behavior problems.

Many parents, whether they specifically ask for help with managing their children, or if the clinician detects problems before the parents actually come in for help, are asking the question, "Who's to blame for the way that my child behaves?" with the implicit answer that "they are." So, whenever behavior problems are encountered, it is wise for the clinician to spend time addressing this question. Most parents, regardless of their educational level or socioeconomic status, have not had one hour of training in child-rearing. If they have a college degree in the social sciences, they may have had a course in child development, and psychology and sociology majors have usually had several courses in child psychology, but ordinarily these courses do not provide any practical answers to the questions and problems most commonly faced by parents. This point needs to be made to the parents, that they have done the best job that they knew how to do, that they did what most parents would have done in the same situation, and that (and this is very important) the technology does not exist for determining who is to blame for the way that a particular child behaves. We know that parents do influence their children, but so do neighbors, relatives, friends, siblings, etc. The only important thing in the management of behavior problems is, "Who cares enough to do something about the problems?" The answer to this question is usually "the parents." The parents need to be assured that there are procedures that you, the clinician, can teach them, that will result in demonstrable changes in the way that their children behave. But, since children are literally constantly learning, the parents need also to be aware that their child's behavior can and will revert to the original problems if they do not maintain a high degree of compliance with the suggested treatment regimens. Most pediatric clinicians are aware of the sometimes dismal compliance that they can expect from parents with something as simple as following the directions for administration of an antibiotic—procedures for managing behavior problems are identical in that, if the parents don't use the procedures, they cannot expect to see any change. The issue of compliance needs to be discussed, albeit briefly, with the parents, prior to suggesting any management procedures.

Along a similar vein, the clinician needs to be aware that pleasant interaction between parents and children begets pleasant interaction and unpleasant interaction begets unpleasant interaction. A very typical pattern seen in the pediatric clinic is the mother of poorly behaved children who is usually doing an incredible number of things around the house that both take up a lot of her time and are things that the children could be doing. The mother makes all the beds, picks up all the clothes, clears the kitchen table, picks up all the toys, etc., to the point where the mother doesn't have any time to do any fun or recreational things with her children because she is spending all of her time being a maid, a cook, and a housekeeper. She also frequently spends an inordinate amount of time with vain attempts to get the children to help with the housework. Some husbands will even aggravate this by suggesting, or insisting, that the mother's job is to take care of the house and that she is shirking her responsibility when she tries to get the children to help her. The sad result of this situation is that the mother does not have time to take the children to the library or to a park, or whatever else might be enjoyable to both mother and child.

Conceptually, the most important thing to remember about child-rearing is that children learn a great deal from what they see and hear their parents do. Parents frequently ask very practical questions like, "How can I have a conversation on the telephone without my son or daughter constantly interrupting me?" "Why can't I go to the grocery store without it turning into a battle with my son?" "How do I get David to behave like a human being when we have to go someplace in the car?" The answers to these and other similar questions lie in the general, day-to-day interactions between the parents and the child. In the case of the mother wanting to be able to make telephone calls, the answer is really pretty simple. When mom is on the telephone and the children are playing nicely or watching TV quietly, mom ignores them. This teaches the children that if they behave themselves when mom is on the telephone, she will ignore them. However, if one of the children succeeds in getting his brother or sister to cry, or scream, or run up to mom to tattle, then mom will usually say, "Just a minute!" and put the phone down. In doing so, she teaches the children that they have to do something wrong in order to get mom off the telephone. Whoever heard of a mother saying, "Just a minute!" and putting the phone down in order to tell the children how pleased she is with the way they are conducting themselves? This would, in fact, teach the children that mom appreciated the fact that they were behaving themselves while she spoke to a friend on the phone. This would reduce, over time, the number of problems that mom had while she was on the phone. The same point applies to the children's behavior in the grocery store (cf. Barnard, Christophersen, and Wolf, 1977) or in the automobile—the parents teach their children how to behave by the way that they interact with them. If the parents usually interact with their children only when they have misbehaved, then the children will misbehave more often. However, if the parents interact with their children both when they are behaving appropriately and inappropriately, then the children will tend to behave much better. The following set of guidelines have been used in a pediatric clinic for several years in order to help to get some important points about parent-child interaction across to parents.

TEN GUIDELINES FOR LIVING WITH CHILDREN[2]

1. "Catch 'em being good." The single most important rule in living with a child is to work very hard to praise or attend to the child when he or she is being appropriate (not when *you* feel like it!). Being appropriate includes everything (depending on the parents' personal preference) from playing quietly with siblings to doing homework to being a good sport.

2. "Let them help you." The second most important rule is to let your children help you to do the variety of activities involved in everyday living. This is much better than you doing the job or task by yourself because it's too difficult for the child to do. Most children enjoy helping their parents and can learn a great deal while doing so. The "helping" might just consist of simulated "work" in your vicinity, but it's still good to have them with you.

3. Monitor your children. When your child is playing quietly—catch him being good! Don't fall into the old trap that you don't want to disturb them. Check on your child frequently (at first, every ten minutes or so; then gradually decrease your monitoring to every 30 minutes or so) so you can give him lots of *feedback* on what he's doing. But, don't disrupt activities which you wish to encourage; a 5- to 10-second interaction is all that is necessary.

4. Home routines and responsibilities should be (within reason) orderly and predictable. Don't let toddlers decide their own timetables. You should decide on a reasonable bedtime and stick to it. Don't do all the housework yourself. Your most important job is that of a teacher. Don't use all of your time being a maid, cook, etc.

5. Discipline and enforcement of discipline should be as matter of fact as possible. A child who breaks a rule should pay for it in whatever way you enforce broken rules. Once a child has paid for a broken rule, no part of the incident should *ever* be mentioned again. It is much better to have a child sit in a kitchen chair or sit on the sofa for 3 or 4 minutes than to be spanked. Spank a child only if he gets up from the chair. Spank only *once*. The first spank is for the child; all the rest are for you. Try placing a younger child in the crib until he is quiet for 5 or 10 seconds; then go in and pick him up. Don't be reluctant to have a child sit on the chair ten or fifteen times in one day if it is deserved.

[2]© 1976. Reprinted with permission of the author, Edward R. Christophersen, Ph.D.

6. Lectures belong in lecture halls, not in homes. Do *not* lecture your children—not even under the guise of reasoning with them. Threats and nagging are useless in dealing with children. In fact, if anything, threats probably make children worse—not better. Talking with your children is important; however, be careful that you avoid talking with them only at times of crisis, problems, etc. Rather, spend your time talking with them when things are pleasant and running smoothly. For example, if you and your child are working together or going somewhere together, that's a perfect time to talk with your child. With smaller children, talking to them a lot is a good way to get language development started. Just try carrying on a running description of what you're doing.

7. Show sympathy when you discipline. When a child has to miss a movie, a trip to McDonald's or an opportunity to play a game with a friend because of some misbehavior, you should be sympathetic, but don't give in. Make sure that this sympathy doesn't last over a minute.

8. Prompting and modeling or imitating. Children learn by what they see and hear you and others do. If your child breaks one of the house rules and you handle the whole issue matter-of-factly, then your child will learn that problems can be handled matter-of-factly. If you scream when you're mad, you can probably expect your children to follow that example. Therefore, it's important to show your children that you can handle problem situations without losing your cool.

9. Be a mother, not a martyr. Find a *good* babysitter or preschool and use it—not as an escape, but as a breather. (Fathers, by the way, make excellent babysitters.) It's very desirable for a mother to spend some time with adults with no children around. If your child spends most of his waking hours with a babysitter, you can expect him to behave a lot like that babysitter—so choose babysitters carefully.

10. Parents are teachers. Whether you program it or not, whether you intend it or not, you teach your children through your interaction with them. If you only pick them up when they are crying, you teach them to cry more often. Particularly with younger children, what you do is much more important than what you say.

When counseling parents on the management of behavior problems, it is a good idea, when possible, to provide the parents with either a written handout (for problems that occur with a high enough frequency to merit the cost of printing a handout) or at least jot down your suggestions on a piece of paper so that the parents have a permanent reminder of what it was you said in the clinic. For example, with the ten guidelines above, the clinician should provide a copy for the parents and go over each of the guidelines, briefly, to make sure that the parents understand the points that you're trying to make. Beyond this, there are some points that require actual demonstration in order to assure that the parents can adequately follow through with your instructions. With guideline 5 on discipline, for example, Dr. Hunter Leake, Mrs. Susan Rainey, and this writer have developed a procedure whereby we actually practice placing the child on a chair in a "make believe" situation in the clinic to show the parents and the child exactly what we mean. This is begun with a question to the child such as, "How would you like it if your mommy didn't yell at you as much?" Usually, the child, with a little prodding, will admit that he or she would like that. Then the clinician asks, "Have you ever done anything that your mommy and daddy didn't like?" Usually, the child answers, "No!" which results in our asking the follow-up questions, "Not even once?" and then, "Once, when you were little?" which is usually adequate to get the child to admit that, "yes," once, when he was little, he did do something that mommy didn't like. Then, the clinician says, "The next time that you do something that your mommy doesn't want you to do, she's going to ask you to go sit in the chair. When she does, I want you to go over to the chair like this," and the clinician takes the child by the hand and walks him over to the clinic chair, gently puts the child on the chair and proceeds with the demonstration. "Now, there are two rules when you're on the chair. One is that the time does not begin until after you stop crying. If you feel like it you can cry when mommy asks you to sit in the chair, but your time does not start until after you are quiet." (We usually recommend that the parents use a maximum of 1 minute in the chair for each year of age, so a 3-year-old would stay a maximum of 3 minutes. However, *never* ask a child to sit for more than 5 minutes after he is quiet). Then, we say, "When does your time start?" Some of the children are able to verbalize that the time starts when they are quiet, but some are too young. The verbalization really does not make much difference. The important thing is to demonstrate to the parents and to the child that discipline can be handled matter-of-factly, without getting mad. Then the child is told the second rule, "If you get up from the chair before the timer rings, I have to give you one hard spank. Do you want to get up and I'll give you one hard spank and then you'll know the rule?" At this time, look at the parents, one at a time, and ask them if it is all right for you to administer one spank. Inevitably, both parents say, "Okay." We have only had two or three children who have gotten up at this time. But, if they do get up, the clinician has to administer one spank and replace the child on the chair. Then the two rules are restated, exactly as they were the first time, including the questions, and answers are solicited from the child. Rare, indeed, is the child who, in the clinic, will get up the second time. After years of experience using this procedure, we have found that once parents begin using the "chair" for discipline, they rarely spank their children for any reason.

This use of what is called "practicing" in the clinic greatly aids the clinician in the effort to educate the parents, because, with the use of practicing, the clinician knows that the parents and the child know how to use the chair routine before they are sent home from the clinic to try it on their own. Obviously, practicing can be used with many of the instructions that a clinician might have for the parents and the child. For example, if the clinician is engaged in a discussion with the parents about the first guideline, "Catch 'em being good," and the child is behaving appropriately while the discussion is taking place, then the clinician needs to model this behavior for the parents by praising the child, or messing up his hair, etc. In this way, the clinician is *teaching* with both words and actions.

In addition to the general "Guidelines for Living with Children," the parents can also be provided with specific handouts for the problems that they are reporting having with their child. An example of one of these handouts, the one that goes along with the discipline example just outlined above follows.

TEMPER PROBLEMS/NONCOMPLIANCE[3]
GUIDELINES FOR PARENTS

If you are having problems getting your child to follow instructions the first time or if your child tantrums if you tell him "no," the following procedures can help you teach your child how to follow instructions appropriately without tantruming.

1. *Praise* your child every time he follows instructions.
2. Only give instructions once.
3. If your child does not comply with your instruction the first time that you give it, then: place the child in time-out (kitchen chair, steps, etc.—*no closets or dark rooms*).
   a. Carry the child (if needed) to the chair in such a way that it cannot look at you.
   b. State the rule, "Whenever you don't follow instructions, you have to sit in the chair."
   c. Place the child on the chair.
   d. After the child is quiet, set a timer (a portable kitchen timer is best) for 2 (toddler) or 5 (school age) minutes—never more than 5 minutes.
   e. If the child gets up give him one spank and put him back in the chair. As soon as he is quiet, reset the timer for 2 or 5 minutes.
   f. When the timer rings, ask the child if he wants to get up.
   g. If the child says, "no" or starts fussing or crying, wait for him or her to be quiet, then reset the timer.
   h. When the child is through with time-out, encourage him to engage in a pleasant and/or acceptable activity.

Individual clinicians will obviously have some guidelines that they prefer to use more than others, and some clinicians may recommend different methods of discipline for different families. The important point to

---

[3] © Reprinted with permission of the authors, Susan K. Rainey, Edward R. Christophersen, and Hunter C. Leake, 1976.

remember is that the parents cannot possibly carry out your instructions properly if they have not had adequate instruction and if you do not provide them with some brief written guidelines to follow. The requirement that you have written handouts to give to the parents has a second benefit in that you cannot prepare a handout until you have it clear in your mind exactly how you think each problem area should be handled. After using a particular handout for several months in the clinic, it is then possible to modify the handout, based on the feedback that you receive from the parents that you have given it to, to make it easier for the parents to follow the procedures that you recommend. Most clinicians who have used the handouts that we have supplied have been surprised by the fact that, in spite of the many differences that exist between the families seen in the clinic, the handouts do work with almost all of their families. This fact, in itself, is encouraging, because it suggests that behavior problems are not as elusive as we once thought they were—a set of procedures that work with several hundred families, as is the case with the handout provided above for temper problems/noncompliance, certainly suggests that essentially the same mechanisms are involved with each of these families.

One additional point needs to be made here about the management of behavior problems through the pediatric clinic—frequent telephone contact is an important adjunct to the rest of the procedures spelled out above. We usually count on calling a family the day after a clinic visit to see if they have any questions or if they have run into any problems with the recommended procedures. If this is done as a routine procedure over a period of time, the same questions come up with subsequent families and so the clinician can acquire the skills for answering the parents' questions without spending an inordinate amount of time on the telephone. Failure to use adequate telephone follow-up is probably the most common reason that clinicians do not have more success in their attempts to manage behavior problems. It is naive to think that one 20-minute appointment is sufficient to teach parents how to derive more enjoyment from their parenting efforts. The clinician who is interested in managing behavior problems simply has no choice but to make this commitment to follow families by phone until most of the problems are ironed out. (This writer suspects that parental compliance with instructions for administering antibiotics would be greatly enhanced if the clinician would take the extra couple of minutes to telephone the mother or father to see that they were still administering the medication properly!)

REFERRAL OF BEHAVIOR-DISORDERED CHILDREN

As Rainey and Christophersen (1976) stated in a recent article, "One of the most difficult parts of working with behavior problems is knowing when to refer the family for more intensive therapy. It is very easy to let yourself go ahead with a case that may be too difficult because you want to be of assistance to a family."

Fortunately, behavioral pediatrics has a sound scientific base, which provides the pediatric clinician with sufficient information to answer the question, "Should I manage this case myself or should I refer it to someone else?" If the referring complaint (or a problem detected early, before the parent has identified it as a complaint) is something that has been adequately investigated and clearly defined procedures for management have been published, then the clinician who is familiar with the procedures may proceed with intervention. Examples of such problem areas include: bedtime, mealtime, dressing (Christophersen, 1977b), temper tantrums, noncompliance (Bernal, 1970; Rainey and Christophersen, 1976), sleep disturbances (Wright, Woodcock, and Scott, 1970), enuresis (Azrin, Sneed, and Foxx, 1973; Olness, 1975), toilet training (Azrin and Foxx, 1974; Christophersen, 1977b), habit disorders (Azrin and Nunn, 1973), and encopresis (Wright, 1973; Christophersen and Rainey, 1976).

Christophersen (1973) reviewed a number of comprehensive programs for dealing with moderate to severe behavior problems of children. The reader is referred to Christophersen, Barnard, Ford, and Wolf (1976), Patterson (1974), Berkowitz and Graziano (1972), Patterson, Reid, Jones, and Conger (1975), Mash, Handy, and Hamerlynck (1976), and Mash, Hamerlynck, and Handy (1976) for descriptions of these programs. Each of these program descriptions are, in principle, quite similar to the procedures recommended in the present manuscript for effecting behavioral change in children. They share the common features of (1) using the parents as the change agent, (2) giving the parent concrete suggestions for ways of altering their interaction with their children that usually result in therapeutic change in the children, and (3) a strong deemphasis on the role of punishment in managing behavior problems.

If, on the other hand, the referring complaint is something that has not been adequately investigated, or represents an area where the clinician suspects more severe pathology, then the family should obviously be referred to an appropriate mental health professional. Problems that, to this author's knowledge, have not been adequately investigated include chronic lying, stealing, fire setting, and active aggression. Obviously, families with histories of psychoses, autism, and drug abuse usually cannot be dealt with through a pediatric setting.

There are also mitigating circumstances that should discourage the pediatric clinician from attempting to manage problems that would normally be well within their scope (Rainey and Christophersen, 1976). These include families that have multiple problems (e.g., temper tantrums, mealtime and bedtime problems). The reason for this is that each of these problems may tend to interfere with the management of the other problems.

Parents who are known to the clinician to be noncompliant may need more prompting to use the suggested procedures than can be done realistically. If the clinician has had problems in the past with getting parents to adhere to specific medical treatment regimens, then managing behavior problems would probably meet with similar kinds of resistance.

In families where there are four or more children who are all assessed to have behavior problems, the pediatric clinician would be well advised to refer them to an appropriate professional. Frequently, the parents in such a situation need more support than is possible, realistically, through the pediatric clinic.

If the clinician ascertains that the parents are having marital problems that are severe enough to interfere with the family's day-to-day functioning, then the parents should probably be referred to an appropriate counselor, with management of the behavior problems postponed until the marital problems are resolved.

CONCLUDING REMARKS

The point that I made in the introduction needs to be reiterated. The primary focus of behavioral pediatrics is on prevention and early detection of behavioral and developmental problems. This *is* the province of the primary health care provider. The provision of psychiatric, psychological, or social work services can certainly be included in a pediatric practice, but doing so is beyond the scope of most pediatric clinicians. When the clinician is conducting a well-child visit or is providing anticipatory guidance (both of which were probably adequately covered in the respective pediatric training program), it is a relatively simple matter to encourage and include discussion about the "normal" problems that "normal" parents experience during their exercise in child-rearing. Frequently, these problems stem from a lack of or ineffective parenting techniques (Friedman, 1975). The interested pediatric clinician can, through reading and seminars and workshops, become quite well versed in the management of commonly encountered pediatric behavior problems, such that this service can routinely be rendered as a part of their well-child care.

REFERENCES

Azrin, N. H., & Foxx, R. *Toilet training in less than a day: How to do it.* New York: Simon and Schuster, 1974.

——, and Nunn, R. G. Habit reversal: A method of eliminating nervous habits and tics. *Behavior Research and Therapy,* 1973, *11,* 619–628.

——, Sneed, T. J., & Foxx, R. M. Dry bed training: Rapid elimination of childhood enuresis. *Behavior Research and Therapy,* 1974, *12,* 147–156.

Barnard, J. D., Christophersen, E. R., & Wolf, M. M. Teaching children appropriate shopping behavior through parent training in the supermarket setting. *Journal of Applied Behavior Analysis,* 1977, *10,* 49–59.

Becker, W. C., & Becker, J. W. *Successful parenthood: How to teach your child values, competence and responsibility.* Chicago: Follet, 1974.

Berkowitz, B. P., & Graziano, A. M. Training parents as behavior therapists: A review. *Behavior Research and Therapy,* 1972, *10,* 297–317.

Bernal, M. E. Training parents in child management. In R. Bradfield (Ed.), *Behavior modification and the learning disorders.* San Rafael, Cal.: Academic Therapy Publications, 1970, 41–67.

Brazelton, T. B. Crying in infancy. *Pediatrics,* 1962, *29,* 579–588.

Christophersen, E. R. Children's behavior during automobile rides: Do car seats make a difference? *Pediatrics,* 1977, *60,* 69–74.

———. *Little people: Guidelines for common sense child rearing.* Lawrence, Ks.: H & H Enterprises, 1977.

———. Behavior modification in a family setting. In D. P. Hymovich and M. U. Barnard (Eds.), *Family Health Care.* New York: McGraw-Hill, 1973.

———, and Barnard, J. D. Management of behavior problems: A perspective for pediatricians. *Clinical Pediatrics,* 1978, *17,* 122–124.

———, Barnard, J. D., Ford, D., & Wolf, M. M. The family training program: Improving parent-child interaction patterns. In E. J. Mash, L. C. Handy, & L. A. Hamerlynck, (Eds.), *Behavior modification approaches to parenting.* New York: Brunner/Mazel, 1976.

———, Rainey, S. K., & Leake, H. C. Simultaneous evaluation of ambulatory behavior disorders by the pediatrician and the pediatric psychologist. *Proceedings of the Ambulatory Pediatric Association,* Toronto, Canada, June, 1975 (Abstract).

Dudding, G. *The first year, beginning the parenting process.* Kansas City, Kans.: University of Kansas, Dept. of Pediatrics, 1975.

Friedman, S. B. (Ed.). *The pediatric clinics of North America.* London: Saunders, 1975.

Kenny, T. J., and Clemmens, R. L. *Behavioral pediatrics and child development.* Baltimore: Williams and Wilkins, 1975.

Mash, E. J., Hamerlynck, L. A., & Handy, L. C. (Eds). *Behavior modification and families.* New York: Brunner/Mazel, 1976.

———, *Behavior modification approaches to parenting.* New York: Brunner/Mazel, 1976.

Olness, K. The use of self-hypnosis in the treatment of childhood nocturnal enuresis. *Clinical Pediatrics,* 1977, *14,* 273–279.

Patterson, G. R. Interventions for boys with conduct problems: Multiple settings, treatments, and criteria. *Journal of Consulting and Clinical Psychology,* 1974, *42,* 471–481.

———, Reid, J. B., Jones, R. R., & Conger, R. E. *A social learning approach to family intervention: Families with aggressive children.* Eugene, Oreg.: Castalia, 1975.

Quilitch, H. R., & Risley, R. R. *A mother and her infant: An ecological study.* Overland Park, Kans.: KPA, 1971.

Rainey, S. K., and Christophersen, E. R. Behavioral pediatrics: The role of the nurse clinician. *Issues in Comprehensive Pediatric Nursing,* New York: McGraw Hill, 1976, 19–29.

Sostek, A. M., Anders, T. F., & Sostek, A. J. Diuranal rhythms in 2- and 8-week old infants: Sleep-waking state organization as a function of age and stress. *Psychosomatic Medicine,* 1976, *38,* 250–256.

Spock, B. *Baby and Child Care.* New York: Pocket Books, 1976.

White, B. *The first three years of life.* Englewood Cliffs, N.J.: Prentice-Hall, 1975.

Williams, C. D. The elimination of tantrum behaviors by extinction procedures. *Journal of Abnormal and Social Psychology,* 1959, *59,* 269.

Wright, L. Handling the encopretic child. *Professional Psychology,* 1973, *16,* 137–144.

———, Woodcock, J., and Scott R. Treatment of sleep disorders in a young child. *Southern Medical Journal,* 1970, *63,* 174–176.

CHAPTER TWENTY-FIVE

LEGAL ASPECTS OF NURSING AND MEDICINE

LEE J. DUNN

A good deal of the difficulty (real and perceived) that arises in the law/ nursing interface occurs because of a lack of knowledge of the basic legal concepts, rights, responsibilities, and liabilities of nurses with respect to their colleagues, other health care providers, and their patients. This is especially true in the area of professional negligence (or "malpractice"), where interest has been heightened by the alleged threat of great verdicts being levied against penniless nurses. Therefore, before discussing a few of the legal aspects of primary nursing care (it would take volumes to discuss the topic thoroughly), it is important to discuss the basic legal relationship between the nurse and the patient and what acts or omissions can breach the duties that arise from that relationship. It should be stated and understood from the beginning that a great many of the problems or incidents that develop into malpractice actions could be avoided simply through the application of common sense to the practice of nursing, and by the nurse treating the patient as the nurse would want to be treated were the roles reversed. The fact that an individual is licensed to practice nursing does not in itself place the nurse in a privileged status with respect to the patient.

STANDARD OF CARE

The cornerstone of the nurse/patient relationship is the precept that every individual has a right not to be touched in any way or for any reason without having given consent (*Schloendorff*, 1914). Any unauthorized touching constitutes at least a technical battery (*Younts,* 1970), and this fact is true regardless of the motivation of the individual doing the touching. Therefore, a nurse, even though motivated by a desire to treat and/or help a patient, commits a battery if the treatment rendered was not consented to. Assuming for the moment that the treatment rendered was consented to, once treatment is begun the nurse is under the legal obligation to render "ordinary and reasonable care" to the patient (*Ybarra,* 1944). Such care is more fully defined as that degree of skill and care that a similarly trained nurse would render under the same or similar circumstances (*Woods,* 1938). No nurse is required either to render the best possible nursing care or to be the best nurse in the community. Rather, the nurse is only required to meet the standard of practice that the ordinary and reasonable nurse in that community meets. The determination as to what constitutes ordinary and reasonable care is made by nurses themselves, who, if a question as to the competence of an individual nurse were to come before the court, would testify as to what they knew the standard of care to be in the community in which this nurse practiced. (Contrary to popular belief, therefore, the standard is established by peer professionals and not by nonprofessionals.) Notice within the definition of the standard of care the term "similarly trained." This is important to understand, because nurses who received specialized training and/or function in a specialized area of nursing are held to the standard met by similarly situated nurses and/or that which they profess to possess (*Webb v. Jorns,* 1971). Accordingly, for example, a nurse who practices solely in intensive care units or who is a Certified Registered Nurse Anesthetist would be held to the standard of other nurses performing the same kind of function. Therefore, a nurse who provides primary family health care, to the extent that that area of specialization reflects or requires specialized training or skill, will be held to the standard practiced in the community in that specialty.

STAYING WITHIN THE PRACTICE OF NURSING

One of the problems that nurses frequently encounter as they practice within a profession whose role is rapidly changing is balancing on the thin line between practicing nursing and practicing medicine. Since nurses who provide primary health care may be the first health care provider to encounter an individual who needs to be seen by a physician, there is the strong possibility of the nurse stepping over that line and practicing medicine. The nurse should always know exactly what is permitted under the nursing practice act of the state. A small number of states have expanded the role of the nurse by allowing the performance of actions previously reserved to the physician (Bullough, 1975, pp. 153–170). Most states, however, do not. Therefore, the nurse who encounters a nonemergency patient in a state in which the more traditional boundaries between medicine and nursing continue to exist should not attempt to diagnose a patient's condition, especially if that diagnosis is acted upon without the prior assessment of a physician. Obviously, nurses should evaluate the patient's condition and advise a physician as to their opinion, but they should be very careful not to take action that by law they are not permitted to take. Although it does not necessarily reflect the nature and extent of health care being provided in the 1970s, the primary legal relationship into which the patient enters in the health care delivery system is the physician/patient relationship (Morris and Moritz, 1971). This is not to say that the physician is solely liable for the negligence of those who assist him. On the contrary, nurses will be liable for personal acts of negligence if they deviate from the previously explained standard of care (Ybarra and Kambas, 1944, pp. 135–145). However, it should be understood that the repository of the vast bulk of the legal responsibilities in the delivery of primary family health care is the physician/patient relationship. It is the physician's responsibility to diagnose and treat the patient (Morris and Moritz, 1971, pp. 135–191, 325–477). The physician may utilize or employ the resources of others in executing professional duties, but cannot delegate to anyone else the legal responsibility not only to provide competent medical care, but also to see to it that the patient is not exposed to such unnecessary risks as medical treatment rendered by one who does not have the competence or who is not licensed to render such treatment (Morris and Moritz, 1971, pp. 135–191, 325–477).

STANDING ORDERS

One of the most common ways in which physicians get into difficulty in this area is by writing broad standing orders in an attempt to allow a nurse, a physician's assistant, or some other health care provider broad parameters within which to work. The difficulty with this practice is that physicians do not have the authority to permit someone to practice medicine on their patients without their supervision (Morris and Moritz, 1971, pp. 135–191, 325–477) and cannot compromise the responsibility to continue to render treatment by causing an agent to do their job for them. Obviously, medicine is frequently practiced on patients by persons other than physicians, but this technical violation of the law is obviated by the physician's presence and/or approval of the nonphysician's actions before they are executed. Most state licensing laws provide that actions that would otherwise constitute the unauthorized practice of medicine when performed by a layman are permissible when performed under the supervision or under the direction and control of a licensed physician. Assuming for the moment that the physician has exercised caution in writing standing orders and has not, by writing excessively broad or vague standing orders, put the nurse into the difficult position of being compelled to practice medicine in order to render any treatment at all, but has told the nurse specifically what should be done in the event the nurse observes certain conditions or anomalies, the nurse is then free to practice nursing and not run afoul of the law. A nurse should never render care under standing orders that are so broad and/or vague that the nurse, in effect, is practicing without guidance or without restriction. This is especially important to the primary care nurse, who often must act without immediate physician support.

TELEPHONE TREATMENT

One of the easiest ways for both doctors and nurses to get into difficulty is through use of the telephone. Telephone contact between a nurse, who is in the presence of the patient and who can relate what is observed to the physician, often eliminates difficulties concerning not only the unauthorized practice of medicine, but also the incorrect or insufficient transmission of data to the physician prior to treatment. However, the use of the telephone can be and has been misused to the detriment of patients and the legal status of health care providers.

Generally speaking, neither physicians nor nurses should use the telephone to diagnose or treat a patient who is unknown to them or who is suffering from a condition that has not previously been diagnosed or treated by them. Nor should a physician or nurse act on information transmitted over the telephone when neither has seen the patient nor can attest to the actual condition of the patient. Obviously, if the physician or nurse has been treating a patient for a particular condition for some time, and the telephone is being used to maintain contact with the patient or another health care provider, treatment can be rendered on the basis of information so obtained or imparted. However, as a general rule, in the nonemergency situation, prescription medication should never be administered to a patient without a physician's prior written order. Obviously, this is a difficult rule to observe in practice, but primary family health care nurses must be very careful not to administer medications when they consider the prescription to be somehow incorrect or inappropriate. No professional can ever walk away from his or her own knowledge, and if for some reason a prescription or any aspect of treatment is thought to be incorrect, the nurse should always question the physician, and, if the nurse's doubt persists, an entry concerning the nature of the challenge and its resolution should be entered in the patient's treatment record. Refusal to follow a physician's order is an extreme response, which should only be undertaken in cases in which the life or health of the patient is gravely threatened. It is the physician's responsibility to provide the patient with competent medical care, and, in order to insure that such care is rendered and to protect the legal status of the nurse, the nurse should, if at all possible, obtain the signature of the patient's physician before a telephone medication order is filled and the medication is administered, or before any extraordinary care is rendered.

ABANDONMENT

Once treatment has been commenced, the nurse is generally held to be the agent or employee of the physician, and, therefore, is the extension of the physician. Under one or more legal doctrines, nurses, to the extent that they remain within the scope of their professional responsibility, bind the physician by their actions. Under the employer/employee, or master/servant, principal/agent, or "Borrowed Servant" doctrines, a nurse, whether actually employed or (if not actually employed) whose professional actions are controlled or could have been controlled by a physician, can be considered to be acting under the physician's supervision and control, and, therefore, the physician will be liable for the nurse's negligence (Morris and Moritz, 1971, pp. 368–376.) Physicians have a duty to maintain treatment as long as the medical need of the patient exists, and a breach of that duty constitutes abandonment (*Miller v. Dore,* 1959; *Rodgers v. Lawson,* 1948). Whether or not a nurse could be liable for abandonment is an issue that has yet to be resolved. Clearly, however, if a nurse, in direct contravention of a physician's orders, failed to provide treatment that a patient required, the nurse would be singularly liable, at least for negligence (*Goff v. Doctors General Hospital,* 1958). Conversely, if the nurse failed to provide adequate nursing care as a result of a physician's failure to assess correctly the continuing medical need of the patient, the nurse would not necessarily be personally liable to the patient. The nurse has the right to rely upon the professional competence of the physician.Therefore, if the nurse, consistent with ordinary and reasonable care, fails to appreciate the medical need of a patient (a need that the physician should have recognized but did not), the nurse would not be liable for any resulting injury to the patient.

PATIENT'S RIGHT OF PRIVACY

The development of the law with respect to a patient's right to privacy has experienced a tremendous expansion in the last several decades, and quite often the question arises as to whether or not medical or nursing care in and of itself can constitute an invasion of privacy (Morris and

Moritz, 1971, pp. 141–144). Generally speaking, it does not. The primary element that a nurse needs to worry about with respect to invasion of privacy is the unauthorized granting of access to others to the information generated by the doctor/patient or nurse/patient relationship. Regardless of the nature or the amount of confidential information that a nurse obtains about a patient, the nurse does not run the risk of invading the patient's privacy as long as the information gathered is reasonably related to the evaluation and treatment of the patient's condition and is not divulged in an unauthorized manner to a third party who has no right to that information, for example, someone whom the patient has not expressly consented to being allowed access to the interchange of information with the health care provider.

TREATMENT OF MINORS

The treatment of minors is an unnecessarily complicated issue in that, once again, it is an issue about which there is considerable misunderstanding (Dunn, 1975). The most practical way to approach the issue is from the perspective of a general rule to which there are certain exceptions. The general rule is that the parent and the parent *alone* can consent to the treatment of a minor child. [Within the definition of the word "parent" this writer includes a guardian or some other individual who has been appointed by the court to act as or in the palce of a parent (Prosser, 1971).] As was the case in our discussion of assault and battery, any touching of a child, for whatever reason, that has not been consented to by the child's parent is at least a technical battery (*Fiske v. Stone,* 1968). Therefore, other than in one of those exceptional situations that we will shortly discuss, the nurse should always remember to obtain the consent of the parent prior to rendering treatment to a minor in a nonemergency setting.

The major exception to the previously stated general rule is that of the "emancipated minor." "Emancipated minor" is a legal term that means, in effect, that in certain circumstances the minor is emancipated from the requirement of having to obtain parental consent prior to receiving medical care, and, conversely, the physician or nurse is similarly emancipated from having to obtain parental consent (Dunn, 1975). The problem with the "emancipated minor" is that the definition or criteria for emancipation differ markedly from state to state. In some states minors are considered to be emancipated if they live apart from or are financially independent of their parents. In other states minors are considered to be emancipated for the treatment of certain diseases or conditions if they are suffering from or suspected to be suffering from those diseases or conditions at the time the consent issue arises. Since there are such marked differences between the states, the nurse should take great care to know precisely what the law in a given state is with respect to the treatment of minors.

Moreover, simply obtaining the consent of an adult prior to the rendering of treatment to a minor will not necessarily be sufficient if that adult does not have the authority to give such consent (*Moss v. Rishworth,* 1920). In the absence of specific authorization of the parent, no adult should be considered capable of giving a valid consent to the treatment of a minor in the nonemergency situation.

LIABILITY IN EMERGENCY SITUATIONS

Once again we are confronted with an issue about which there is significant misunderstanding. All too often health care providers assume that the rendering of treatment in an emergency situation exposes them to liability and increases the possibility that they will be sued for malpractice, even though the care rendered was gratuitous and performed under difficult circumstances. Their fears are unfounded. Distinguishing for the moment between the emergency situation within the medical setting and those arising outside the medical setting, it should be clearly understood that the law presumes that a competent, lucid adult, when faced with the choice between life and death or between illness and health, would consent to whatever treatment is necessary in order to maintain life or health. Accordingly, when that individual is unable to give such consent because he is medically or legally incapable of doing so, the law implies that the consent has been given (*Wall v. Brim,* 1943). Therefore, medical treatment necessary to maintain the life or health of a patient can be rendered without the consent of the patient, provided two criteria are met. First, the patient must truly be in need of prompt medical treatment in order to maintain life or health, and, second, the patient must be incapable of giving consent (*Salgo v. Leland Stanford,* 1957). The absence of either of these two criteria renders the situation a nonemergency and requires the consent of the patient before treatment can be rendered. The situation just described was meant primarily to reflect emergency situations arising within the medical setting, in which the nurse's opportunity and ability to evaluate the medical needs of the patient and the patient's ability to give consent can be presumed to be better than in situations arising outside the medical setting. The former situations do not seem to create the fear and doubt in the minds of physicians and nurses that situations arising outside the medical setting present. There is a widespread misunderstanding that the rendering of treatment to an accident victim outside the medical setting is unwise because of the exposure to malpractice litigation it presents.

Once again, this is untrue. However, in response to this fear, nearly all the states have enacted statutes that protect different classes of health professionals who render care in a variety of different "emergency" situations (Morris and Moritz, 1971, pp. 356–357). In addition, in the last 10 years an amazing patchwork of statutes has been enacted by the states that presume to protect a variety of professionals and paraprofessionals in a variety of situations, but do not necessarily cover all statuses. Therefore, the nurse should be sure to know exactly what the situations in a state provide and protect.

However, it should also be understood that there is not a single reported case in any American jurisdiction in which a health care provider has been successfully sued for rendering care in an emergency. The "crisis" that spurred the enactment of so many of the "Good Samaritan" statutes never has existed and does not now exist. As long as nurses render reasonable care, and by this is meant that they perform procedures or render care that are within their competence to perform, practically speaking they will not be exposed to liability. This does not mean that nurses are free to render any treatment or perform any procedure, including those with which they are unfamiliar. On the contrary, nurses should only perform those procedures or render that treatment with which they are familiar and comfortable. However, the nurse should not fail to render treatment because of a fear of liability. Remembering the basic precept that the nurse is under no legal obligation to treat anyone, and that any treatment rendered in such a situation is totally a voluntary act, in the emergency situation the nurse would be well advised to act under the maxim of "when in doubt, treat."

COOPERATION OF THE PATIENT

Finally, the nurse should remember that patients have an obligation to participate and cooperate in their treatment, to follow the advice of those who are treating them, and not to worsen their condition by unreasonable unilateral action (Louisell and Williams, 1973, pp. 246–250). Uncooperative patients should be advised of this fact and told that the physician and nurse neither can nor will be responsible for injuries or adverse results caused by their failure to cooperate. Continued lack of cooperation should be recorded in writing and the patient should be advised that a failure to assist in one's own treatment could constitute grounds for termination of the physician/patient relationship. Nurses should remember that they alone cannot and should not attempt to terminate the physician/patient relationship and, generally speaking, isolated acts of nonparticipation are not sufficient grounds for such a termination.

CONCLUSION

At the beginning of this chapter it was observed that the use of common sense can be of great value in the law/nursing interface. This is true with respect to both the nurse/patient and nurse/colleague relationship. Knowing (not guessing or assuming) what the law is, treating patients as the nurse would want to be treated personally, and practicing common sense with respect to protecting and preserving one's own legal and professional status can go a long way toward freeing the nurse from much of the unnecessary concern currently surrounding the law/nursing interface and, therefore, permit the nurse to practice better nursing.

REFERENCES

Bullough, B. *The law and the expanding nursing role.* New York: Appleton-Century-Crofts, 1975.

Dunn, L. J. The availability of abortion, sterilization, and other medical treatment for minor patients. 44 *U.M.K.C.L. Rev.* 1 (1975).

Fiske v. Stone, 8 Ariz. App. 585, 448 P. 2d 429, 1968.

Goff v. Doctors General Hospital, 166 Cal. App. 2d 314, 333 P.2d 29, 1958.

Louisell D., & Williams, H. *Medical malpractice.* New York: Matthew Bender, 1973, 246–250.

Kambas v. St. Joseph's Mercy Hospital, 33 Mich. App. 127, 189 N. W.2d 879.

Miller v. Dore, 148 A.2d 692, 1959.

Morris, C., & Moritz, A. *Doctor and patient and the law* (5th ed.). St. Louis: C. V. Mosby, 1971, 135–145.

Moss v. Rishworth, 222 S.W. 225, 1920.

Prosser, W. *Handbook of the Law of Torts* (4th ed.). 102-03, 1971.

Rodgers v. Lawson, 170 F.2d 157, 1948.

Salgo v. Leland Stanford Jr. Univ. Brd. of Trustees, 154 Cal. App. 2d 560, 317, P.2d 170, 1957.

Schloendorff v. Society of the New York Hospital, 211 N.Y. 125, 105 N.E. 92, 1914.

Wall v. Brim, 138 F.2d 478, 1943.

Webb v. Jorns, 473 S.W.2d 328 (Tex.Civ.App.), 1971.

Woods v. Miller, 158 Or. 444, 76 P.2d 963, 1938.

Ybarra v. Spangard, 25 Cal. 2d 486, 154 P.2d 687, 1944.

Younts v. St. Francis Hospital and School of Nursing, Inc., 205 Kan. 292, 469 P.2d 330, 1970.

INDEX

INDEX